# Cochlear Implants
## A Practical Guide
### Second Edition

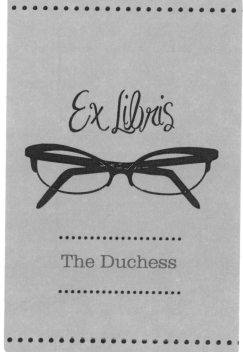

# Cochlear Implants

## A Practical Guide

### Second Edition

*Edited by*

**Huw R. Cooper**

and

**Louise C. Craddock**

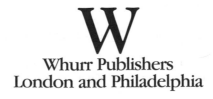

**Whurr Publishers**
London and Philadelphia

*Other Wiley Editorial Offices*

John Wiley & Sons Inc., 111 River Street, Hoboken, NJ 07030, USA
Jossey-Bass, 989 Market Street, San Francisco, CA 94103-1741, USA
Wiley-VCH Verlag GmbH, Boschstr. 12, D-69469 Weinheim, Germany
John Wiley & Sons Australia Ltd, 42 McDougall Street, Milton, Queensland 4064,
Australia
John Wiley & Sons (Asia) Pte Ltd, 2 Clementi Loop #02-01, Jin Xing Distripark,
Singapore 129809
John Wiley & Sons Canada Ltd, 22 Worcester Road, Etobicoke, Ontario, Canada
M9W 1L1

Wiley also publishes its books in a variety of electronic formats. Some content that
appears in print may not be available in electronic books.

A catalogue record for this book is available from the British Library

ISBN -13        978-1-86156-481-8
ISBN -10        1-86156-481-3

Printed and bound in Great Britain by TJ International Ltd, Padstow, Cornwall

This book is printed on acid-free paper responsibly manufactured from sustain-
able forestry in which at least two trees are planted for each one used for paper
production.

# Contents

# Contributors

**Paul J. Abbas**, PhD, Departments of Speech Pathology and Audiology, Otolaryngology, Head and Neck Surgery, University of Iowa, Iowa City, IA 52242, USA

**Thomas J. Balkany**, MD, FACS, FAAP, Hotchkiss Professor and Chairman, Department of Otolaryngology, University of Miami, Florida, USA

**Mrs Jean Briggs**, Stoke-on-Trent, Staffordshire, UK

**Steve C. Branin**, University of Iowa, Department of Otolaryngology Head and Neck Surgery, University of Iowa, Iowa City, IA 52242, USA

**Carolyn J. Brown**, PhD, Departments of Speech Pathology and Audiology, Otolaryngology, Head and Neck Surgery, University of Iowa, Iowa City, IA 52242, USA

**Graeme M. Clark**, AO, FAA, FTSE, MB, PhD (Sydney), HonMD (Hannover), HonMD (Sydney), HonDSc (Wollongong), HonDEng (CYC Taiwan), FRCS (Edin. & Lond.), FRACS, Laureate Professor of Otolaryngology, University of Melbourne, Director, Bionic Ear Institute, 384–388 Albert St, East Melbourne, VIC 3002, Australia

**Mrs Jennie Clewes**, Stourbridge, West Midlands, UK

**Huw R. Cooper**, MSc, Consultant Audiological Scientist, Midlands Adult Cochlear Implant Programme, Centre for Hearing and Balance Assessment, Rehabilitation and Research, University Hospital Birmingham, UK

**Louise C. Craddock**, MSc, CCC-A, Audiological Scientist, Cochlear Implant Programme Co-ordinator, Midlands Adult Cochlear Implant Programme, Centre for Hearing and Balance Assessment, Rehabilitation and Research, University Hospital Birmingham, UK

**Colin L.W. Driscoll**, MD, Department of Otorhinolaryngology, Mayo Clinic, Rochester, Minnesota, USA

**Camille C. Dunn**, University of Iowa, Department of Otolaryngology Head and Neck Surgery, University of Iowa, Iowa City, IA 52242, USA

**Adrien A. Eshraghi**, MD, MSc, Assistant Professor, Department of Otolaryngology, University of Miami, Florida, USA

**Claire A. Fielden**, MSc, Audiological Scientist, Midlands Adult Cochlear Implant Programme, Centre for Hearing and Balance Assessment, Rehabilitation and Research, University Hospital Birmingham, UK

**Bruce J. Gantz**, MD, University of Iowa, Department of Otolaryngology Head and Neck Surgery, University of Iowa, Iowa City, IA 52242, USA

**Michael B. Gluth**, MD, Department of Otorhinolaryngology, Mayo Clinic, Rochester, Minnesota, USA

**John M. Graham**, FRCS, Consultant Otologist, Director of Cochlear Implant Programme, Royal National Throat, Nose and Ear Hospital, Gray's Inn Road, London, UK

**David B. Grayden**, PhD (Melbourne), BE(Hons), BSc, Research Fellow, Bionic Ear Institute, 384–388 Albert St, East Melbourne, VIC 3002, Australia

**Mrs Tricia Kemp**, Southwest London, UK

**John F. Knutson**, PhD, Department of Psychology, University of Iowa, Iowa City, IA, USA

**William Noble**, University of New England, Australia

**Mary Joe Osberger**, PhD, Advanced Bionics Corporation, Valencia, CA, 3 Azalea Drive, Nanuet, NY 10954 USA

**Aaron J. Parkinson**, Cochlear Americas, Englewood, CO, USA

**Geoff Plant**, Rehabilitation Specialist, Med-El Medical Electronics, Fürstenweg 77a, A-6020 Innsbruck, Austria; The Hearing Rehabilitation Foundation, 35 Medford Street, Somerville, MA 02143, USA

**David W. Proops**, FRCS, Consultant ENT Surgeon, University Hospital Birmingham NHS Foundation Trust, Queen Elizabeth Hospital, Edgbaston, Birmingham, UK

**Richard T. Ramsden**, FRCS, Department of Otolaryngology, Manchester Royal Infirmary, Manchester, UK

**Amy McConkey Robbins**, MS, Communication Consulting Services, Indianapolis, IN, USA

**Jay T. Rubinstein**, MD, PhD, University of Iowa, Department of Otolaryngology Head and Neck Surgery, University of Iowa, Iowa City, IA 52242, USA

**Jennifer L. Smullen**, MD, Clinical Fellow of Neurotology, Department of Otolaryngology, University of Miami, Florida, USA

**Timothy Stanley**, Teignmouth, Devon, UK

**Jacqueline Stokes**, MSc, Cert AVT, Auditory-Verbal UK, Oxford, UK

**Patricia G. Trautwein**, AuD, Advanced Bionics Corporation, Valencia, CA, USA

**Richard S. Tyler**, PhD, University of Iowa, Department of Otolaryngology Head and Neck Surgery, University of Iowa, Department of Speech Pathology and Audiology, University of Iowa, Iowa City, IA 52242, USA

**Elizabeth Tyszkiewicz**, MSc, Cert AVT, Auditory-Verbal UK, Oxford, UK

**Blake S. Wilson**, Research Triangle Institute International, PO Box 12194, Research Triangle Park, NC 27709, USA

**Shelley A. Witt**, University of Iowa, Department of Otolaryngology Head and Neck Surgery, University of Iowa, Iowa City, IA 52242, USA

# Preface

The first edition of this book, edited by Huw Cooper, was published in 1991 and became a popular and widely read textbook for what was then a relatively new and developing field. Since then, the field of cochlear implantation has moved forward on all fronts and the time had clearly come for a second edition. Progress in this field is rapid and, while we have attempted to include the latest techniques, technology and research in this book, it is likely that there will be yet newer aspects that will come to light after the book is published. We have intended this book to be a collection of the 'state of the art' opinions, and the authors are some of the leading authorities in the world on their chosen topic areas. Some chapters have been rewritten by the original authors from the first edition. Others are new authors to this book, but all contribute many years of experience and expertise in the field. We are indebted to our colleagues from the United States, Australia and the United Kingdom for their extensive and outstanding contributions.

This book is intended for use by professionals in the field of implants, in audiology in general, by students, other trainees and those with an interest in deafness.

# About the editors

**Huw R. Cooper, MSc, Consultant Audiological Scientist**, after obtaining his Master's degree in audiology at Southampton University in 1983, joined the team at University College Hospital, London, where he initially worked on tinnitus research. He was then closely involved in the set-up and development of the new UCH/RNID Cochlear Implant Programme, which led the way in establishing cochlear implantation in the UK. Since 1991, he has managed the audiology services at University Hospital Birmingham, including overseeing the growth and development of the Midlands Adult and the Birmingham Children's Cochlear Implant Programmes. His research interests include Neural Response Telemetry and Auditory Perceptual Grouping, on which topic he is currently working towards a PhD. Huw lives just outside Birmingham with his wife and three teenage children.

**Louise C. Craddock, MSc, CCC-A, Audiological Scientist**, originally trained as a teacher of hearing-impaired children and taught in London for twelve years before obtaining her MSc in Audiology at the University of Washington in Seattle. Since then she has worked on the UCL Adult and Nuffield Paediatric Cochlear Implant Programmes in London and is now the Co-ordinator of the Midlands Adult Cochlear Implant Programme in Birmingham. She has a research interest in objective measures in cochlear implantation, particularly in Neural Response Telemetry, and has published and presented her work in this area. Louise lives in Birmingham with her husband and two young daughters.

# Introduction

HUW R. COOPER AND LOUISE C. CRADDOCK

> I had come alive again. I was not on the outside looking in – I was in.
>
> Jean Briggs, cochlear implant recipient

> Without his cochlear implant, Matthew would not be who he is today. With the implant, his life is in full swing and the sky's the limit.
>
> Jennie Clewes, mother of a cochlear implant recipient

In the introduction to the first edition of this book, Mark Haggard said, 'Cochlear implants have not merely become an accepted treatment for sensory deafness, they have come of age.' To continue his theme, it would be fair to say that fourteen years after that edition cochlear implants have not only come of age but are now fully matured. The knowledge, experience and understanding of this fascinating field have grown hugely over the intervening years and Chapter 1 gives an overview of the process over time of this 'coming of age'. What was once a relatively new direction for hearing rehabilitation is now thoroughly established in the mainstream of audiology.

Mark Haggard also discussed the objections to cochlear implantation from some groups. Those of us who have been involved in the field over the years may have first-hand experience of the sometimes strongly held views of those people who disagree with the whole concept of cochlear implantation, particularly in children. Although there remain some who will continue to object in principle, most would probably now accept that deafened adults should be able to benefit from the available technology. Chapter 4 addresses the importance of a thorough assessment and the technological challenges this presents. As the technology has advanced and outcomes have improved, the importance of deciding who might benefit from an implant becomes even more crucial, and these aspects are addressed in Chapter 6, while Chapter 3 refers to the importance of making these clinical decisions as part of an interdisciplinary team. However, the benefit an individual can gain from his or her implant depends on the support they have from the rehabilitation professionals on the implant team, and this is the subject of Chapter 13. The positive impact implantation has on a deaf person is expressed most eloquently in the sections in Chapter 17 written by two of our cochlear implant recipients.

However, the implantation of children remains controversial, despite the overwhelming evidence that has accumulated of the positive benefits and amazing results that can be achieved. It is now a generally accepted fact that children who are given an implant at a young age can, in many cases, thrive in mainstream education and the hearing world, and develop good spoken language. The routine implantation of young children only became widespread in the 1980s, and so it is only recently that the long-term outcomes for this group are becoming apparent. The effects of discovering that a child is profoundly deaf and the journey the whole family takes towards the implant — and the life-changing experience this is for all involved – are explored in Chapter 18. For the professionals involved, this group is also the most challenging to work with. The assessment and habilitation of profoundly deaf children who receive implants are covered in Chapters 5 and 14, while Chapter 7 explores the related issues of the psychological aspects of deafness and cochlear implantation.

Other, sometimes startling, developments in the field have emerged since the first edition. The quality of hearing and speech discrimination performance expected from current implants far exceeds the typical results fourteen years ago, and the advances in speech processing strategies are discussed in Chapter 2. Smaller, ear-level speech processors are now routinely used and it is likely that completely implantable systems will become available in the future. Chapter 16 looks at this and other future developments, including some astonishing predictions for the possibilities of implant systems.

The surgical process has become more and more refined and there is now a greater expectation that residual hearing may be preserved, with a reduction in cochlear trauma during surgery. The complexity of the medical and surgical assessment has increased and the surgery itself has become more intricate, and Chapters 8 and 10 contain details of both these stages in the patient pathway. Of course, the pre-operative assessment and the surgery itself both rely on information provided by the radiological evaluation, and this is included in Chapter 9 with many superb images of the cochlear structures in the normal and abnormal ear.

As the technology advances and outcomes improve, the type of patient seen by implant teams has changed. The importance of binaural hearing has been the subject of much research and, as shown in Chapter 15, the potential benefits of bilateral implants and other forms of spatial hearing are now becoming more apparent. Moreover, implant teams are now working with patient groups – the very young or those with additional disabilities – where there is a greater reliance on the use of objective measures during the assessment and after implantation. The value of these methods and how they may be applied clinically when programming the device are addressed in Chapters 11 and 12.

As in any speciality, there is a great deal of terminology and technical expressions and most have been clearly defined within each chapter. In addition, readers will find an excellent glossary of many of the terms used in the field of cochlear implants in Chapter 2 by Blake Wilson.

In summary, we hope that this new edition will provide the interested reader with a comprehensive insight into the current 'state of the art' in the exciting and varied field of cochlear implants. Those of us lucky enough to work in this field will have experienced at first hand the massive changes to the lives of deaf people that can be achieved. It has been a privilege to work with such an outstanding group of authors and hugely satisfying to be able to bring their great expertise together into one book.

# CHAPTER 1

# Implant design and development

DAVID B. GRAYDEN AND GRAEME M. CLARK

## Introduction

The cochlear implant is an electronic device that is implanted under the skin with electrodes positioned in the cochlea to stimulate the auditory nerve. Electrical currents induce action potentials in the auditory nerve fibres and these are transmitted to the brain. It thus bypasses damaged or missing hair cells within the cochlea that would normally code sound. It consists of a receiver-stimulator, which receives power and decodes instructions for controlling the electrical stimulation, and an electrode array, which has electrodes placed near the auditory nerve (generally in the cochlea) to stimulate residual auditory nerve fibres.

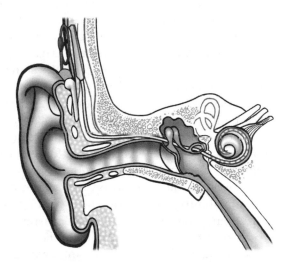

**Figure 1.1** The cochlear implant. The microphone, implant processor and transmission coil are outside the skin. The receiver-stimulator is implanted in the mastoid bone. The electrode array is threaded into the scala tympani of the cochlea.

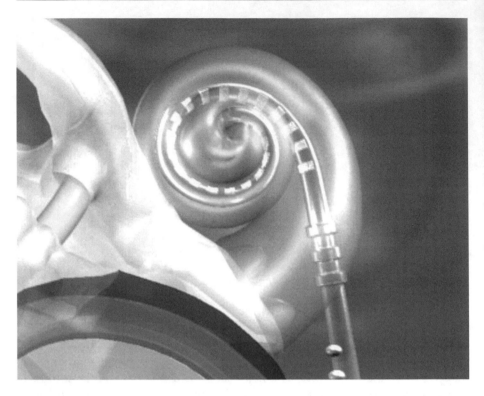

**Figure 1.2** Close-up of a banded electrode array in the scala tympani of the cochlea (courtesy of Cochlear Europe Ltd).

In addition, there is an external component (speech processor) that contains a microphone and device for picking up and processing incoming sound to create a set of stimuli for the electrodes. The processed signal, which contains temporal and spatial patterns of stimulation, is transmitted to the implanted receiver that decodes the signal and controls an electrical current on each electrode. While these components are common to all existing systems, the methods of processing the sounds, transmitting the information to the implant and stimulating the electrodes vary from system to system. Also, there are many different electrode arrays available. Initial systems had single electrodes, but for speech understanding multiple implanted electrodes are required. Multiple electrodes provide the ability to present information on more than one channel by dividing the acoustic signal into portions that have meaningful differences, such as different frequency bands. The electrode arrays have different shapes and are designed to be placed within the scala tympani.

This chapter gives a history of cochlear implants, working through the initial design problems and how they were overcome. The important design principles are then described, as well as the differences that may exist between different implants that are not critical to their usefulness, but offer alternatives to the recipients. Finally, a description of the present implants that are available is presented. Further modifications are anticipated in the future.

## 1950s and 1960s

Lundberg performed the first attempt at direct electrical stimulation of the auditory nerve in 1950 (Gisselsson, 1950). The perceived sound from sinusoidal stimulation was only noise. Djourno and Eyriès (1957) placed a telecoil on the frayed end of the auditory nerve and stimulated it with pulses of current. The patient was able to distinguish words in a small closed set, but could not achieve open-set speech recognition. Closed-set speech recognition is a test of whether a person can perceive a word from a small, defined list of words. Open-set speech recognition is the ability to perceive any words, although usually large sets of monosyllabic or bisyllabic words, or words in sentences, are used in testing. A second patient was implanted with an electrode placed extracochlearly near the promontory but also could not recognize speech (Zollner and Keidel, 1963). In 1961, House and Urban (1973) implanted electrodes into three people for short periods. The patients experienced some hearing sensations. Michelson (1971) implanted a number of profoundly deaf patients with multiple electrodes but only stimulated one pair of electrodes with a single channel of information. The patients were able to perceive environmental sounds and control their own voices better, but unaided speech recognition was not achieved.

Doyle et al. (1964) made the first attempt to stimulate the auditory nerve with multiple electrodes. Four electrodes were placed in the middle ear on the surface of the cochlea of one volunteer, but this did not produce a spatial distribution of stimulated auditory nerve fibres. Speech recognition was not possible, but the volunteer did achieve some perception of pitch and rhythm.

Simmons and colleagues performed a study where six electrodes were implanted in the modiolus aiming to stimulate nerves tonotopically (Simmons, 1966), which is stimulation of each electrode with a different frequency band. On each electrode, a pitch change was perceived as the rate of stimulation was changed up to a maximum of 300 pulses/s. In addition, pitch varied with electrode position, supporting the possibility that excitation could be localized to sets of auditory nerve fibres that correspond to different characteristic frequencies. At this stage, some speech processing was attempted, but speech recognition was not achieved.

In the 1960s, many experts believed that a cochlear implant for speech perception was not possible (Clark, 2000). The criticisms were largely based on physiological and biological arguments, and these were addressed by experiments with electrical stimulation in the experimental animal and the application of appropriate implant designs in humans.

## 1970s

In the 1970s, the number of implant designs grew rapidly, with many varieties of single- and multiple-channel devices constructed and implanted. They provided varying degrees of hearing, from providing perception of sound to open-set speech recognition.

An Austrian device, developed at the Technical University of Vienna, had eight intracochlear (inside the cochlea) electrodes in four stimulating pairs plus a pair of extracochlear (outside the cochlea) electrodes but only used single-electrode sound processing strategies (Hochmair and Hochmair-Desoyer, 1983). Some open-set speech recognition was obtained for two patients.

A single-channel approach was developed in London using extracochlear stimulation of the auditory nerve (Douek et al., 1977). The implant was stimulated with electrical currents corresponding to glottal vibrations picked up from a microphone placed beside the larynx. This aided speech (lip) reading and improved the user's own vocalizations.

The House Ear Institute in Los Angeles, USA, developed a single-electrode scheme for stimulation in the scala tympani (Danley and Fretz, 1982). Open-set speech recognition was not achieved, but the users obtained an increased perception of some speech features and environmental sounds, and were able to improve the modulation of their own voices (Hannaway, personal communication, April 1996).

At the University of California, San Francisco, a single electrode was placed through the round window into the scala tympani of four patients (Michelson, 1971). It was reported that any residual hearing in the operated ears was lost. Some closed-set speech recognition was possible in two patients.

Animal research demonstrated a number of principles of electrical stimulation that led to important design decisions in cochlear implants. Neurons in the auditory brainstem showed a limitation in synchronous firing in response to electrical stimulation above 200–300 pulses/s, although some responded in time to stimuli with rates of up to 500 pulses/s (Clark, 1969). Auditory nerve responses also tended to plateau at 500 pulses/s (Moxon, 1971). Thus, it was demonstrated that providing pitch information using rate of stimulation on a single electrode was impossible for speech, which requires a range of 100 Hz to at least 3000 Hz. A place coding mechanism, where different frequency bands were represented on different sets of auditory nerve fibres, was thus seen as necessary, and this could best be achieved with multiple electrodes (Clark, 1969).

In order to access sites that would allow separate stimulation of groups of auditory nerve fibres, it would be necessary to place the electrodes in positions that were closest to different groups of spiral ganglion cells and their dendrites. The most promising location was in the scala tympani. Simmons (1967) demonstrated that it was possible to insert electrodes through the round window without causing degeneration of the cochlea.

Clark et al. (1975a) demonstrated that electrodes could be inserted along the scala tympani with little trauma provided the basilar membrane or the spiral lamina were not damaged.

It was the introduction of multiple-electrode devices that provided open-set speech understanding for many of those who were implanted. The Chorimac multiple-channel devices, developed in Paris, France, had eight and later twelve channels. The electrodes were inserted into the scala tympani through individual holes drilled in the lateral wall of the cochlea (Chouard and MacLeod, 1976; Chouard, 1980). After training, postlinguistically deafened users were able to achieve some phoneme discrimination with electrical stimulation alone and some closed-set word recognition.

The other major multiple-channel device implanted in the 1970s was the Australian ten-channel device, developed at the University of Melbourne, providing a large increase in speech reading ability and some open-set speech recognition using electrical stimulation alone (Tong et al. 1980; Clark and Tong, 1981). Stimulating different electrodes caused a dull perception of sound at the apical end and a sharp perception at the basal end, near the round window, that could best be described as timbre. This allowed a successful speech processing strategy to be implemented known as the F0/F2 strategy, where the voicing pitch (F0) was represented by rate of stimulation and the second formant (F2), one of the resonance frequencies created in the vocal tract, was represented by choice of electrode to stimulate.

## 1980s

The success of multiple-channel implants in the late 1970s provided the impetus for more research and development. The development of single-channel devices also continued at that time. The Vienna device was developed industrially by 3M, but little open-set word recognition was obtained (Bredberg et al., 1987). The single-channel implant developed at the House Ear Institute in Los Angeles was also developed commercially by 3M (Fretz and Fravel, 1985). Users could identify environmental sounds and discriminate some vowels, but could not understand speech at conversational levels (Tyler et al., 1987; Gantz et al., 1989). The Czechoslovak Academy of Sciences developed a single-channel system placed in the round window. It provided an aid to patients in speech reading, pitch perception and hearing environmental sounds, but did not achieve speech recognition (Valvoda et al., 1987). The Department of Otolaryngology in Bordeaux, France, implanted a single-channel extra-cochlear implant (Negrevergne et al., 1987). It, too, provided rhythm and intonation but not speech recognition.

In Australia, Cochlear Proprietary Limited, now Cochlear Limited and its subsidiary in the USA, Cochlear Corporation, commenced clinical trials in 1982 of the Nucleus multiple-channel implant. Place coding of frequency was performed on 22 electrodes. An international trial was commenced in 1983 for the US Food and Drug Administration (FDA). A study of 40 users showed significant and substantial improvements in speech reading, and in speech understanding with electrical stimulation alone (Dowell et al., 1986). The F0/F2 strategy and WSP-II wearable speech processor were approved by the FDA in October 1985 as safe and effective for postlinguistically deaf adults. In 1986, the F0/F1/F2 strategy and WSP-III processor were approved by the FDA for use with postlinguistically deaf adults.

In Antwerp, Belgium, the LAURA multiple-electrode implant system was developed at the University of Louvaine (Peeters et al., 1987). The eight-channel electrode array and packaging of the implant progressed through a number of developments and changes as testing revealed important design considerations. A stimulation scheme similar to that of the Nucleus device was used.

The Chorimac-8 (eight channels) and Chorimac-12 (twelve channels) devices were developed in France by Bertin St Antoine and the University of Paris in the late 1970s and 1982, respectively. The electrodes continued to be implanted through fenestrations in the cochlea. There were some improvements in vowel recognition, voicing perception and closed-set word recognition (Fugain et al., 1984).

The University of Utah Symbion Ineraid multiple-channel device stimulated four electrodes in the cochlea (Eddington, 1980). Open-set sentence perception was achieved (Dorman et al., 1989), but pre-market approval from the FDA was not granted, primarily due to concerns with the percutaneous (connection through the skin) plug that was used to connect the external circuitry to the implant.

A large number of patients were implanted with a multiple-electrode extracochlear device developed in Cologne-Düren, Germany. The eight electrodes were placed in the wall of the cochlea in small holes (Banfai et al., 1984). A small percentage of the users showed signs of developing open-set speech perception.

The 1980s also saw the first use of cochlear implants in children. The House/3M single-channel implant was trialled in children in 1980. The children were able to recognize environmental sounds and discriminate different speech patterns (Thielemeir et al., 1985), and a few of them obtained some open-set speech recognition (Berliner et al., 1989).

The Australian Nucleus multiple-channel device was first implanted in a child in 1985. The child was 14 years old and obtained some help from the device in speech reading (Clark et al., 1987a). Cochlear Pty Ltd and the University of Melbourne developed a new implant that was smaller and had a magnet inserted in the receiver and transmitter coils to aid in aligning them. Initial results suggested that children born deaf or deafened early in life could achieve speech recognition ability similar to postlinguistically deaf adults (Dawson et al., 1989). A large proportion (50%) could obtain open-set speech recognition (Dawson et al., 1992). In

1990, the device was approved by the FDA as safe and effective for children from 2 to 18 years of age.

Thus, in the 1980s the cochlear implants moved from experimental to clinical devices approved for use in children and adults. Over 4000 people had received the Nucleus system alone. The 1990s saw the emergence of three new companies – Advanced Bionics, Med-El and MXM – and an expansion in the number and types of implants available. The major implant developments in the 1990s were increasing rates of stimulation, different numbers of electrodes, telemetry to obtain information from the implant about its condition and of neural responses, and the introduction of perimodiolar arrays that brought the electrodes closer to the modiolus at the centre of the cochlea.

# Implant design

There are a large number of components that make up a cochlear implant. Each of these components must be designed to provide optimal performance and to be safe in the environment of the head and cochlea. The following discussion looks at different design considerations for cochlear implants.

### Reliability

The electronics for the receiver-stimulator package, its electronics and the electrode array must be reliable. It must be able to cope with repeated small movements over long periods of time with no wire breakages resulting from metal fatigue, especially at the point where the electrode array emerges from the receiver-stimulator. For this reason the wires are usually longer than required and spiralled to allow movement without stress. This was also necessary for the growth of implanted children (Dahm et al., 1993). The prosthesis should be robust enough to reduce the chance of damage by impact, such as a blow to the head. Implantation in the mastoid bone prevents the receiver-stimulator from protruding from the head and provides some protection from knocks and bumps. Cochlear Pty Ltd and the University of Melbourne developed their smaller ('mini') receiver-stimulator for use with young children, and the CI-24 implant for implantation in infants and children under 2 years of age. All of the cochlear implant manufacturers strive to make the implant packages as small as possible, and each new generation of implant is thinner and smaller.

### Biocompatibility

The insertion of the electrode array must not cause excessive damage to the cochlea. Provided the basilar membrane or spiral lamina are not damaged or infection does not occur, electrodes can be inserted in the scala tympani without causing the loss of auditory neurons (Clark, 1977; Leake-Jones and Rebscher, 1983). Clark et al. (1975a) discovered that an array of uniform stiffness could be inserted into the apical and middle turns of the cochlea and pushed towards the basal turn more easily than from the basal turn pushed upward from the round window. However, the least trauma occurred when an electrode array with graded stiffness was inserted upward from the basal turn of the cochlea and holes were not drilled in the wall of the cochlea (Clark et al., 1979). Investigation of the use of relatively stiff wire electrodes, in particular the 3M/House electrode arrays, showed that there was significant insertion trauma resulting in damage to the basilar membrane, Reissner's membrane and the osseous spiral lamina (Johnsson et al., 1982). Such trauma leads to neuronal loss and new bone growth.

The implanted components must be biocompatible and not lead to long-term adverse tissue damage. The use of platinum alloys, certain silicone rubbers and titanium achieves this goal (Clark, 1987). In addition, it was found that the array should not fit snugly in the scala tympani as this was shown to be traumatic (Sutton et al., 1980), causing significant loss of auditory neurons in the basal turn (Schindler and Merzenich, 1974), but rather should only fill the middle of the scala tympani (Clark, 1977; Leake-Jones and Rebscher, 1983).

The electronics package must be impervious to body fluids. Salts and tissue that enter the implant will cause electronic failure. The most vulnerable area is where the wires exit the receiver-stimulator package to pass through to the cochlea. It was the advent of pacemaker-sealing technology pioneered by the Australian firm Telectronics that provided the containment necessary for the early successful implants.

**Placement of the electrode array**

The electrodes may be placed in the cochlea (intracochlear) or outside the cochlea (extracochlear). Early researchers were divided about the best location for placing auditory prosthesis electrodes for stimulation of the auditory nerve. At this stage, the four major commercial manufacturers of implants designed them for placing in the scala tympani of the cochlea. Early research at the University of Melbourne found that the most effective site for localized stimulation of the auditory nerve was the scala tympani (Black and Clark, 1980). Other early devices were designed for insertion into the scala tympani, including single-channel devices (Michelson, 1971; Hochmair and Hochmair-Desoyer, 1983; Fretz and Fravel, 1985) and multiple-channel devices (Eddington, 1980).

The electrodes of the Chorimac device were each inserted into separate holes drilled through the wall of the cochlea into the scala tympani (Pialoux et al., 1979). Insulating material was inserted between the fenestra in an attempt to further localize current flow to different portions of the auditory nerve. This practice continued with the Chorimac-8 (Chouard and MacLeod, 1976) and Chorimac-12 (Chouard et al., 1985) devices. However, with this method of insertion there is more fibrous tissue and new bone growth in the cochlea (Clark et al., 1975b). This approach was later found suitable for ossified cochleae by implanting with split arrays where the electrodes are separated into two or three separate sections and inserted through the round window and/or one or two holes drilled into the wall of the cochlea (Bredberg et al., 2000).

Other groups approached the insertion of electrodes within the cochlea with more caution. Work by Douek et al. (1977) implanted single electrodes in the mastoid cavity as they were concerned that intracochlear electrodes would damage auditory nerve fibres. The electrode was placed on the promontory of the cochlea and was able to produce auditory nerve stimulation to represent the frequency of voicing. Other single-channel implants were also implanted extracochlearly (Fraser, 1987; Negrevergne et al., 1987). The multiple-channel implant developed at Cologne-Düren was implanted outside the cochlea by placing the electrodes in small holes drilled in the wall of the cochlea, but not all the way through it (Banfai et al., 1984). This method was chosen on the grounds that it was less traumatic and would minimize the loss of spiral ganglion cells.

**Power and data transmission**

The transmission of power and data to the implant is preferably transcutaneous (through intact skin) rather than percutaneous (direct electrical connection) as the latter is prone to lead to infection. Where a percutaneous connection was used (Pialoux et al., 1979; Eddington, 1980) infection tended to develop around the plug. The connector was also prone to damage from bumping, fingering and other body movements, and was not aesthetically pleasing to patients.

There were several methods considered and used for transmitting data and power to an implant by transcutaneous means. The most common means of transmitting the power is via an inductively coupled link from an external coil to the receiver-stimulator (Djourno and Eyriès, 1957; Michelson, 1971; Clark et al., 1977). However, it is important that the method of transmission should not cause tissue damage. The use of very high frequencies carries the risk of over-exposure to non-ionizing radiation. Generally, it is best to keep the carrier frequency as low as possible and energy absorption within established limits as set by national standards boards. The data is transmitted in most devices by the modulation of the carrier wave. The data to be transmitted must specify which electrode to stimulate, the mode of stimulation, amplitude, pulse width and interpulse separation.

**Localization of current**

For place coding with multiple-channel devices, the current must be localized to separate groups of auditory nerve fibres. Three modes of stimulation are possible in implants: bipolar, common ground and monopolar. In bipolar stimulation, current flows between a pair of electrodes. Merzenich and Reid (1974) and Black and Clark (1980) found that current could be localized to separate groups of fibres using bipolar stimulation. Common ground stimulation occurs when current flows between one electrode and all of the other electrodes in the array, the latter having been connected together electronically. Black and Clark (1980) demonstrated that common ground stimulation also localized current to separate groups of auditory nerve fibres. Monopolar stimulation occurs when the current flows between one electrode in the array and one or more other electrodes placed outside the cochlea. Animal experiments showed that monopolar stimulation is not as localized as bipolar and common ground stimulation. However, psychophysical studies demonstrated that users could scale pitch just as well with monopolar stimulation as with the other two modes (Busby et al., 1994). Monopolar stimulation is commonly used in contemporary implants because the amount of current required to elicit perceptible stimulation is less than bipolar stimulation, thus reducing current density and increasing battery life.

**Safety**

Electrical stimulation must be charge-balanced to minimize DC currents, which can lead to electrode corrosion, production of toxic products and neural and tissue damage. One method of ensuring this is to short-circuit the electrodes together after stimulation to remove any residual current. The Nucleus 22 implant used shorting of electrodes, but high rates of stimulation could not be used as this would not leave sufficient time for the shorting to occur. Placing capacitors in series with the electrodes is another method of minimizing DC current, as they are effectively open circuits to zero-frequency currents. All currently available devices use capacitors for this purpose. The Nucleus 24 devices also use short-circuiting.

Charge density must be kept low. Charge density is the amount of charge passing through an area, so a current passing through a small area has a larger charge density than the same amount of current passing through a large area. If charge density is too high, there will be electrolytic changes at the electrode tissue interface and release of gas and toxic products. Thus, there is a danger of using electrodes that are too small, as a reduced area will increase the charge density.

**Array design**

The receiver-stimulator should be designed so that the stimulus parameters can be varied to allow the patient to use alternative speech processors and speech processing schemes as they are developed. This is preferable to replacing the implant with a more up-to-date model. Nevertheless, the array should be easy to remove and another inserted without causing

trauma and adverse effects. This may be necessary if the implant electronics fail, the device is damaged or if removal is required because of
severe infection. The original University of Melbourne device and the first
Nucleus device had connectors to join the receiver-stimulator to the electrode array. This allowed the receiver-stimulator package to be removed if
necessary without disturbing the electrode array. However, it was found
that with banded electrodes the array was smooth and free fitting so it
could be easily removed and replaced (Clark et al., 1987b). In the next
generation implant the connector was not used. Other electrode configurations could be more problematic. Those with protruding ball
electrodes, such as the Symbion/Ineraid device, could be difficult to
remove from the scala tympani as they could be tightly bound by fibrous
tissue or bone. Explantation sometimes caused wires to break and the
balls to be left in situ (Gray et al., 1993).

The number of electrodes is one of the main variables between different implant designs. Single-channel devices only stimulated one
electrode, and have only rarely provided open-set speech recognition for
users. Multi-channel devices have four to 22 electrodes as described earlier in this chapter, and have been able to provide open-set speech
understanding with electrical stimulation alone to many children and
adults. In addition, some implants include one or more extracochlear
electrodes to use as a return path for monopolar stimulation. Early studies with the Nucleus CI-22 device showed that the more electrodes in use
for an individual, the better the performance in speech recognition
(Deguine et al., 1993). For the Nucleus F0/F2 and F0/F1/F2 strategies,
open-set CID word-in-sentence scores improved with the use of
increased numbers of electrodes, and the SPEAK strategy benefited when
using 20 electrodes rather than eight for speech perception in noise
(Blamey et al., 1992). Lawson et al. (1996) found that an upper limit
when using the CIS strategy was seven or eight electrodes. Another benefit of more electrodes is that the pattern of stimulation may be altered
if there is reduced neural population in certain regions of the cochlea
compared to others or if certain electrodes cause stimulation of the facial
nerve (McKay et al., 1994).

The depth of insertion of multiple-channel implants also varies. Studies
with the Nucleus CI-22 and CI-24 devices demonstrated that speech perception ability correlates positively with the depth of electrode insertion
(Deguine et al., 1993; Yukawa et al., 2004).

The rate of stimulation defines the number of electrical current pulses
per second that may be presented across the electrode array. Each new
generation of a cochlear implant device has usually allowed for higher
rates of stimulation. Higher rates may improve the representation of temporal information by providing finer amplitude variations through finer
control of the rate and population of nerves excited (Rubinstein et al.,
1999). However, high rates of stimulation must reach a limit to utilize the
excitation properties of neurons. Paolini et al. (2001) have found with

intracellular recordings from the brainstem that their response becomes random above 1800 pulses/s. This is barely time enough between pulses for the nerve membrane to recover. Furthermore, preliminary studies in the Department of Otolaryngology by Linahan et al. (1999) indicated that at double those rates there is the possibility of neuronal loss. It therefore behoves clinicians and scientists not to proceed with very high rates of stimulation unless there is clear evidence physiologically, psychophysically and with safety studies that this should be carried out clinically.

**Telemetry**

Telemetry allows information to be transmitted from the device to an external system. Information, such as voltages generated by an active electrode, can be measured to help determine the state of the cochlea in that region, such as pathological changes in nearby tissue. As tissue forms, impedance increases, and so greater voltages are required to generate a fixed current. Another measure is the compound action potential of the auditory nerve, which indicates how much neural activity the stimulation is causing. This information can be used to estimate threshold and maximum stimulation levels in infants and young children. The systems may also be used to measure the spread of excitation and other parameters, allowing more detailed information to be obtained regarding performance of different implant configurations (e.g. Cohen et al., 2003).

**Perimodiolar arrays**

Early cochlear implant designs were free-fitting, allowing easy insertion into the scala tympani through small holes made in the wall of the cochlea. Because of the spiral shape of the cochlea, the electrodes tended to lie along the outer wall of the cochlea near the spiral ligament. This placed them as far away as they could be from the spiral ganglion cells and any peripheral processes that might still exist. Shepherd et al. (1993) demonstrated that the placement of the electrodes in the scala tympani affected the thresholds and the localization of current. The thresholds were lowest when the electrodes were closer to the peripheral processes of the spiral ganglion cells and there was evidence of more localized current flow when the electrodes were closer to the spiral ganglion cells. Placing the electrodes closer to the modiolus (perimodiolar) would provide the opportunity to produce better place coding of frequency. In addition, the amount of current needed to stimulate the neurons should be less since the electrodes would be closer to their target cells.

One way to cause the electrode array to lie closer to the modiolus is for the array to be precurved and have a method to make it curl once it had been inserted. This requires a mechanism to hold it straight prior to insertion and then allow it to resume its curled shape after insertion. Research commenced in developing perimodiolar arrays at the University of

Melbourne/Bionic Ear Institute in 1989. The array was refined by the Cooperative Research Centre (CRC) for Cochlear Implant Speech and Hearing Research (1992–99) and then the CRC for Cochlear Implant and Hearing Aid Innovation (1999–). The array was precurved to fit the curvature of the inner wall of the scala tympani. It was held straight during insertion for approximately 8 mm beyond the round window before being released and further advanced into the cochlea. Releasing the electrode too early resulted in the array curling back on itself. X-rays of the first three patients showed that the precurved array was closer to the modiolus than a typical straight array, although the distance was not uniform for two patients (Clark, 2003a).

An alternative array was developed by Cochlear Pty Limited. It was a straight array with a Teflon strip attached to the tip. After insertion, the strip could be pressed forwards to force the tip to move in towards the modiolus. However, this approach was abandoned when it was found that the Teflon strip could cause considerable damage to the basilar membrane (Clark, 2003a).

The final design developed by Cochlear Ltd and the CRCs used a platinum stylet passed along the centre of the array to hold it straight. During insertion, the stylet could be withdrawn allowing the array to reassume its curled position. This array was called the Contour array. The array was tested by inserting it into twelve temporal bones. It was found that the average insertion depth was deeper than the straight electrode array (Saunders et al., 2002) and that the probability of insertion-induced trauma was the same as the straight array.

The Advanced Bionics Clarion array was precoiled to 'hug' the modiolus and was inserted using an insertion tool that held the array straight for the first 8 mm. As with the Australian precurved arrays, the distance from the modiolus varied and it tended to lie in the centre of the scala tympani (Roland et al., 2000). Further development led to the HiFocus I array, which used a separate, unattached positioner that was inserted after the array in order to press the array into the modiolus, and the HiFocus II array, which had a positioner attached 10 mm from the tip of the array. However, these arrays caused severe damage to the basilar membrane and osseous spiral lamina when tested in human temporal bones (Richter et al., 2002). In addition, the closed space between the positioner and array could prevent tissue from growing between them and make it easier for infection to pass through to the cochlea and produce labyrinthitis and meningitis. The Advanced Bionics Corporation ceased using the positioner as a precaution against this risk. The US Centres for Disease Control and Prevention and the US Food and Drug Administration showed that the use of the positioner was associated with a greater risk of contracting post-implantation bacterial meningitis for children implanted before the age of 6.

Psychophysical studies demonstrated that thresholds and maximum comfortable levels of stimulation were lower the closer the electrodes were to the inner wall of the cochlea (Saunders et al., 2002). It was also shown that the dynamic range increased, that there were more usable steps in loudness and that electrode place could be discriminated better with reduced distance from the modiolus (Cohen et al., 2001, 2003).

# Present multi-channel implants

## Advanced Bionics Corporation

The Clarion® cochlear implant was developed by the University of California in San Francisco, the Research Triangle Institute in North Carolina and the Advanced Bionics Corporation in California. This has since been developed into the CII Bionic Ear™ implant, which received approval from the FDA in 2000. It is a pre-coiled array with sixteen electrodes that terminate in square electrode contacts designed to direct current towards the modiolus (called 'HiFocus Electrodes'). The receiver circuitry and coil are integrated into a single case made of zirconia ceramic material. The case has dimensions of 31 mm x 25 mm x 6 mm. The device has an information update rate of 90,000 updates per second and a stimulation rate of 83,000 pulses/s across the electrodes. The implant allows simultaneous and non-simultaneous stimulation in monopolar or bipolar configurations with a number of different processing and stimulation strategies. It also incorporates Neural Response Imaging for measurement of compound action potentials and telemetry about the performance of the device. It must be stressed, however, that there is presently no physiological evidence that stimulus rates above 1800 pulses/s are any more effective.

In July 2003, the HiRes™ 90K implant was released. It is essentially the same as the CII Bionic Ear™ implant except that the packaging has been altered to make it more suitable for young children. The electronics are packaged in a titanium case and the coil has been placed outside in the package but in the same flexible silicone housing. The case is now 28 mm x 56 mm x 5.5 mm, i.e. it is narrower and thinner but longer than the CII.

## Cochlear Ltd, Cochlear Corporation

The Nucleus® 24 cochlear implants and their precursors were developed by the University of Melbourne, the Cooperative Research Centre (CRC) for Cochlear Implant Speech and Hearing Research, the CRC for Cochlear Implant and Hearing Aid Innovation and Cochlear Ltd (formerly Cochlear Pty Ltd). The Nucleus® 24 Contour™, Nucleus® 24 M and the Nucleus® 24k have 22-channel electrode arrays. The Contour is a precurved electrode array designed to hug the modiolus. All electrode arrays are going to find some obstruction to their advancement at the distal end of the basal turn. This is because the dimensions narrow and there is a risk that the tip of the electrode may jam and cause buckling of the array. For that reason a soft tip has been developed to negotiate the region in a more flexible way. The electrodes are half-bands situated on the inner side of the array to direct current towards the modiolus. The 24M and 24k implants have straight arrays, though the 24k is a later development that has a smaller receiver body. In addition, the Nucleus 24 Double Array has two separate electrode arrays with eleven electrodes each for ossified cochleae. The receiver is encased in titanium and the receiving coil beside it. It has a maximum depth of 6.9 mm, with width 22 mm plus some extra width of the coil and length of 50.5 mm. The device can be stimulated at 14,400 pulses/s across the electrodes with monopolar or bipolar stimulation with no upper limit on a single electrode. The device incorporates Neural Response Telemetry for measurement of compound action potentials and telemetry about the performance and behaviour of the device. The magnet in the receiving coil may be surgically removed to allow MRI scanning up to 1.5 Tesla.

### Med-El

The Combi 40+ Cochlear Implant System was developed by the Technical University of Vienna and Med-El. It has a straight electrode array with 24 electrodes arranged as connected pairs to give twelve-channel monopolar stimulation. The array is designed for placement as deep as 31 mm in the scala tympani, which is about two turns of the cochlea. In addition, there are two other electrode arrays for use in cases of cochlear ossification: the C40+S, which is only 12 mm long compared to 26 mm for the standard version, for shallow insertions, and the C40+GB, which is a dual array with five channels on one array and seven on the other, for insertion into two drilled canals. The receiver circuitry and coil are integrated into a single ceramic case that is very similar in size and shape to the Advanced Bionics CII implant, though it is only 4 mm thick. The device can stimulate at 18,000 pulses/s across the electrodes with no upper limit on each channel. The device incorporates telemetry for testing the functionality of the implant. MRI up to 1.5 Tesla is possible.

### MXM

The Digisonic multi-channel cochlear implant was developed by Bertin/CHU St Antoine and MXM from the Chorimac devices by Pialoux et al. (1979). It has a straight, free-fitting electrode array with 15 band-like electrodes over 24 mm length. In addition, the Digisonic Multi-Array has three electrode arrays with large surface electrodes for implantation in the totally ossified cochlea. Stimulation is common ground with the amplitude of stimulation fixed and pulse duration varied to alter the level of stimulation. The package is circular and convex, with a diameter of 28.5 mm and maximum depth of 5.5 mm.

# Conclusion

Cochlear implants have developed from a device that was considered impossible for speech recognition and useful only for the perception of sound to an established clinical device for restoring hearing to profoundly and severely hearing-impaired children and adults. There are now four major companies that produce cochlear implants that are capable of advanced stimulation of the auditory nerve. Cochlear Ltd alone by 2003 had provided 50,000 implants for adults and children worldwide. There is considerable competition and each company is spending much on research and development. We will certainly be seeing new, improved devices coming onto the market in the future. It remains, however, to be seen whether devices that stimulate faster, have more electrodes and reach deeper into the cochlea offer advantages. Fully implanted devices with no external speech processor are expected. Further advances are likely in the fields of tissue engineering, nanotechnology and micromechanics as well as neuroscience (Clark, 2003b). The electrode needs to be closer to a greater number of auditory nerves to better reproduce more advanced speech processing strategies, in particular simulations of the physiology. This requires a finer temporal-spatial pattern of activity. The electrodes may lie in the scala tympani but directed with control of bending to lie favourably under the spiral lamina. In addition, they will need to be able to release neurotrophins to preserve the neural elements or promote the regeneration of the peripheral fibres. Alternatively, it may be possible to place electrodes in the scala media. However, before doing so a number of key issues need to be resolved, particularly the loss of neural activity from a mixing of the perilymph and endolymph and also the need for the spread of neurotrophins through the tight junctions.

# References

Banfai P, Karczag A, Luers P (1984) Cochlear implants. Clinical results: the rehabilitation. Acta Oto-Laryngologica (suppl. 411): 183–94.

Berliner K, Tonokawa L, Dye L et al. (1989) Open-set speech recognition in children with a single-channel cochlear implant. Ear and Hearing 10: 237–42.

Black R, Clark G (1980) Differential electrical excitation of the auditory nerve. Journal of the Acoustical Society of America 67: 868–74.

Blamey P, Pyman B, Gordon M et al. (1992) Factors predicting postoperative sentence scores in postlinguistically deaf adult cochlear implant patients. Annals of Otology, Rhinology and Laryngology 101: 342–8.

Bredberg G, Ossean-Corp B, Lindstrom B (1987) Results from 10 patients with extracochlear 3M/Vienna single electrode implant. In: P Banfai (ed.), Cochlear implant: Current situations. International Cochlear Implant Symposium, Düren, Germany, pp. 175–77.

Bredberg G, Lindstrom B, Lopponen H et al. (2000) A new approach for the treatment of ossified cochleas. In: S Waltzman, N Cohen (eds), Cochlear Implants. New York: Thième Medical Publishers Inc.

Busby P, Whitford L, Blamey P et al. (1994) Pitch perception for different modes of stimulation using the cochlear multiple-electrode prosthesis. Journal of the Acoustical Society of America 95: 2658–69.

Chouard C (1980) The surgical rehabilitation of total deafness with the multi-channel cochlear implant: indications and results. Audiology 19: 137–45.

Chouard C, MacLeod P (1976) Implantation of multiple intracochlear electrodes for rehabilitation of total deafness: preliminary report. Laryngoscope 86: 1743–51.

Chouard C, Fugain C, Meyer B et al. (1985) The Chorimac-12. A multichannel cochlear implant for total deafness: description and clinical results. Acta Oto-Rhino-Laryngologica Belgica 39: 735–48.

Clark G (1969) Middle ear and neural mechanisms in hearing and the management of deafness. Thesis (PhD), University of Sydney.

Clark G (1977) An evaluation of per-scalar cochlear electrode implantation techniques: an histopathogical study in cats. Journal of Laryngology and Otology 91. 185–99.

Clark G (1987) The University of Melbourne Nucleus Multi-Electrode Cochlear Implant. Basel: Karger.

Clark G (2000) The cochlear implant: a search for answers. Cochlear Implants International 1: 1–17.

Clark G (2003a) Cochlear Implants: Fundamentals and Applications. New York: Springer-Verlag.

Clark G (2003b) Research directions for future generations of cochlear implants. Keynote Address for 4th Congress of Asia Pacific Symposium on Cochlear Implant and Related Sciences, 4–6 December 2003.

Clark G, Tong Y (1981) Multiple-electrode cochlear implant for profound or total hearing loss: a review. Medical Journal of Australia 1: 428–9.

Clark G, Hallworth R, Zdanius K (1975a) A cochlear implant electrode. Journal of Laryngology and Otology 89: 787–92.

Clark G, Kranz H, Minas H et al. (1975b) Histopathological findings in cochlear implants in cats. Journal of Laryngology and Otology 89: 495–504.

Clark G, Black R, Dewhurst D et al. (1977) A multiple-electrode hearing prosthesis for cochlear implantation in deaf patients. Medical Progress through Technology 5: 127–40.

Clark G, Patrick J, Bailey Q (1979) A cochlear implant round window electrode array. Journal of Laryngology and Otology 93: 107–9.

Clark G, Blamey P, Busby P et al. (1987a) A multiple-electrode intracochlear implant for children. Archives of Otolaryngology 113: 825–8.

Clark G, Pyman B, Webb R et al. (1987b) Surgery for safe insertion and reinsertion of the banded electrode array. Annals of Otology, Rhinology and Laryngology 96 (suppl. 128): 10–12.

Cohen L, Saunders E, Clark G (2001) Psychophysics of a prototype peri-modiolar cochlear implant array. Hearing Research 155: 63–81.

Cohen L, Richardson L, Saunders E et al. (2003) Spatial spread of neural excitation in cochlear implant recipients: comparison of improved ECAP method and psychophysical forward masking. Hearing Research 179: 72–87.

Dahm M, Shepherd R, Clark G (1993) The postnatal growth of the temporal bone and its implications for cochlear implantation in children. Acta Oto-Laryngologica (suppl. 505): 1–39.

Danley M, Fretz R (1982) Design and functioning of the single-electrode cochlear implant. Annals of Otology, Rhinology and Laryngology (suppl. 91): 21–6.

Dawson P, Blamey P, Clark G et al. (1989) Results in children using the 22 electrode cochlear implant. Journal of the Acoustical Society of America 86 (suppl. 1): 81.

Dawson P, Blamey P, Rowland L et al. (1992) Cochlear implants in children, adolescents and prelinguistically deafened adults: speech perception. Journal of Speech and Hearing Research 35: 401–17.

Deguine O, Fraysse B, Uziel A et al. (1993) Predictive factors in cochlear implant surgery. Advances in Oto-Rhino-Laryngology 48: 142–5.

Djourno A, Eyriès C (1957) Prosthèse auditive par excitation électrique à distance du nerf sensorial à l'aide d'un bobinage inclus à demeure. Presse Médicale 35: 14–17.

Dorman M, Dankowski K, McCandless G (1989) Consonant recognition as a function of the number of channels of stimulation by patients who use the Symbion cochlear implant. Ear and Hearing 10: 288–91.

Douek E, Fourcin A, Moore B et al. (1977) A new approach to the cochlear implant. Proceedings of the Royal Society of Medicine 70: 379–83.

Dowell R, Mecklenburg D, Clark G (1986) Speech recognition for 40 patients receiving multichannel cochlear implants. Archives of Otolaryngology 112: 1054–9.

Doyle J, Doyle J, Turnbull F (1964) Electrical stimulation of eighth cranial nerve. Archives of Otolaryngology 80: 388–91.

Eddington D (1980) Speech discrimination in deaf subjects with cochlear implants. Journal of the Acoustical Society of America 68: 885–91.

Fraser J (1987) UCH/RNID cochlear implant programme – an overview: patient selection and surgical technique. In: P Banfai (ed.), Cochlear Implant: Current Situations. International Cochlear Implant Symposium, Düren, Germany, pp. 273–9.

Fretz R, Fravel R (1985) Design and function: a physical and electrical description of the 3M House cochlear implant system. Ear and Hearing 6: 14S–19S.

Fugain C, Meyer B, Chabolle F et al. (1984) Clinical results of the French multi-channel cochlear implant. Acta Oto-Laryngologica (suppl. 411): 237–46.

Gantz B, Tye-Murray N, Tyler R (1989) Word recognition performance with single-channel and multichannel cochlear implants. American Journal of Otology 10: 91–4.

Gisselsson L (1950) Experimental investigation into the problem of humoral transmission in the cochlea. Acta Oto-Laryngologica (suppl. 82): 16.

Gray R, Baguley D, Harries M et al. (1993) Profound deafness treated by the Ineraid multichannel intracochlear implant. Journal of Laryngology and Otology 107: 673–80.

Hochmair E, Hochmair-Desoyer I (1983) Percepts elicited by different speech coding strategies. Annals of the New York Academy of Sciences 405: 268–79.

House W, Urban J (1973) Long-term results of electrode implantation and electronic stimulation of the cochlea in man. Annals of Otology, Rhinology and Laryngology 82: 504–17.

Johnsson L, House W, Linthicum F (1982) Otopathological findings in a patient with bilateral cochlear implants. Annals of Otology, Rhinology and Laryngology 91: 74–89.

Lawson D, Wilson B, Zerbi M et al. (1996) Speech processors for auditory prostheses, Third Quarterly Progress Report. NIH contract No1-DC-5-2103.

Leake-Jones P, Rebscher S (1983) Cochlear pathology with chronically implanted scala tympani electrodes. Annals of the New York Academy of Sciences 405: 203–23.

Linahan N, Tykocinski M, Shepherd RK et al. (1999) Physiological and histopathological effects of chronic monopolar stimulation on the auditory nerve using very high stimulus rates. Proceedings of the Australian Neuroscience Society. (Australian Neuroscience Meeting. Hobart, 31 January–3 February 1999) 10: 181.

McKay C, McDermott H, Clark G (1994) The beneficial use of channel interaction for the improvement of speech perception for multichannel cochlear implants. Australian Journal of Audiology 15: 20–1.

Merzenich M, Reid M (1974) Representation of the cochlea within the inferior colliculus. Brain Research 77: 397–415.

Michelson R (1971) Electrical stimulation of the human cochlea: a preliminary report. Archives of Otolaryngology 93: 317–23.

Moxon E (1971) Neural and mechanical responses to electrical stimulation of the cat's inner ear. Thesis (PhD), Cambridge, MA: MIT.

Negrevergne M, Dauman R, Lagourgue P et al. (1987) Extra-cochlear implant Prelco. In: P Banfai (ed.), Cochlear implant: Current situations. International Cochlear Implant Symposium, Düren, Germany.

Paolini A, Fitzgerald J, Burkitt A et al. (2001) Temporal processing from the auditory nerve to the medial nucleus of the trapezoid body in the rat. Hearing Research 159: 101–16.

Peeters I, Marquet J, Offeciers E et al. (1987) The Laura cochlear prosthesis development description. In: P Banfai (ed.), Cochlear Implant: Current situations. International Cochlear Implant Symposium, Düren, Germany.

Pialoux P, Chouard C, Meyer B (1979) Indications and results of the multichannel cochlear implant. Acta Oto-Laryngologica 87: 185–9.

Richter B, Aschendorff A, Lohnstein P et al. (2002) Clarion 1.2 standard electrode array with partial space filling positioner: radiological and histological evaluation in human temporal bones. Journal of Laryngology and Otology 116: 507–13.

Roland J, Fishman A, Alexiades G et al. (2000) Electrode to modiolus proximity: a fluoroscopic and histologic analysis. American Journal of Otology 21: 218–25.

Rubinstein J, Wilson B, Finley C et al. (1999) Pseudospontaneous activity: stochastic independence of auditory nerve fibers with electrical stimulation. Hearing Research 127: 108 18.

Saunders E, Cohen L, Aschendorff A et al. (2002) Threshold, comfortable level and impedance changes as a function of electrode-modiolar distance. Ear and Hearing 23(1): 28S–40S.

Schindler R, Merzenich M (1974) Chronic intracochlear electrode implantation: cochlear pathology and acoustic nerve survival. Annals of Otolaryngology 83: 202–15.

Shepherd R, Hatsushika S, Clark G (1993) Electrical stimulation of the auditory nerve: the effect of electrode position on neural excitation. Hearing Research 66: 108–20.

Simmons F (1966) Electrical stimulation of the auditory nerve in man. Archives of Otolaryngology 84: 2–54.

Simmons F (1967) Permanent intracochlear electrodes in cats. Tissue tolerance and cochlear microphonics. Laryngoscope 77: 171–86.

Sutton D, Miller J, Pfingst B (1980) Comparison of cochlear histopathology following two implant designs for use in scala tympani. Annals of Otology, Rhinology and Laryngology 89: 11–14.

Thielemeir M, Tonokawa L, Petersen B et al. (1985) Audiological results in children with a cochlear implant. Ear and Hearing (suppl. 6): 27S–35S.

Tong Y, Clark G, Seligman P et al. (1980) Speech processing for a multiple-electrode cochlear implant hearing prosthesis. Journal of the Acoustical Society of America 68: 1897–9.

Tyler R, Tye-Murray N, Preece J et al. (1987) Vowel and consonant confusions among cochlear implant patients: do different implants make a difference? Annals of Otology, Rhinology and Laryngology 96 (suppl. 128): 141–4.

Valvoda M, Betka J, Hruby J (1987) The first experience with cochlear implantations in Czechoslovakia. In: P Banfai (ed.), Cochlear Implant: Current situations. International Cochlear Implant Symposium, Düren, Germany, pp. 235–7.

Yukawa K, Cohen L, Blamey P et al. (2004) Effects of insertion depth of cochlear implant electrodes upon speech perception. Audiology and Neuro-Otology 9: 163–72.

Zollner F, Keidel W (1963) Gerorvermittlung durch elektrische erregung des nervous acousticus. Archiv Ohr Nas Kehlkopfheilk 181: 216–23.

# CHAPTER 2

# Speech processing strategies

BLAKE S. WILSON

## Introduction

Speech processing strategies for cochlear implants transform a micro-phone or other input into electrical stimuli. Ideally, the stimuli represent the essential elements of the input in a way that they can be perceived and utilized by the patient.

Progress in the development of processing strategies has led to great strides forward during the past 25 years in the performance and widespread application of cochlear implants. Over the course of that relatively short period, implants have become the standard treatment for deafness and severe hearing loss. The main purpose of this chapter is to describe strategies in current use and to indicate some possibilities for further improvements in performance. Detailed descriptions of prior strategies, as well as histories of developments leading up to the current strategies, are presented elsewhere (Loizou, 1998, 1999; Wouters et al., 1998; Clark, 2000; Wilson, 2000a, 2004; David et al., 2003; Brown et al., in press). Designs of other components in implant systems – including the microphone, tran-scutaneous or percutaneous link and the implanted electrodes – are described in Wilson (2004). A broad overview of implant design can be found in a recent article by Dorman and Wilson (2004).

A glossary of commonly used terms and abbreviations is presented at the end of this chapter.

## Aspects of normal hearing

Aspects of normal hearing are illustrated in the top panel of Figure 2.1. Sound waves traveling through air reach the tympanic membrane via the ear canal, causing vibrations that move the three small bones of the middle ear. This action produces a piston-like movement of the stapes, the third

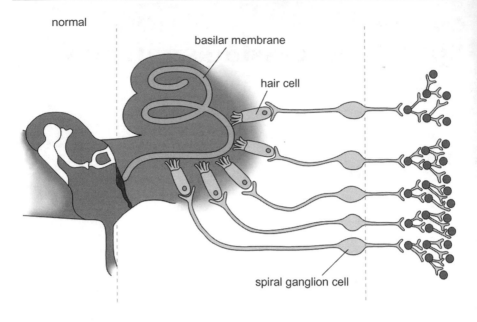

normal

basilar membrane

hair cell

spiral ganglion cell

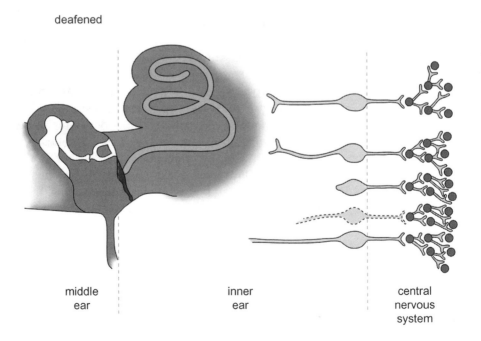

deafened

middle
ear

inner
ear

central
nervous
system

**Figure 2.1** Illustrations of anatomical structures in the normal and deafened ears. Note the absence of sensory hair cells in the deafened ear. Also note the incomplete survival of spiral ganglion cells and of neural processes peripheral to cells that are still viable. The illustrations do not reflect the details of the structures and are not to scale. (From Dorman and Wilson (2004), and used with the permission of the American Scientist and Sigma Xi.)

bone in the chain. The 'footplate' of the stapes is attached to a flexible membrane in the bony shell of the cochlea called the oval window. Inward and outward movements of this membrane induce pressure oscillations in the cochlear fluids, which in turn initiate a traveling wave of displacement along the basilar membrane (BM), a highly specialized structure that divides the cochlea along its length. This membrane has graded mechanical properties. At the base of the cochlea, near the stapes and oval window, it is narrow and stiff. At the other end of the cochlea, near the apex, the membrane is wide and flexible. These properties give rise to the traveling wave and to points of maximal response according to the frequency or frequencies of the pressure oscillations. For an oscillation with a single frequency, displacement increases up to a particular point along the membrane and then drops precipitously. High frequencies produce maxima near the base of the cochlea, whereas low frequencies produce maxima near the apex.

Motion of the BM is sensed by the inner hair cells (IHCs) in the cochlea, which are attached to the top of the membrane in a matrix of cells called the organ of Corti. Each hair cell has fine rods of protein, called stereocilia, emerging from one end. When the BM moves at the location of a hair cell, the rods are deflected as if hinged at their bases. Such deflections in one direction increase the release of a chemical transmitter substance at the base (other end) of the cells, and deflections in the other direction inhibit the release. The variations in the concentration of the chemical transmitter substance can inhibit or increase discharge activity in nearby neurons according to the direction of the deflections. Changes in neural activity thus reflect events at the BM. These changes are transmitted to the brain via the auditory nerve, the collection of all neurons that innervate the cochlea.

## Anatomical considerations for implants

A cutaway drawing of the implanted cochlea is presented in Figure 2.2. The figure shows a partial insertion of the electrode array into the scala tympani (ST). This is characteristic of all available ST implants. No array has been inserted further than about 30 mm from the cochleostomy or round window, and typical insertions are much less than that, e.g. 18–26 mm. (The total length of a typical human cochlea is about 35 mm.) In some cases, only shallow insertions are possible, such as when bony obstructions in the lumen of the ST impede further insertion. Different electrodes in the implanted array may stimulate different subpopulations of cochlear neurons. As noted above, neurons at different positions along the length of the cochlea respond to different frequencies of acoustic stimulation in normal hearing. Implant systems attempt to mimic or reproduce this tonotopic encoding by stimulating basal electrodes (first turn and lower part of the drawing) to indicate the presence of high-frequency sounds and by stimulating electrodes at more apical positions (deeper into the ST and ascending along the first and second turns in the drawing) to indicate the presence of

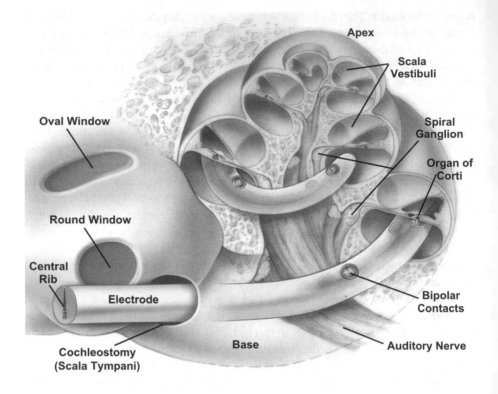

**Figure 2.2** Cutaway drawing of the implanted cochlea. The electrode array developed at the University of California at San Francisco is illustrated (Loeb et al., 1983). That array includes 8 pairs of bipolar electrodes, spaced at 2 mm intervals and with the electrodes in each pair oriented in an 'offset radial' arrangement with respect to the neural processes peripheral to the ganglion cells in the intact cochlea. Only four of the bipolar pairs are visible in the drawing, as the others are 'hidden' by cochlear structures. This array was used in the UCSF/Storz and Clarion 1.0 devices. (From Leake and Rebscher (2004), and used with the permission of Springer-Verlag.)

sounds with lower frequencies. Closely spaced pairs of bipolar electrodes are illustrated here, but arrays of single electrodes that are each referenced to a remote electrode outside of the cochlea also may be used. (Indeed, this is the most common arrangement for present-day implants.) Choices and tradeoffs in the design of electrodes are described in Wilson (2004). In general, such choices, along with the condition of the implanted cochlea, can affect the spatial specificity of neural excitation in the vicinity of each stimulus site. An important goal of electrode design is to maximize the number of largely non-overlapping populations of neurons that can be addressed with the electrode array. Present evidence suggests, however, that no more than 4–8 independent sites may be available using current designs, even for arrays with as many as 22 electrodes (Lawson et al., 1996; Fishman et al., 1997; Wilson, 1997; Kiefer et al., 2000; Friesen et al., 2001; Garnham et al., 2002). That is, a high number of electrodes does not guarantee a high number of

largely non-overlapping excitation fields. The many issues related to electrode design, along with prospects for the future, are discussed in the
references cited above and in other recent papers (Cohen et al., 2001; Frijns
et al., 2001; Gstoettner et al., 2001; Balkany et al., 2002; Badi et al., 2003;
Hillman et al., 2003).

Figure 2.2 shows a complete presence of hair cells (in the organ of
Corti) and a pristine survival of cochlear neurons. However, the number
of hair cells is zero or close to it in the deafened cochlea. In addition, survival of neural processes peripheral to the ganglion cells (the 'dendrites',
projecting from the ganglion cells to the organ of Corti) is rare in the deafened cochlea (e.g. Hinojosa and Marion, 1983). Survival of the ganglion
cells and central processes (the axons) ranges from sparse to substantial.
The pattern of survival is in general not uniform, with reduced or sharply
reduced counts of spiral ganglion cells in certain regions of the cochlea.
In all, the neural substrate or 'target' for a cochlear implant can be quite
different from one patient to the next. A detailed review of these observations and issues is presented in Leake and Rebscher (2004).

The anatomical situation faced by designers of implant systems is illustrated further in the bottom panel of Figure 2.1. In the deafened cochlea,
the hair cells are largely or completely absent, severing the connection
between the peripheral and central auditory systems. The function of a
cochlear prosthesis is to bypass the hair cells by stimulating directly the
surviving neurons in the auditory nerve. In general, a substantial fraction
of neurons survive even in cases of prolonged deafness and even for viru-
lent etiologies such as meningitis (Hinojosa and Marion, 1983; Miura et al.,
2002; Leake and Rebscher, 2004). However, the distribution of cells along
the length of the cochlea may be 'patchy', with good survival in some
regions and poor survival in others. Such latter regions may produce gaps
or 'holes' in the hearing produced with implants (Kasturi et al., 2002;
Shannon et al., 2002). Finally, the degree of myelination among surviving
neurons may vary strongly within and across patients. Myelinated neurons
usually exhibit greater sensitivity and more-rapid recovery from prior stimulation than non-myelinated neurons (see a review in Abbas and Miller,
2004). Thus, the pattern and physiology of surviving neurons in the
implanted cochlea are likely to be quite different from patient to patient.
This is a sometimes-neglected but important aspect of implant design.

## Processing strategies in current use

Present strategies for representing speech information with cochlear
implants are listed in Table 2.1. They include the continuous interleaved
sampling (CIS; see Wilson et al., 1991), spectral peak (SPEAK; see Skinner et
al., 1994; Seligman and McDermott, 1995; Patrick et al., 1997), advanced
combination encoder (ACE; see Arndt et al., 1999; Vandali et al., 2000; Kiefer
et al., 2001), $n$-of-$m$ (corresponding to selection of $n$ among $m$ channels for

**Table 2.1** Processing strategies in current use[a]

| System[b] | CIS | n-of-m | ACE[c] | SPEAK | SAS | PPS[d] | HiRes[e] |
|---|---|---|---|---|---|---|---|
| COMBI 40 | • | | | | | | |
| COMBI 40+ | • | • | | | | | |
| PULSAR[f] | • | | | | | | |
| LAURA | • | | | | | | |
| CI22 | | | | • | | | |
| CI24M, CI24R[g] | • | | • | • | | | |
| Clarion 1.2 | • | | | | • | • | |
| Clarion CII | • | | | | • | • | • |
| HiRes 90K[h] | • | | | | | • | • |

a Systems are listed in the leftmost column and the strategies used with each are indicated in the remaining columns. See text for full names of the strategies. Note that the strategies indicate broad categories and the details of implementations for a given strategy can vary (sometimes widely) across systems.

b The COMBI 40 system was manufactured by Med-El GmbH of Innsbruck, Austria; the COMBI 40+ and PULSAR systems are manufactured by that company now; the LAURA system was recently manufactured by Philips Hearing Instruments and before then by Antwerp Bionic Systems, in Antwerp, Belgium (manufacture of this system has been discontinued); the CI22 system was manufactured by Cochlear Ltd. of Sydney, Australia, up until 1997; the CI24M and CI24R systems are manufactured by that company now; the Clarion 1.0 and 1.2 systems were manufactured by Advanced Bionics Corporation of Sylmar, CA, USA; and the Clarion CII and HiRes 90K systems are manufactured by that company now.

c As indicated in this chapter and described more thoroughly in Wilson (2000a), the ACE strategy can be regarded as a close variation of the n-of-m strategy.

d The PPS strategy also has been called the 'multiple pulsatile sampler', or MPS, strategy.

e As described in this chapter, the HiRes strategy is a close variation of the CIS strategy.

f The PULSAR system was introduced in the spring of 2004 and has greater hardware capabilities than the COMBI 40+ implant, e.g. it can support higher rates of stimulation and has better current sources. The CIS strategy has been used in conjunction with the PULSAR in initial clinical trials in Europe. The hardware is capable of supporting many additional strategies, and evaluations of alternative strategies are planned (see www.medel.com and Zierhofer, 2003).

g The CI24M, CI24R (CS) and CI24R (CA) systems differ only in the type of electrode arrays that are used and the size of the implanted receiver/stimulator package. The CI24M uses the N22 array and the CI24R (CS) uses the Contour array with removable stylet. The CI24R (CA) uses the Contour 'Advanced' array that includes a bevelled and flexible tip at the basal end of the array (the 'softip' electrode array) and is inserted at surgery using an 'advance off-stylet' technique. The N22 is a straight array and the Contour is a curved array, designed to conform to the inner wall of the scala tympani. The same receiver/stimulator package is used in the CI24R (CS) and CI24R (CA) systems, and that package is smaller than that of the CI24M system. The internal electronics are identical among the systems.

h The HiRes 90K system has a smaller receiver/stimulator than the Clarion CII system. The electronics for the receiver/stimulator are the same for the two systems.

stimulation in each 'sweep' across channels; see Wilson et al., 1988; McDermott et al., 1992; Lawson et al., 1996; Ziese et al., 2000), simultaneous analog stimulation (SAS; see Battmer et al., 1999; Kessler, 1999; Osberger and Fisher, 2000), paired pulsatile sampler (PPS; see Kessler, 1999; Zimmerman-Phillips and Murad, 1999; Loizou et al., 2003), and 'high resolution' (HiRes; see Firszt, 2004; Koch et al., 2004) strategies. As described in many of the references above, each of these strategies can support relatively high levels of speech reception (at least in quiet) for a majority of users. However, a wide range of outcomes persists with any of the strategies, with some users obtaining only a small if any benefit from their implants.

Among the listed strategies, the CIS, ACE, and HiRes strategies are the 'default' choices for the most recent versions of the Med-El, Cochlear, and

Advanced Bionics devices, respectively. Use of those strategies is far more prevalent than use of the other strategies in present clinical practice.

All of the strategies represent the spectral content of a sound by place of stimulation in the cochlea. Beyond this central concept, the strategies vary in many respects, including number of processing channels, channel-to-electrode assignments, representation of temporal variations within channels, stimulus waveforms, the type of compression used to map the wide dynamic range of sound onto the narrow dynamic range of electrically evoked hearing, and whether particular aspects of a sound are selected for stimulation. The approach taken by each of the strategies is described in the subsections below.

## CIS

As indicated in Table 2.1, the CIS strategy is available as a processing option for all implant systems in current use except for the CI22 system, which offers the SPEAK strategy only. CIS also is among the simplest of the strategies.

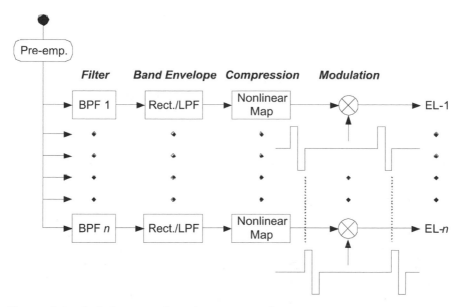

**Figure 2.3** Block diagram of a CIS processor. The CIS strategy uses a pre-emphasis filter (Pre-emp.) to attenuate strong components in speech below 1.2 kHz. The pre-emphasis filter is followed by multiple channels of processing. Each channel includes stages of bandpass filtering (BPF), envelope detection, compression, and modulation. The envelope detectors generally use a rectifier (Rect.) and lowpass filter (LPF). A Hilbert Transform or a half-wave rectifier without the lowpass filter also may be used. Carrier waveforms for two of the modulators are shown immediately below the two corresponding multiplier blocks. The outputs of the multipliers are directed to intra-cochlear electrodes (EL-1 to EL-n) via a transcutaneous link or a percutaneous connector. (From Wilson et al. (1991) and used with the permission of Macmillan Publishers Ltd.)

A block diagram of a CIS processor is presented in Figure 2.3. Inputs from a microphone (or other source) and optional automatic gain control (AGC) are directed to a pre-emphasis filter, which attenuates frequency components below 1.2 kHz at 6 dB/octave. This pre-emphasis helps relatively weak consonants (with a predominant frequency content above 1.2 kHz) compete with vowels, which are intense compared to most consonants and have strong components below 1.2 kHz.

The output of the pre-emphasis filter is directed to a bank of bandpass channels. Each channel includes stages of bandpass filtering, envelope detection, compression, and modulation. Envelope detection typically is accomplished with a rectifier, followed by a lowpass filter. Alternatives include use of a Hilbert Transform (e.g. Helms et al., 2001) or use of a half-wave rectifier without the filter (Firszt, 2004; Koch et al., 2004). A logarithmic or power-law transformation is used to map the relatively wide dynamic range of derived envelope signals onto the narrow dynamic range of electrically evoked hearing. The outputs of the compression stages are used to modulate trains of biphasic pulses. The logarithmic transformation produces a normal or nearly normal growth of loudness with increases in sound level (Eddington et al., 1978; Zeng and Shannon, 1992; Dorman et al., 1993). The modulated pulses for each channel are sent to a corresponding electrode in the cochlea, either through a percutaneous connector or through transmission of instructions to an implanted receiver/stimulator via a transcutaneous link. (All presently available implant systems use the latter method, including each of the systems listed in Table 2.1.) Stimuli derived from channels with low center frequencies for the bandpass filter are directed to apical electrodes in the implant, and stimuli derived from channels with high center frequencies are directed to basal electrodes in the implant. This arrangement mimics at least the order, if not the precise locations, of frequency mapping in the normal cochlea, with high-frequency sounds exciting neurons at basal locations and low-frequency sounds exciting neurons at apical locations.

CIS processors may use any number of channels. Typical implementations use between 8 and 16, although both lower and higher numbers have been used. The highest number of effective channels for most patients may asymptote at about 8, as noted above. Some patients, however, may benefit from a higher number (e.g. Frijns et al., 2003), and this may depend on the particular type of electrode array used, its position with respect to excitable tissue, the patient's pattern of nerve survival in the implanted cochlea, the condition of the patient's central auditory nervous system, or some combination of these factors.

The operation of a simplified implementation of CIS is illustrated in Figure 2.4. A block diagram of a 4-channel processor without the pre-emphasis filter, AGC, or mapping stages is shown at the top of the figure, and waveforms corresponding to steps in the processing are shown beneath the block diagram. The waveforms include those for an input signal and for the outputs of all stages in the simplified processor. The

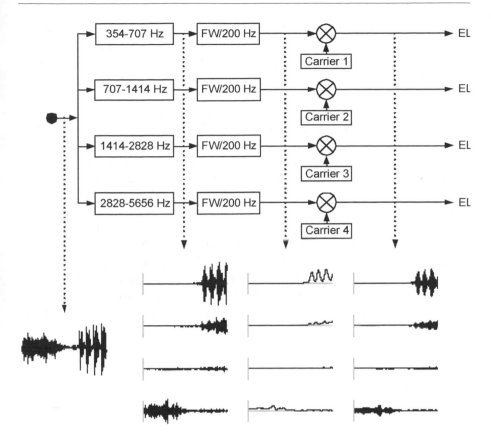

**Figure 2.4** Block diagram and waveforms for a simplified implementation of a CIS processor. The block diagram is shown at the top and corresponding waveforms at the bottom. Four channels of processing and stimulation are shown. Each channel includes a bandpass filter with the indicated frequency range (3 dB down points, with a 36 dB/octave attenuation beyond the 3 dB points), an envelope detector with a full-wave rectifier and a lowpass filter with a 3 dB down point at 200 Hz (and 24 dB octave attenuation beyond the 3 dB point), and a multiplier for modulation of a train of biphasic pulses with the output of the envelope detector. Waveforms at the bottom include, from left to right, the input, the outputs of the bandpass filters, the outputs of the envelope detectors, and the outputs of the multiplier blocks. The waveforms in each column are arranged in the order of the channels in the block diagram, with the waveforms in the top row corresponding to the channel with the lowest frequency range for the bandpass filter, the next row corresponding to the channel with the 707–1414 Hz range, and so forth. The input is a 100-millisecond snippet from the speech sound 'asa', which includes the terminal part of the 's' and the initial part of the final 'a'. Actual implementations of CIS processors include a pre-emphasis filter before the bank of bandpass filters and a compressive mapping table between the envelope detector and the multiplier block in each channel. Actual implementations also typically include more than four channels.

input in this example is a 100-millisecond snippet from the speech sound 'asa', that includes the terminal portion of the 's' and the initial portion of the final 'a'. Each bandpass filter is one octave in width. Together the filters span the range from 354 to 5656 Hz. The envelope detectors include a full-wave rectifier followed by a lowpass filter with a cut-off frequency of 200 Hz and with a 24 dB/octave attenuation beyond the cut-off (a fourth-order filter). The derived envelope signals (third column of waveforms) modulate trains of biphasic pulses to produce the stimuli (final column of waveforms). The trains are offset in time with respect to one another, so that no stimulus pulse for one channel overlaps a pulse for any other channel. Electrodes 1–4 range from apical to basal positions in the implant.

CIS processors use relatively high rates of stimulation to represent rapid temporal variations within channels. The pulse rate must be higher than twice the cut-off frequency of the lowpass filters (in the envelope detectors) to avoid aliasing effects (Rabiner and Shafer, 1978). Results from recordings of auditory nerve responses to sinusoidally amplitude-modulated pulse trains indicate that the rate should be even higher – four to five times the cut-off frequency – to avoid other distortions in the neural representations of the modulation waveforms (Wilson et al., 1994a; Wilson, 1997, 2000b). A typical CIS processor might use a pulse rate of 1000 pulses/s/electrode or higher, in conjunction with a 200 Hz cut-off for the lowpass filters.

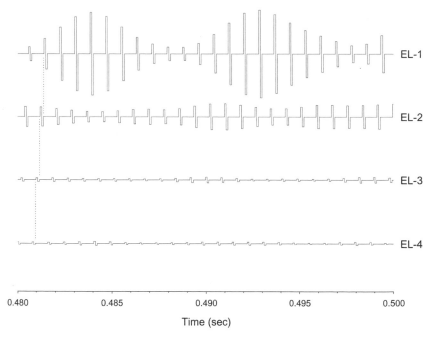

**Figure 2.5** Final 20 ms of the stimuli shown in Figure 2.4 (rightmost column of waveforms). Vertical dotted lines show relative timing of the pulses across electrodes. In this case, a base-to-apex order is used, with stimulation of basalmost electrode 4 (EL-4) first, electrode 3 (EL-3) next, electrode 2 (EL-2) next, and apicalmost electrode 1 (EL-1) last. This sequence is repeated at the outset of each cycle of stimulation across electrodes. The pulse duration is 90.7 microseconds/phase. Sequential pulses are separated by a 22.7 microsecond gap. The pulse rate for each electrode is 1225/s.

The final 20 milliseconds of the stimuli from the simplified implementation of CIS (Figure 2.4) is shown in Figure 2.5. This expanded display shows the interlacing and order of stimulus pulses across electrodes. In this particular implementation, stimulus pulses are delivered in a non-overlapping sequence from the basalmost electrode (EL-4) to the apicalmost electrode (EL-1). The rate of pulses on each electrode may be varied through manipulations in the duration of the pulses and the time between sequential pulses. Any ordering of electrodes may be used in the stimulation sequence, such as an apex-to-base order or a staggered order (i.e. an order designed to produce on average the maximum spatial separation between sequentially stimulated electrodes). The default choice of update order varies among implant systems, e.g. a staggered order is used for the COMBI 40 and 40+ systems whereas an apex-to-base order is used for the CI24M and Clarion devices.

Unlike some prior processing strategies for implants, no specific features of speech – such as the fundamental or formant frequencies – are extracted or represented with CIS processors. Instead, envelope variations in each of the multiple bands are presented to the electrodes through modulated trains of interleaved pulses. The rate of stimulation for each channel and electrode does not vary between voiced and unvoiced sounds. This 'waveform' or 'filterbank' representation does not make any assumptions about how speech is produced or perceived.

A key feature of the CIS, $n$-of-$m$, ACE, and SPEAK strategies is the interlacing of stimulus pulses across electrodes. This eliminates a principal component of interaction among electrodes that otherwise would be produced through vector summation of the electric fields from different (simultaneously stimulated) electrodes (Eddington et al., 1978; White et al., 1984; Favre and Pelizzone, 1993; Boëx et al., 2003; de Balthasar et al., 2003; Bierer and Middlebrooks, 2004). Such interaction, if allowed to stand, would be expected to reduce the salience of channel-related cues.

An additional aspect of the CIS, $n$-of-$m$, and ACE strategies is relatively high cut-off frequencies for the lowpass filters in the envelope detectors, along with rates of stimulation that are sufficiently high to represent the highest frequencies without aliasing or other distortions. The cut-off frequencies generally are in the range of 200–400 Hz, although higher effective cut-offs are used in the 'HiRes' variation of CIS (see separate section on HiRes below). This 200–400 Hz range encompasses the fundamental frequency of voiced speech sounds and rapid transitions in speech such as those produced by stop consonants. The range also does not exceed the perceptual space of typical patients. In particular, most patients perceive changes in frequency or rate of stimulation as changes in pitch up to about 300 Hz or 300 pulses/s, respectively (e.g. Shannon, 1983; Tong et al., 1983; Townshend et al., 1987; Zeng, 2002). Further increases in frequency or rate do not produce further increases in pitch for a majority of patients, for loudness-balanced stimuli. Some subjects have higher pitch saturation limits, as high as about 1000 Hz, but these subjects may be the exception rather than the rule (Hochmair-Desoyer et al., 1983; Townshend et al., 1987; Wilson et al., 1997). Thus, a representation of frequencies much beyond 300 Hz probably would not convey any additional information that could be perceived or utilized by typical patients.

Reference to Figure 2.3 indicates a relatively high number of parameters for CIS processors, including number of channels, the overall range of frequencies spanned by the channels, how the bandpass frequencies are distributed within that range, whether a full- or half-wave rectifier is used in the envelope detectors, the cut-off frequency for the lowpass filter in the envelope detectors, whether some other method is used to derive the envelope signals, the endpoints and shape of the compressive mapping function, the duration of stimulus pulses, the rate of stimulus pulses at each electrode, and the order in which electrodes are stimulated. Effects of manipulations in the values for each of these parameters have been measured (e.g. Loizou et al., 2000). In general, optimal or nearly optimal results for speech reception usually are obtained with at least 6 channels, an overall bandpass from about 300 to 7000 Hz, a logarithmic distribution of bandpass frequencies within that range (at least for 12 or fewer channels, see below), either a full- or half-wave rectifier, a cut-off frequency of 50 Hz or higher for the lowpass filters in the envelope detectors (or 200 Hz or higher for natural-sounding speech), a logarithmic mapping function, relatively brief pulses (e.g. 40 $\mu$s/phase or less), and relatively high pulse rates at each electrode (e.g. 1500 pulses/s/electrode or higher). Effects of update order appear to vary among patients. In addition, use of a Hilbert Transform to derive the envelope signals can produce a better result than the combination of a rectifier and lowpass filter, at least for the COMBI 40 and COMBI 40+ implant systems (Helms et al., 2001). The best choices for many of these values can vary somewhat among patients. They can also vary among implant devices that have different capabilities in supporting choices across wide ranges (e.g. some devices do not support relatively high pulse rates). In some cases, a selection of a high number of channels can actually degrade performance compared with a selection of a lower number (e.g. Frijns et al., 2003). A possible explanation for this is that selection of a number higher than the maximum number of effective channels may merely increase electrode interactions without producing any compensating increase in transmitted information.

**PPS**

As mentioned above, manipulations in the rate of stimulation can affect the performance of CIS processors. Some representative data are presented in Figure 2.6, which includes data from all published and some unpublished studies as of March 2000 (Lawson et al., 1996; Brill et al.,

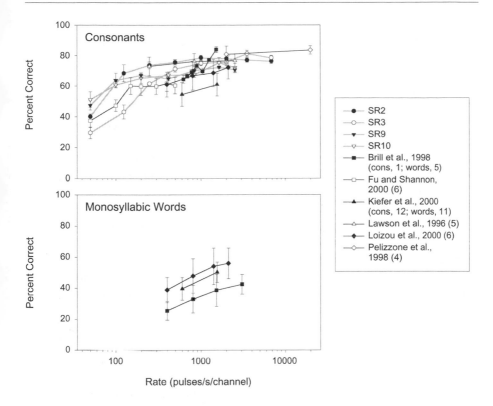

**Figure 2.6** Results from all published and several unpublished studies as of March 2000 showing effects of changes in rate of stimulation for CIS processors having 4 or more channels. Individual subjects SR2, SR3, SR9, and SR10 are from the study of Wilson et al. (2000), and their scores are connected by the grey lines. Scores from other studies are connected by the black lines. The numbers in the parentheses following the citations in the legend indicate the number of subjects. Error bars show standard errors of the means. Details of the experimental conditions for each study are presented in Wilson et al. (2000), and of course in the cited primary references.

1998; Pelizzone et al., 1998; Fu and Shannon, 2000; Kiefer et al., 2000; Loizou et al., 2000; Wilson et al., 2000). The methods and experimental conditions for each of the studies are described in Wilson et al. (2000). In general, the results indicate quite large increases in speech reception scores with increases in rate from very low values up to about 300 pulses/s/electrode (see top panel of Figure 2.6) and further significant increases in scores with further increases in rate at least up to about 1500 pulses/s/electrode (see especially the bottom panel of Figure 2.6). In addition, the figure indicates that effects of rate manipulations can vary among subjects (see the individual data for subjects SR2, 3, 9, and 10 in the top panel of the figure) and across tests (compare the two panels in the figure). For example, results for subject SR3 show significant improvements in consonant identification with increases in rate up to about 3500 pulses/s/electrode, whereas results for subject SR2 show improvements with increases in rate only up to 500 pulses/s/electrode. Group scores for recognition of monosyllabic words improve with increases in rate over the tested ranges for each of the three studies.

Results obtained in subsequent studies have been generally consistent with the findings shown in Figure 2.6, i.e. increases in rate up to about 1500 pulses/s/electrode or higher produce increases in speech reception scores, especially for speech presented in competition with noise (Büchner et al., 2003; Frijns et al., 2003). In addition, the results have demonstrated large gains in performance for some subjects with very high rates (3000–5000 pulses/s/electrode), along with decrements in scores for other subjects using the same high rates (Büchner et al., 2003, 2004). In all, increases in rate up to 1500 pulses/s/electrode or somewhat higher produce increases in speech reception scores for most subjects. Further increases in rate produce further increases in scores for some but certainly not all subjects. On average, increases beyond 3000 pulses/s/electrode do not appear to provide a significant advantage, at least in the studies conducted to date.

The PPS strategy was motivated by the initial findings indicating benefits of relatively high rates of stimulation for CIS processors. PPS is identical to CIS except that pairs of distant electrodes are stimulated simultaneously, with the pairs presented in a non-simultaneous sequence. This approach doubles the rate of stimulation at any one electrode compared with CIS, while possibly minimizing interactions between the simultaneously stimulated electrodes by choosing electrodes in each pair that are far apart. Thus, the trade-off with PPS is between possible benefits of the higher rate (for individual patients) versus increased interactions for the simultaneously stimulated electrodes.

PPS was developed for use with the Clarion 1.2 implant system. That system does not support an especially high pulse rate for CIS processors. For example, the maximum rate for an 8-channel CIS processor is about 800 pulses/s/electrode (Kessler, 1999), which is far below the 1500 pulses/s/electrode generally needed for optimal performance. Doubling the rate with PPS moved the rate into a more effective zone, according to results like those presented in Figure 2.6.

Loizou et al. (2003) have compared CIS, PPS, and other strategies using within-subjects controls. They found that two of their nine subjects achieved a higher score in a test of consonant identification with PPS than with CIS (running at a rate of about 800 pulses/s/electrode), and that one of those subjects and another achieved a higher score in a test of sentence recognition using PPS.

Frohne-Büchner and coworkers also have compared CIS as implemented in the Clarion CII device (see the section on the HiRes strategy below) and a 'paired pulsatile' variation of that strategy with the same device (Frohne-Büchner et al., 2003). The Clarion CII can present pulses much faster than the Clarion 1.2. For example, a pulse rate of about 2800 pulses/s/electrode can be supported with the Clarion CII for a 16-channel CIS processor. The paired-pulsatile variation can support rates as high as about 5600 pulses/s/electrode for the same number of channels.

Results from this latter study showed a large reduction in scores when the Clarion CII implementation of PPS was used instead of the Clarion CII implementation of CIS (both of these implementations have been given the name 'HiRes' by the Advanced Bionics company). The drop in scores was especially marked for tests of speech reception in competition with noise. For these subjects, the rate available for the CIS implementation already was quite high, and thus the further increase in rate provided with the PPS implementation may not have produced any further benefit. Instead, the PPS implementation may have merely exacerbated electrode interactions, with little or no gain produced by the increase in rate.

### n-of-m and ACE

The CIS, n-of-m, and ACE strategies share (1) non-simultaneous stimulation and (2) high cut-off frequencies for the envelope detectors. The principal difference between CIS and the other strategies is that the channel outputs are 'scanned' in the latter strategies to select the n channels with the highest envelope signals prior to each frame of stimulation across electrodes. Stimulus pulses are delivered only to the subset of m electrodes that correspond to the n selected channels. This 'peak picking' scheme is designed in part to reduce the density of stimulation while still representing the most important aspects of the acoustic environment. The deletion of low-amplitude channels for each frame of stimulation may reduce the overall level of masking across electrode and stimulus regions in the implanted cochlea. To the extent that the omitted channels do not contain significant information, such 'unmasking' may improve the perception of the input signal by the patient. In addition, for positive signal-to-noise ratios, selection of the highest peaks in the spectra may emphasize the primary speech signal with respect to the noise.

An n-of-m approach also may offer a significant advantage for implant systems with a relatively low overall rate of stimulation across electrodes, as set by the design of the transcutaneous transmission link. In particular, stimulation of some electrodes among many allows for a higher pulse rate at the selected electrodes, compared with the highest possible rate for the condition in which all or most electrodes are stimulated, as with typical implementations of CIS. A likely trade-off in choosing an n-of-m approach is between possible benefits of increasing rate on the one hand versus deleting information that may be important (e.g. for maintaining a continuous representation of envelope information within bands or for representing weak consonant sounds) on the other hand.

The n-of-m and ACE strategies are quite similar in design. The n-of-m approach was first described in 1988 (Wilson et al., 1988) and has been refined in several lines of subsequent development (e.g. McDermott et al.,

1992; Lawson et al., 1996; McDermott and Vandali, 1997). Current implementations include those listed in Table 2.1, along with laboratory
implementations. Comparisons between $n$-of-$m$ (or ACE) versus CIS have
indicated roughly equivalent performances for the two (e.g. Lawson et al.,
1996; Ziese et al., 2000) or better performance for the $n$-of-$m$ approach
(Kiefer et al., 2001). The results have varied from subject to subject and
also among different implementations of the strategies, using the COMBI
40+, CI24M, or CI24R systems, or laboratory hardware and software.

Some implementations of the $n$-of-$m$ strategy use high values of $m$. In
the ACE implementation, for example, $m$ may be as high as 22. In such
cases, frequencies for the bandpass filters are distributed along a linear
scale for frequencies below about 1000 Hz and along a logarithmic scale
for the higher frequencies. This allocation of frequencies follows the mel
scale in normal hearing (Zwicker and Fastl, 1990) and (1) avoids the spec-
ification of very narrow filters for the analysis channels with the lowest
center frequencies and (2) increases the resolution (decreases the width)
of the filters for the analysis channels with intermediate center frequencies, in the region of 500–1500 Hz. This 'linear-logarithmic' map may be
better than the logarithmic map only, for the reasons just mentioned.
However, the mapping of frequencies in the human cochlea (Greenwood,
1990), and the widths and frequency coordinates of 'critical bandwidths'
or 'equivalent rectangular bandwidths' in normal hearing (Moore and
Glasberg, 1983; Glasberg and Moore, 1990), all closely approximate a logarithmic function, at least for frequencies above about 300 Hz. Thus, a
closer mimicking of the normal tonotopic pattern might be achieved with
a purely logarithmic distribution of frequencies even for a high number of
analysis channels.

In the ACE strategy, a linear distribution of frequencies is used up to
about 1300 Hz, and a logarithmic distribution is used from that point up
to the maximum frequency. A purely logarithmic distribution might be
better, but this possibility has not been tested to date.

In typical fittings of ACE processors, $m$ ranges from 20 to 22 and $n$
ranges from 6 to 16 (Arndt et al., 1999; Skinner et al., 2002a). In acoustic
simulations of $n$-of-$20$ processors, Dorman et al. (2002) have found that
the $n$ required to reach asymptotic performance varies according to
whether recognition of vowels, consonants, or words in sentences is
measured and also whether the speech items are presented in competition with noise. For their normal-hearing subjects, an $n$ of 9 was required
to reach asymptotic performance for recognition of the words presented
in competition with noise (at the S/N of 0 dB). Asymptotic performance
for all other tests was attained with lower values for $n$. For all tests, a $10$-
of-$10$ processor produced results that were statistically indistinguishable
from the $9$-of-$20$ processor. Together these findings suggest that (1) $n$
should be at least 9 for a $n$-of-$20$ processor and (2) 9–10 channels,
whether presented in an $n$-of-$m$ or $m$-of-$m$ format, are sufficient for high
levels of speech understanding. Of course, present implant systems do

not in general support even 10 effective channels. In addition, possible differences in performance due to differences in pulse rate for the selected electrodes in an $n$-of-$m$ processor could not be evaluated with the normal-hearing subjects in Dorman et al.'s study.

Work to evaluate and refine $n$-of-$m$ processors is still in progress (e.g. Tyler et al., 2000). The choices of $n$ and $m$ probably are important, as the $m$ electrodes most likely should be perceptually distinct for the best performance (limiting the number for practical electrode arrays) and $n$ should be high enough to include all essential information but lower than $m$ to provide any increase in rate for the selected $n$ electrodes, or to provide any release from masking by eliminating low-level stimuli. More fundamentally, there may be better ways to choose the $n$ channels and electrodes for each frame of stimulation. Flanagan (1972), for example, describes various alternative procedures for identifying the channels for analogous 'peak picking' vocoders (vocoders are described in the Terminology and glossary section). Those procedures were more effective for vocoders than a simple selection of maxima, and they might be more effective for implants as well. Loizou (1998) also notes likely deficiencies in selection of the $n$ channels in $n$-of-$m$ processors for cochlear implants. In particular, he points out that multiple maxima, are often identified for strong or broad peaks in the spectra of input sounds, which exhausts the number of maxima available to represent other important peaks in the spectra. A procedure to encode the most important peaks or features of the spectra for a given $n$ may be more effective than simply identifying the $n$-highest envelope signals.

## SPEAK

The SPEAK strategy uses an adaptive $n$-of-$m$ approach, in which $n$ may vary from one stimulus frame to the next. The input is filtered into as many as 20 bands, with a linear distribution of bandpass frequencies up to about 1850 Hz and a logarithmic distribution thereafter. Envelope signals are derived as in the CIS, $n$-of-$m$, and ACE strategies above, with an envelope cut-off frequency of 200 Hz. The number of bandpass channels selected in each scan (the adaptive $n$) depends on the number of envelope signals exceeding a preset 'noise threshold' and on details of the input such as the distribution of energy across frequencies. In many cases, 6 channels are selected. However, the number can range from 1 to a maximum that can be set as high as 10. Cycles of stimulation, which include the selected channels and associated electrodes, are presented at rates between 180 and 300/s. The amount of time required to complete each cycle depends on the number of electrodes and channels included in the cycle ($n$) and the pulse amplitudes and durations for each of the electrodes. In general, the inclusion of relatively few electrodes in a cycle allows relatively high rates, whereas inclusion of many electrodes reduces the rate.

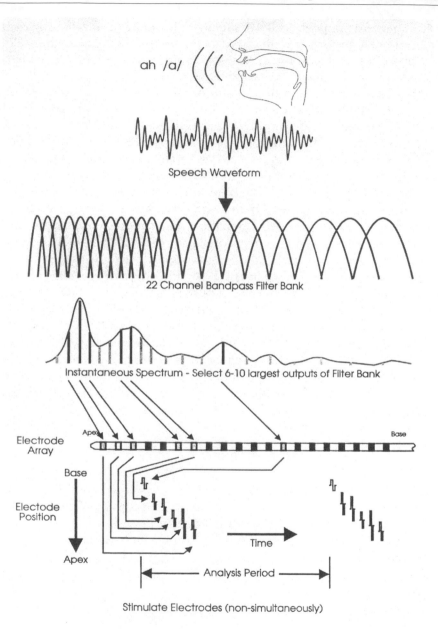

**Figure 2.7** Key steps in the SPEAK processing strategy. Speech inputs are directed to a bank of up to 20 bandpass filters and envelope detectors. The envelope signals are scanned just prior to each cycle of stimulation across electrodes. Between 1 and 10 of the highest-amplitude signals are selected in each scan, depending on the overall level and spectral composition of the input. Electrodes associated with the selected envelope signals (and bandpass channels) are stimulated in a base-to-apex order. (From Patrick et al., 1997, and used with the permission of Thomson Delmar Learning, a part of the Thomson Corporation and purchaser of the Singular Publishing Group, Inc., the original publisher of this illustration.)

A diagram illustrating the operation of the SPEAK strategy is presented in Figure 2.7. The speech input is directed to a bank of bandpass filters and envelope detectors, whose outputs are scanned for each cycle of stimulation. In this diagram, six channels are selected in each of two scans, and the corresponding electrodes are stimulated sequentially in a base-to-apex order. The diagram does not illustrate the compressive mapping of envelope signals onto pulse amplitudes.

The SPEAK strategy was initially designed for use with the CI22 implant system. The transcutaneous link in that system is relatively slow, e.g. the maximum cycle rate for 6 channels of stimulation is about 400/s under ideal conditions (Crosby et al., 1985; Shannon et al., 1990). This limitation constrained the design of the strategy such that the average rate was set at about 250 cycles/s, and the range of rates between 180 and 300/s, as noted above.

A variation of the SPEAK strategy was implemented for use with the CI24M implant system, when it became available in 1996. This variation, SPEAK II, uses the same rates and overall processing strategy, but (1) delivers its outputs to monopolar electrodes rather than to bipolar pairs and (2) selects between 6 and 9 peaks among the bandpass channels in each cycle of stimulation, as opposed to the 1–10 peaks in the original version of the strategy. In addition, the times of pulse presentations may be randomized, or 'jittered', in the SPEAK II processor to reduce the possibility of perceiving the low carrier rate as a continuous tone. (The average rate approximates 250 pulses/s at each of the selected electrodes, and this rate is below the pitch saturation limit for many patients, which might lead to a clear pitch percept without the jittering.)

The rates used in the SPEAK strategy, in combination with the 200 Hz cut-off for the envelope detectors, are substantially lower than the minimum required to prevent aliasing and other distortions. For the average rate of 250 pulse/s/selected electrode, the representation of frequencies in the modulation waveforms above 125 Hz is subject to aliasing effects, and the representation of frequencies in the range of one-fourth to one-half the pulse rate probably is distorted to a lesser extent (Busby et al., 1993; McKay et al., 1994; Wilson et al., 1994a; Wilson, 1997).

Results from recent comparisons of the SPEAK and ACE strategies generally have indicated superiority of the latter (e.g. Arndt et al., 1999; Kiefer et al., 2001; Pasanisi et al., 2002; Skinner et al., 2002b; David et al., 2003). The performance of the SPEAK strategy may be affected by (1) relatively low rates of stimulation, (2) aliasing and other distortions arising from the use of low rates in conjunction with a high cut-off frequency for the envelope detectors, or (3) both of these factors. At present, the ACE strategy is regarded by many clinicians as the default or 'first choice' strategy for the CI24M and CI24R implant systems (Kiefer et al., 2001; Skinner et al., 2002b; Brown et al., in press).

## SAS

The SAS strategy was derived from a compressed analog (CA) strategy (Eddington, 1980; Merzenich et al., 1984), originally used with the Ineraid and the University of California at San Francisco (UCSF)/Storz cochlear implant systems. Manufacture of these systems was discontinued many years ago. More recently, a variation of the CA strategy was used along with the first commercial implementation of CIS in the Clarion 1.0 implant system. Manufacture of that system also has been discontinued. (The present version of the Clarion device is the HiRes 90K; see Table 2.1.) In contrast to the other strategies described above, the CA and SAS strategies use 'analog' or continuous waveforms for stimuli, instead of biphasic pulses.

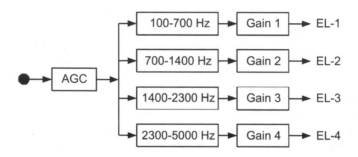

**Figure 2.8** Block diagram of a compressed analog (CA) processor. The CA strategy uses a broadband automatic gain control (AGC), followed by a bank of bandpass filters. The outputs of the filters are adjusted with independent gain controls. Compression is achieved through rapid action of the AGC, and high-frequency emphasis and limited mapping to individual electrodes is accomplished through adjustments of the channel gains. (From Wilson et al., 1991, and used with the permission of Macmillan Publishers Ltd.)

A block diagram of the CA strategy is presented in Figure 2.8. A microphone or other input is compressed with a fast-acting AGC. The AGC output is filtered into contiguous bands that span the range of speech frequencies. In the illustrated implementation, this range includes the fundamental frequencies of voiced speech sounds (note the lower boundary of 100 Hz in the topmost channel). In other implementations, both the lower and upper limits of the frequency range may be higher. The signal from each bandpass filter is amplified and then directed to a corresponding electrode in the implant. The gains of the amplifiers can be adjusted to produce a comfortable loudness for each electrode and to provide at least some high-frequency emphasis. In the default conditions, 4 channels of processing and stimulation were used in the Ineraid and UCSF/Storz systems and 8 channels were used in the Clarion 1.0 system. The Ineraid device used monopolar stimulation in conjunction with widely spaced electrodes (4 mm apart), and the UCSF/Storz and Clarion 1.0 systems used 'offset radial' pairs of bipolar electrodes for each channel of stimulation (Loeb et al., 1983), with 4 mm between the pairs in the UCSF/Storz device and 2 mm between the pairs in the Clarion 1.0 device. The frequency ranges for the bandpass filters shown in Figure 2.8 were the default settings for the Ineraid device.

The compression provided by the AGC can reduce the dynamic range of the input to approximate the dynamic range of electrically evoked hearing. The dynamic range of stimulation also can be restricted with a clipping circuit before or after the amplifiers, for some or all of the bandpass channels (Merzenich et al., 1984; Merzenich, 1985). Of course, such 'front end' compression with the AGC introduces spectral components that are not present in the input. The severity of this distortion depends on the time constants of the AGC (attack and release) and the compression ratio of the AGC (e.g. White, 1986). Thus, a balance must be met between sufficient compression for mapping the wide dynamic range of the input onto the narrow dynamic range of electrically evoked hearing versus the introduction of spurious frequency components, principally in the high-frequency channels.

A further complexity in the fitting of CA processors arises from the differences in dynamic range for electrical sinusoids at low and high frequencies. The dynamic range for low-frequency sinusoids (e.g. at around 100 Hz) can be greater than 30 dB, whereas the dynamic range for high-frequency sinusoids (e.g. at around 5000 Hz) is much narrower, typically 10 dB or less. Thus, an appropriate amount of compression at one frequency (or for frequencies in one bandpass) will not be appropriate for another frequency. This can be compensated to some extent through the manipulation of the amplifier gains and through the use of clipping. For example, a relatively low compression ratio might be selected for the AGC that would be appropriate for the channel with the lowest frequency range for the bandpass filter and would minimize the introduction of spurious components at higher frequencies. Then clipping or lower gains would be used in the channels with higher frequency ranges to keep the percepts from being too loud.

As may be appreciated from the above, the fitting of CA processors can be difficult. The various adjustments interact with each other, and achieving appropriate compression for all channels, along with a high-frequency emphasis, is challenging, if not impossible. In addition, at least some distortion from the AGC is unavoidable. Stimuli produced by a simplified implementation of a CA processor are shown in Figure 2.9. This implementation does not include the AGC or the gain blocks.

As in Figure 2.4, the input is the speech sound 'asa'. The terminal portion of the 's' and the initial portion of the final 'a' are shown. The input is displayed to the left and the outputs are displayed to the right. Each trace is 100 ms in duration.

Figure 2.9 illustrates the fact that CA stimuli represent a large portion of the information in the unprocessed speech input. Spectral and temporal

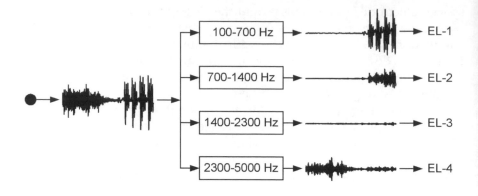

**Figure 2.9** Block diagram and waveforms for a simplified implementation of a CA processor. Four channels of processing and stimulation are shown. Each channel includes a bandpass filter with the indicated frequency range (3 dB down points, with a 36 dB/octave attenuation beyond the 3 dB points). The input waveform is shown to the left of the bandpass filters, and the output waveforms are shown to the right. The input is the same as that used in Figure 2.4. Actual implementations of CA processors include an AGC before the bank of bandpass filters and an amplifier with adjustable gain following each bandpass filter. Some implementations also include a pre-emphasis filter (much like the one used for CIS processors, see Figure 2.3), or adjustable clippers either before or after the gain blocks in one or more (usually basal) channels, or both. CA processors as implemented for use with the Ineraid or UCSF/Storz systems included up to 4 channels of processing and stimulation, and the CA processor implemented for use with the Clarion 1.0 system used up to 8 such channels.

patterns of speech are represented in the relative amplitudes of the stimuli across electrodes and in the temporal variations of the stimuli for each of the electrodes. Fine temporal or frequency variations within channels are preserved in the unprocessed (or lightly processed) bandpass outputs, especially when clipping is not used (even then, zero-crossings information is preserved).

The representation of temporal details is better illustrated in Figure 2.10, which shows the final 20 ms of the output waveforms. The fundamental and first formant frequencies of the 'a' are clearly evident in the time waveform for electrode 1, for example. In contrast, only the overall level in the bandpass and the period of the fundamental are represented with CIS stimuli, as shown in Figure 2.5 for the same input, time segment, and electrode. (The bandpasses for the two processors are different for these illustrations, but making them the same would not alter this basic observation.)

Although a large amount of information is presented with CA stimuli, much of it may not be available to implant patients. As mentioned before, within-channel changes in frequency above about 300 Hz will not be perceived as changes in pitch by many if not most patients. In addition, the simultaneous stimulation of multiple electrodes can produce large

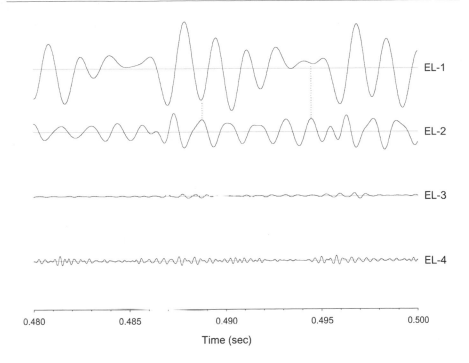

**Figure 2.10** Final 20 ms of the stimuli shown in Figure 2.9 (column of waveforms to the immediate right of the bandpass filters). Vertical dotted lines in the present figure mark instances of likely destructive (first line) and constructive (second line) interference between the stimuli presented at electrodes 1 and 2 (EL-1 and EL-2).

and uncontrolled interactions through vector summation (at sites of neural excitation) of the electric fields from each of the electrodes (e.g. White et al., 1984; Favre and Pelizzone, 1993). The resulting degradation of independence among electrodes would be expected to reduce the salience of channel-related cues.

Interactions may be reduced to some extent through the use of spatially selective electrodes. Indeed, this was the driving concept in the development of CA processors for the UCSF/Storz and Clarion 1.0 systems. However, even such reduced levels of interaction are likely to remain significant (e.g. Boëx et al., 2003), owing to the close spacing between electrodes and the relatively large distance from the electrodes to the spiral ganglion, the closest possible site of stimulation for most if not all implant patients.

The vertical dotted lines in Figure 2.10 mark likely instances of high interaction between the stimuli presented to electrodes 1 and 2. The first dotted line marks a point of likely cancellation between the stimuli (destructive interference) and the second line marks a point of likely summation between the stimuli (constructive interference). Thus, the neural response to the combined stimuli is likely to be much different from the responses that would be elicited with either electrode alone. With combined stimulation, the neural response to stimuli presented at one electrode may be significantly distorted or even counteracted by coincident stimuli presented at the other electrode. Phase is not controlled in CA processors and this may degrade further the representation of channel-by-channel amplitudes, with ongoing variations in summation and cancellation among stimuli from the different electrodes.

A problem encountered with using the CA strategy as implemented with the Clarion 1.0 implant system was that not enough current could be provided to make the stimuli sufficiently loud. This reflected a rather low maximum of voltage that could be supplied for each current source in the implant, the so-called voltage compliance limit, in conjunction with closely spaced pairs of bipolar electrodes that required high currents (and a high voltage compliance) to elicit threshold and suprathreshold percepts. Indeed, the vast majority of patients using the Clarion 1.0 system could not use the CA strategy for this reason (Kessler, 1999), described as 'inadequate loudness growth' with that system and strategy.

The solution was to change the connections between the receiver/stimulator and the intracochlear electrodes such that the longitudinal spacing between electrodes in each bipolar pair was increased from 0.3 mm to 1.7 mm, center to center (radial spacing remained at 0.5 mm). This increase most likely reduced the spatial selectivity of each bipolar pair but also certainly decreased the current levels (and voltage compliance) required for comfortably loud percepts. The new arrangement of electrodes was called the 'enhanced bipolar' coupling mode. This mode reduced the maximum number of available stimulus sites from 8 to 7 but also supported sufficient loudness growth for most patients.

In addition to the change in electrode coupling configuration, various changes were made in the implementation of the processing strategy itself in the Clarion 1.2 system. These changes were made to address likely limitations of the CA strategy as implemented in the Clarion 1.0 system and in the Ineraid and UCSF/Storz systems. The principal changes included (1) insertion of a logarithmic mapping function at the output of each bandpass channel, (2) a sharp reduction in the compression ratio and a lengthening of the time constants for the AGC, and (3) insertion of a preemphasis filter between the microphone (or other) input and the AGC. The first and second of these changes together provided 'back end' rather than 'front end' compression. This greatly reduced the distortions produced by front-end compression, using a relatively high compression ratio for the AGC. It also allowed channel-by-channel adjustments of compression and of target maximum levels for producing comfortably loud percepts. This eliminated any need for clipping circuits and greatly reduced the prior interactions among settings for the AGC and channel gains. The function of the AGC in the new implementation was to provide gentle and relatively slow adjustments in gain according to changes in the acoustic environment, e.g. in moving from a quiet room to a noisy cafeteria. Insertion of the pre-emphasis filter provided the desired emphasis of high-frequency sounds in a precise way and eliminated the need for adjusting channel gains to achieve some approximation to the desired emphasis. In all, these changes simplified the fitting of 'analog' processors. They also supported a better fitting for individual patients.

Because so many changes were made in the analog strategy and in the way its outputs were delivered to the intracochlear electrodes, the strategy was renamed as the SAS strategy to distinguish it from the prior implementations. Present implementations of the SAS strategy include the one described above for the Clarion 1.2 implant and one for the newer Clarion CII implant. The CII implant system includes a new type of electrode array called the 'HiFocus' array. This array has 16 intracochlear electrodes spaced at 1 mm intervals. The electrodes are in-line with each other without any radial offsets. In the initial version of the CII system, a silicone 'positioner' was inserted lateral to the previously inserted electrode array at surgery, to move the array closer to the medial (inner) wall of the ST. In a subsequent version, use of the positioner was discontinued. In either case, a SAS strategy can be implemented using the 'emulation mode' of the CII implant. In this mode, up to 8 channels of processing and stimulation are used. The output for each channel is delivered to a pair of closely spaced electrodes in the intracochlear array (i.e. to longitudinal bipolar pairs).

Prior comparisons between the CA and CIS strategies showed a marked superiority of the latter (e.g. Wilson et al., 1991; Boëx et al., 1996;

**Table 2.2** Comparisons among CIS, PPS, and SAS strategies, as implemented in either the Clarion 1.2 or CII implant systems[a]

| Study | System | Electrode[b] | Subjects | Percent preferring | | |
|---|---|---|---|---|---|---|
| | | | | CIS | PPS | SAS |
| Battmer et al., 1999 | 1.2 | Std | 22[c] | 50 | N/A | 50 |
| Osberger and Fisher, 2000 | 1.2 | Std | 58 | 72 | N/A | 28 |
| Zwolan et al., 2001 | 1.2 | Std | 56 | 50 | 11 | 39 |
| | 1.2 | HiFocus | 56 | 15 | 33 | 52 |
| Stollwerck et al., 2001[d] | 1.2 | Std | 55 | 75 | N/A | 25 |
| Frijns et al., 2002[e] | CII | HiFocus | 10 | 90 | 10 | 0 |

a  Subject preferences are indicated. For studies that included multiple test intervals, results for the final interval are given. See text for full names of the strategies. The PPS strategy was not included in some of the comparison studies, as indicated by the 'N/A' entries in the PPS column.

b  'Std' references the standard electrode array used with the Clarion 1.2 implant system. It is a precurved array based on the original UCSF design (Loeb et al., 1983). 'HiFocus' references the HiFocus electrode array (see text). The positioner was used in both of the listed studies that included subjects with the HiFocus electrode. The positioner was fully inserted in the study of Zwolan et al. and partially inserted in the study of Frijns et al.

c  Two of the subjects could not use SAS, owing to inadequate loudness. The data in the 'per cent preferring' columns reflect findings for the 20 subjects who could use both the SAS and CIS strategies.

d  Within-subject comparisons demonstrated that the subjects performed better with their preferred strategy.

e  The strategies tested in this study were implemented using the 'emulation mode' of the CII system.

Dorman and Loizou, 1997; Pelizzone et al., 1999). More-recent comparisons of the SAS and CIS strategies, as implemented in the Clarion hardware and software, have produced varied results across studies, but generally have demonstrated high levels of performance for some subjects using SAS (Battmer et al., 1999; Osberger and Fisher, 2000; Stollwerck et al., 2001; Zwolan et al., 2001; Frijns et al., 2002). In each of these studies, subjects have been asked to indicate their preference between the SAS and CIS strategies, or among the SAS, CIS, and PPS strategies. The results are listed in Table 2.2. They vary widely across studies. In the study of Battmer et al., half of the subjects preferred SAS to CIS and also achieved scores with SAS that were comparable to the scores achieved by the other subjects with CIS. In the study of Osberger and Fisher, less than 30% of the subjects preferred SAS, but some of those subjects had exceptionally high scores (on average, scores for the SAS and CIS groups were not different at the final, six-month test interval). The subjects preferring SAS had short durations of deafness compared to the CIS group. In the study of Zwolan et al., SAS was compared with both CIS and PPS. In addition, the standard electrode array for the Clarion 1.2 implant was compared with the HiFocus electrode used in conjunction with the same implanted receiver/stimulator and external hardware (this use of the HiFocus array with the 1.2 system presaged its application as the new standard array with the CII system). At the final (again, six-month) test interval, half of the 56 subjects using the standard electrode array preferred CIS, and about 40 and 10% of those subjects preferred SAS and PPS, respectively. For the additional 56 subjects using the HiFocus electrode array, 15% preferred CIS, 52% preferred SAS, and a third preferred PPS. Zwolan et al. attribute this reversal in preference, between the standard and HiFocus arrays, to a closer positioning of electrodes next to the inner wall of the ST with the latter. (Closer positioning, if present, might reduce interactions among electrodes and thereby perhaps allow simultaneous stimulation strategies to become more effective.) In another group of 55 subjects using the 1.2 system and standard array, Stollwerck et al. found that 75% of the subjects preferred CIS over SAS. Among the 10 subjects studied by Frijns et al., nine preferred CIS, one preferred PPS, and none preferred SAS. These subjects used the CII implant and HiFocus electrode array, but with the positioner inserted only along the basal turn (see rationale for this in Frijns et al., 2001, 2002).

Speech reception data also have been collected for at least the preferred strategy for each subject in each of the studies. Controlled comparisons between strategies, balancing experience, and other variables have additionally been made in the study of Stollwerck et al. In broad terms, results from all studies except the study of Frijns et al. (in which none of the subjects preferred SAS) indicated levels of performance for the group preferring SAS that were comparable to those of the group preferring CIS. In addition, some of the subjects in each of the groups had especially high scores. Results from the study of Stollwerck et al. further showed that subjects performed better with their preferred strategy.

The SAS strategy may convey more temporal information (within channels) than the CIS strategy, especially in the apical, low-frequency channels and especially for patients who can perceive changes in frequency as changes in pitch over relatively wide ranges. If so, that advantage may outweigh the likely disadvantage of higher electrode interactions, which would be expected even with a spatially selective electrode array (e.g. Stickney et al., 2001; Boëx et al., 2003).

## HiRes

As mentioned above, HiRes is an implementation of CIS in the CII implant system. It can present biphasic pulses to as many as 16 electrodes in the implant, using monopolar stimulation. For 16 channels of processing and stimulation, pulse rates can be as high as about 2800/s/electrode for pulses presented sequentially across electrodes and as high as about 5600/s/electrode for pulses presented simultaneously to widely spaced pairs of electrodes (as in a PPS processor). The principal differences between HiRes and the prior implementation of CIS in the Clarion 1.2 device are (1) up to twice as many stimulus sites and much higher rates of stimulation, as just noted, (2) use of a half-wave rectifier only for envelope detection in HiRes, and (3) use of a more-sophisticated AGC in HiRes (Firszt, 2004; Koch et al., 2004). A key difference between the 1.2 and CII implants is in the quality of the current sources (Frijns et al., 2002). The sources in the CII implant have rise and fall times that are roughly five times shorter than those in the 1.2 implant. This helps assure full non-simultaneity of pulse presentations for CIS processors. More importantly, the voltage compliance limit is more than twice as high in the CII implant than in the 1.2 implant. This allows stimulation with short-duration pulses (and high rates) without encountering the limit. The increase in the voltage compliance limit and associated maximum currents is a tremendous improvement.

Initial studies to evaluate HiRes have included a clinical trial sponsored by the Advanced Bionics Corporation. In that study (Koch et al., 2004), HiRes was compared with the preferred strategy among the prior CIS, PPS, or SAS strategies for each of 50 subjects, implanted with the HiFocus electrode and positioner across 19 centers in North America. Phase I of the study included use by each subject of their preferred prior strategy for three months. (The prior strategies were implemented using the 'emulation mode' of the CII system.) Phase II included use of HiRes for the subsequent three months. Either the sequential or paired-pulsatile variations could be selected for each subject. Speech reception data were collected at the conclusion of Phase I ('standard' strategies) and at the conclusion of Phase II (HiRes strategy). The speech reception tests included recognition of monosyllabic consonant-nucleus-consonant (CNC) words, recognition of the Central Institute for the Deaf (CID) everyday

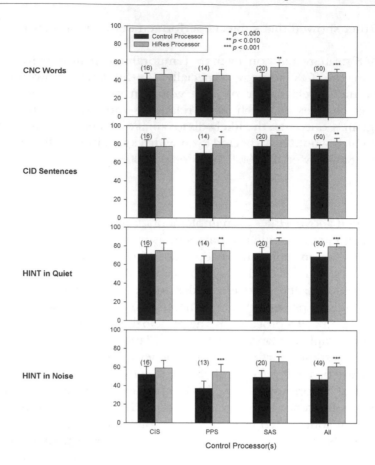

**Figure 2.11** Results from the study of Koch et al. (2004), comparing HiRes to 'standard' strategies, as implemented in the Clarion CII system. The tests with the standard strategies were conducted following three months of use by each of the 50 subjects, and the tests with the HiRes strategy were conducted after three months of subsequent use of that strategy. Each of the subjects was tested with their preferred standard strategy, which they used exclusively or nearly exclusively during the initial three-month period. The number of subjects using each of the standard strategies is indicated in the parentheses. (One of the subjects using the PPS strategy did not take the HINT in Noise test.) One additional subject who preferred and used the SAS strategy did not take the tests with that strategy, at the conclusion of the first interval. The tests included recognition of monosyllabic consonant-nucleus-consonant (CNC) words, recognition of the Central Institute for the Deaf (CID) everyday sentences, recognition of sentences from the Hearing in Noise Test (HINT) presented in quiet, and recognition of HINT sentences presented in competition with speech-spectrum noise at the S/N of +10 dB. The asterisks show results of paired-t comparisons of scores for each standard strategy versus HiRes and for the combined standard strategies (All) versus HiRes, for each test. The standard strategies are labelled as the Control Processors in the figure. They include implementations of the continuous interleaved sampling (CIS), paired pulsatile sampler (PPS), and simultaneous analog stimulation (SAS) strategies. Error bars show standard errors of the means. (Data for this figure were kindly provided by Mary Joe Osberger of the Advanced Bionics Corporation, Sylmar, CA. These same data are presented in different formats in Koch et al., 2004.)

sentences, recognition of sentences from the Hearing in Noise Test (HINT) presented in quiet, and recognition of HINT sentences presented in competition with speech-spectrum noise at the S/N of +10 dB. A preference questionnaire also was given at the conclusion of Phase II.

Results from the speech reception tests are presented in Figure 2.11. The standard strategies are labeled as the control processors in the figure. The first column of bars shows results across tests for the 16 subjects who preferred CIS among the standard strategies, the second column shows results for the 14 subjects who preferred PPS, and the third column shows results for the 20 subjects who preferred SAS. The final column shows results for all 50 subjects and all standard strategies, as compared with HiRes.

**Table 2.3** Results from two-way, repeated-measures ANOVAs of the data presented in Figure 2.11, with tests and processing strategies as the factors

| Factor | CIS/HiRes | PPS/HiRes | SAS/HiRes | All/HiRes |
|---|---|---|---|---|
| Tests | $p < 0.001$ | $p < 0.001$ | $p < 0.001$ | $p < 0.001$ |
| Processors | NS[a] | $p < 0.001$ | $p = 0.003$ | $p < 0.001$ |
| Interaction (tests x processors) | NS | NS | NS | NS |

a Not significant.

Table 2.3 shows the results from two-way, repeated-measures ANOVAs of the data presented in Figure 2.11. The factors included the tests (4 levels) and processing strategies (2 levels). An ANOVA was conducted for each of the standard strategies (as compared with HiRes) and for the combined standard strategies. (These analyses were conducted independently by the author.)

The results demonstrate highly significant differences among tests and between strategies for the PPS, SAS, and combined-strategies comparisons. Differences among tests also are highly significant for the CIS comparisons, but the difference between the CIS and HiRes strategies is not. (Even highly sensitive paired-t comparisons do not show a difference between CIS and HiRes for any of the tests; see Figure 2.11.)

Consistent with these general findings, 90% of the subjects preferred HiRes to their selected standard strategy at the conclusion of Phase II. With further experience in using HiRes, 96% of the subjects ultimately preferred that strategy.

Unfortunately, the study of Koch et al. did not include a crossover design, in which the initially applied strategy would be tested at least once again following the three months of experience with HiRes. HiRes may have benefited in these comparisons through the accumulation of learning effects, first with the standard strategy and then with HiRes, for a total of six months in listening with an implant, all the time with relatively good strategies. Thus, one cannot conclude from these present results that

HiRes is better than the standard strategies. However, the results suggest this possibility (at least for PPS, SAS, and the collected standard strategies) and certainly show that HiRes supports high levels of speech recognition.

The initial studies to evaluate HiRes also have included comparisons of CIS processors using 833 pulses/s/electrode versus processors using about 1400 pulses/s/electrode (Frijns et al., 2003). Each of the nine subjects had used a processor with the lower rate and 8 channels (and electrodes) for a period of three to 11 months. They then were fitted in randomized orders with 8-, 12-, or 16-channel processors using the higher rate. Each of the processors was used for one month prior to testing and then the next processor was fitted. Tests with all processors included recognition of monosyllabic words in quiet and in competition with noise at the S/Ns of $+10$, $+5$, 0, and $-5$ dB. The results demonstrated significant differences in scores between the rates and across the numbers of channels. Some patients achieved their best scores with the higher rate and 8 channels, whereas others achieved their best scores with the higher rate and 12 or 16 channels. These best scores showed a substantial and significant advantage of the higher rate for speech reception in noise, especially at the S/N of $+5$ dB, which is typical of everyday acoustic environments.

Battmer et al. (2002) also have compared the performance of the preferred standard strategy (among CIS, PPS, and SAS) to 8-channel HiRes processors using pulse rates of approximately 1500, 2000, and 3000 pulses/s/electrode. The standard strategies were implemented using the emulation mode of the CII implant system. Each of the ten subjects indicated a preference for one of the strategies at initial fitting and then used that strategy for at least three months. Then each subject was assigned to one of three groups in a crossover study to evaluate HiRes and the different rates. A different order of rates was assigned to each group and each rate was used for a month by each subject. Tests were conducted at the end of each of those months, including recognition of the Hochmair– Schultz–Moser (HSM) sentences in quiet and in noise, at the S/N of $+10$ dB, and recognition of the Freiburger monosyllabic words in quiet. The entire cycle of testing was then repeated for each subject. Thus, each rate was tested twice for each subject, with randomized orders of rates across subjects. Inclusion criteria for the subjects included a fully patent cochlea (no bone growth in the ST) on the implanted side. Although the duration of deafness ranged from 0.75 to 26 years for the subjects, six of the subjects had durations of less than a year.

The results indicated a clear superiority of HiRes over the standard strategies, but no significant differences among the rates. The greatest gains were observed for recognition of monosyllabic words and of HSM sentences in noise. Scores for recognition of sentences in quiet were significantly better with HiRes than with the standard strategies, but also exhibited ceiling effects, with most of the subjects scoring at or near 100% correct using HiRes. For the rate of 2000 pulses/s/electrode, the mean of the scores for recognition of monosyllabic words increased from 55.6% correct to 72.2% correct (SDs 16.2 and 14.2, respectively; $p < 0.01$), and the mean of the scores for recognition of sentences in noise increased from 14.8% correct to 42.4% correct (SDs of 16.6 and 18.9, respectively; $p < 0.01$). Almost identical increases for each test were found for the other rates.

These findings from the studies of Frijns et al. and Battmer et al. indicate high levels of performance with HiRes and with the use of pulse rates at and above about 1400 pulses/s/electrode. This general outcome is consistent with the results of prior studies, such as those shown in Figure 2.6, i.e. increases in speech reception scores with increases in rate up to about 1500 pulses/s/electrode for CIS processors using 4 or more channels. (However, the studies of Frijns et al. and Battmer et al. did not use a crossover design for comparisons between the standard and experimental processors and thus these conclusions about rate effects from those studies must remain tentative.)

In addition to the sequential and 'paired pulsatile' modes for HiRes, the Clarion CII system also can implement a 'virtual channels' variation of CIS, in which perceptual channels are produced between actual electrodes through current steering. In one implementation, a single virtual channel is produced between each pair of adjacent electrodes in the array, for a total of 31 channels (or sites of stimulation), with 16 sites at the actual electrodes and 15 sites between the adjacent pairs. The virtual sites are produced with simultaneous stimulation of the adjacent electrodes, and single-electrode and paired-electrode stimuli are sequenced as in a standard CIS processor. In principle, more sites, and more perceptually distinct sites could be produced using the additional virtual channels. To the extent that an increase in perceptually distinct sites translates to an increase in the number of effective channels, this could be especially helpful for speech reception in noise (e.g. Dorman et al., 1998; Friesen et al., 2001) and for music reception (Smith et al., 2002).

The concept of virtual channels for cochlear implants was introduced by Wilson et al. in the early 1990s (e.g. Wilson et al., 1992, 1994b). Its application now may be beneficial in a 'fixed channel' implementation as described above or in a 'roving channel' implementation, which might be helpful for a fine-grained representation of frequencies that correspond to multiple positions between electrodes (Wilson et al., 2004).

HiRes has become the default strategy for the Clarion CII system. It is also the default strategy for the newer HiRes 90K system, which includes the same electronics in the receiver/stimulator as the CII system, but in a smaller package. However, the electrode positioner is no longer used, owing to a possible association between such use and meningitis (e.g. Arnold et al., 2002). HiRes may be implemented using strictly sequential stimulation across electrodes or simultaneous stimulation of widely spaced pairs of electrodes, with the pairs presented in a non-simultaneous sequence. In addition, virtual sites and channels can be specified for experimental purposes. Between the two standard options for clinical fittings, strictly sequential stimulation is likely to lead to better results for most patients (Frohne-Büchner et al., 2003).

## Outcome data

Results from comparisons between and among processing strategies in current use have been mentioned in the preceding section. In broad terms, many of the strategies support comparably high levels of performance for their users.

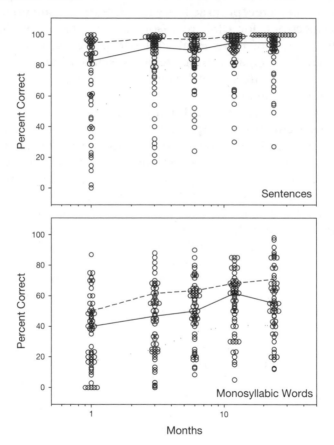

**Figure 2.12** Percent correct scores for 55 users of the COMBI 40 implant and the CIS processing strategy. Scores for recognition of the Hochmair–Schultz–Moser sentences are presented in the top panel, and scores for recognition of the Freiburger monosyllabic words are presented in the bottom panel. The solid line in each panel shows the median of the scores, and the dashed and dotted lines show the interquartile ranges. The data are an updated superset of those reported in Helms et al. (1997), kindly provided by Patrick D'Haese of Med-El GmbH, Innsbruck, Austria. The experimental conditions and implantation criteria are described in Helms et al. All subjects took both tests at each of the indicated intervals following initial fitting of their speech processors. Identical scores at a single test interval are displaced horizontally for clarity. Thus, for example, the horizontal 'line' of scores in the top-right portion of the top panel all represent scores for the 24-month test interval.

Outcome data that exemplify such performance are presented in Figure 2.12. This figure shows scores for 55 users of the COMBI 40 implant system and the CIS processing strategy. Scores for recognition of the HSM sentences are presented in the top panel, and scores for recognition of the Freiburger monosyllabic words are presented in the bottom panel. Results for four measurement intervals are shown, ranging from one month to two years following the initial fitting of the speech processor. The solid line in each panel shows the median of the individual scores and the dashed and dotted lines show the interquartile ranges. The data are a superset of those reported in Helms et al., 1997, that include scores for additional subjects at various test intervals.

Most of the subjects used an 8-channel processor with a pulse rate of about 1500/s/electrode. Some of the subjects used fewer channels and a proportionately higher rate. (All processors used the maximum overall rate of 12120 pulses/s across channels.)

As is evident in the figure, scores are broadly distributed at each test interval and for both tests. However, ceiling effects are encountered for the sentence test for many of the subjects, especially at the later test intervals. Indeed, at 24 months 47 of the 55 subjects score at 75% correct or higher, and 21 of the subjects score at 95% correct or higher.

In addition to the broad distributions of scores, a learning effect is evident in comparing results across intervals. This is seen especially in the lower ranges of scores, e.g. the steady increase in the lower interquartile lines (the dotted lines) in the range of one to 12 months of experience with the implant and CIS.

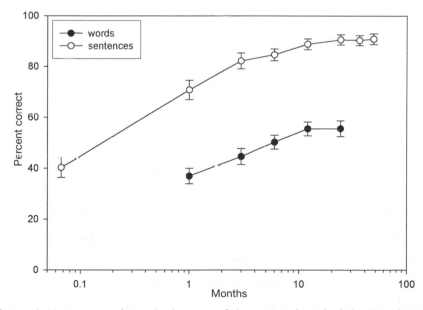

**Figure 2.13** Means and standard errors of the means for 54 of the 55 subjects in Figure 2.12. (One of the subjects did not take the sentence test for the expanded range of intervals in this Figure 2.13.)

The learning effect is even easier to see in plots of mean scores over time, as shown in Figure 2.13 for these same data and a preceding and two subsequent intervals for the sentence test. The mean scores increase for both the sentence and word tests out to 12 months and then plateau thereafter. The mean scores for the sentence test asymptote at about 90% correct, and the mean scores for the word test asymptote at about 55% correct. Such results typify performance with the best of the modern cochlear implant systems and processing strategies.

Recognition of monosyllabic words is a good standard for comparisons among devices and processing strategies. Scores do not encounter possible ceiling effects with any of the present devices or strategies. In addition, floor effects are not generally encountered either, at least with some experience with the implant (see the word scores at 6, 12, and 24 months in the bottom panel of Figure 2.12). The means of scores range between about 40 and 60 for the better of the present devices and strategies, close to or at the point of likely maximum sensitivity of measures.

**Table 2.4** Recognition of monosyllabic words using the default processing strategies of current and widely applied implant systems[a]

| Strategy | System | Study | Subjects | Experience | Mean | SD[b] |
|---|---|---|---|---|---|---|
| ACE | CI24M | Kiefer et al., 2001 | 11 | ≥ 1 mo[c] | 49.8 | 30.9 |
| | | David et al., 2003 | 26 | 12 mo | 55.2 | 11.9 |
| | | Skinner et al., 2002 | 12 | 1.5 mo[d] | 37.9 | 14.9 |
| CIS | COMBI 40 | Helms et al., 1997[e] | 55 | 1 mo | 36.2 | 22.8 |
| | | | | 3 mo | 44.7 | 23.2 |
| | | | | 6 mo | 49.7 | 20.2 |
| | | | | 12 mo | 55.1 | 20.0 |
| | COMBI 40, 40+ | Müller et al., 2002 | 9[f] | ≥ 2 mo | 43.1 | 18.8 |
| | COMBI 40+ | Ziese et al., 2000 | 6 | ≥ 3 mo | 50.9 | 24.0 |
| | COMBI 40 | Hamzavi et al., 2003 | 21 | 12 mo | 40.6 | 9.6 |
| | COMBI 40+ | | 25 | | 41.9 | 7.5 |
| | COMBI 40 | Gstoettner et al., 1998 | 21 | 1 mo | 24.5 | 16.3 |
| | | | | 6 mo | 37.3 | 17.5 |
| | | | | 12 mo | 44.6 | 19.9 |
| HiRes | Clarion CII | Koch et al., 2004 | 51 | 3 mo[g] | 50.0 | 25.1 |

a This table does not include results from unpublished studies or results from studies with children. The table also does not include results from studies in which only a subset of the subjects was tested with a strategy.
b Standard deviation.
c Following 3–6 months of experience with the SPEAK or CIS strategies, as implemented in the CI24M system.
d The ACE, SPEAK, and CIS strategies, as implemented in the CI24M system, were tested. Experience with each strategy was 1.5 months, and the strategies were applied in a counterbalanced order across subjects. Thus, some subjects had 1.5 or 3.0 months of experience with another strategy or other strategies, prior to their experience with ACE.
e Including updated data kindly provided by Patrick D'Haese; see Figure 2.12.
f Mean and SD of 18 unilateral scores, for 9 bilaterally implanted patients.
g Following three months of experience with the CIS, PPS, or SAS strategies, as implemented using the emulation mode of the Clarion CII system.

Published results for the recognition of monosyllabic words are listed in Table 2.4 for the default strategies used in current and widely applied implant systems. In some cases, multiple scores are listed for multiple test intervals in a particular study. Comparisons across studies should be approached with great caution, as results may be affected by (1) the experience of the subjects (as noted above), (2) details of the fittings within each study, (3) the criteria for implantation (e.g. subjects in some studies had more residual hearing than subjects in other studies), (4) the exact test used (one monosyllabic word test can be more or less difficult than another, although all of them are difficult), (5) details of the experimental procedures, and (6) perhaps the skill of the surgeon(s). However, comparisons within studies are generally safe, and comparisons across studies may identify possible 'outliers' and then lead to a more detailed investigation into the possible cause(s).

Table 2.4 shows high scores for each of the default strategies, for comparable amounts of experience. For example, with 12 months of experience, results from the study of David et al. (2003) indicate a mean and standard deviation of 55.2 and 11.9%, respectively, for ACE as implemented in the CI24M system, and results from the study of Helms et al. (1997) indicate a mean and standard deviation of 55.1 and 20.0%, respectively, for CIS as implemented in the COMBI 40 system and with the same amount of experience for the subjects. These mean scores are statistically indistinguishable. Similarly, the mean score for six months of experience with CIS from the study of Helms et al. is statistically indistinguishable from the mean score for six months of aggregated experience with one of the standard strategies (first three months) and HiRes (subsequent three months), as implemented in the Clarion CII system (Koch et al., 2004). (The mean score for three months of experience with CIS as implemented in the COMBI 40 system also is statistically indistinguishable from the mean score for 6 months of aggregated experience with one of the standard strategies and HiRes as implemented in the Clarion CII system.)

In addition, strong learning effects are indicated in the results from the studies listed in Table 2.4 with multiple test intervals. Such effects have been discussed in connection with the study conducted by Helms et al. (1997), with its 8 test intervals for sentences and 5 test intervals for monosyllabic words (Figures 2.12 and 2.13). Learning effects also are clearly seen in the results reported by Gstoettner et al. (1998), across the test intervals of one, six and 12 months, for monosyllabic words.

No one of the default strategies listed in Table 2.4 'pops out' as the best of the three. This may not be altogether surprising in view of facts that two of them use a CIS approach (the CIS and HiRes strategies), and one of them uses an $n$-of-$m$ approach that is similar to CIS in important ways, e.g. the same filter banks, envelope detectors, mapping functions, and non-simultaneous sequencing of stimulus pulses across electrodes. Good implementations of each of these default strategies generally lead to relatively high levels of speech reception performance for most patients.

A recent trend in implant design is to move in the direction of progressively higher rates of stimulation. The Clarion CII, CI24M, COMBI 40+, and PULSAR implant systems all support higher rates than their predecessors. (The PULSAR is the newest system from Med-El GmbH.) Such increases in supported rates, in conjunction with high compliance voltages that allow stimulation with short-duration pulses, are likely to be helpful for most patients and for rates up to about 1500 pulses/s/electrode. In addition, higher rates may be helpful to a smaller subset of patients. More research is needed to gauge the size of this latter population precisely and to explore effects of very high rates, e.g. in the range from 3000 to 5000 pulses/s/electrode.

Although the mean scores in Table 2.4 (and Figures 2.11 and 2.13) are high, they also show a large remaining gap between normal and electrically evoked hearing. A listener with normal hearing would score at or near 100% correct in taking the monosyllabic word test, for example. In contrast, the mean and median scores for implant patients, using the most recent processing strategies and implant systems, are around 50% correct for the same test. Some patients achieve quite high scores, approaching those of normal hearing, but most do not.

While not yet perfect by any means, truly remarkable progress has been made in the development of cochlear implants to date, leading up to the present levels of performance. In the course of roughly 20 years, implants have moved from supporting little or no recognition of speech with hearing alone to high levels of recognition. This achievement is among the great success stories of modern medicine. Much work is underway aimed at producing further improvements, as very briefly described in the next section.

## Future directions

This is an especially exciting time in the history of cochlear implants. Quite recently, substantial advances have been made by stimulating both ears with bilateral cochlear implants or by combining electric and acoustic stimulation (EAS) for persons with some residual, low-frequency hearing. Each of these approaches produces large gains in scores for speech reception in noise for a majority of patients. In addition, combined EAS appears to provide a significant advantage for music reception, compared with electric stimulation only. An overview of findings with bilateral implants and with combined EAS is presented in Wilson et al. (2003a).

In addition to these recent advances, work is in progress to (1) provide a much closer mimicking than was previously possible of the signal processing that occurs in the normal cochlea and (2) represent 'fine-structure' or 'fine-frequency' information in a way that it can be perceived and utilized by patients. These new approaches may support further gains in performance, either alone or in combination with other approaches. A useful representation of frequency variations within channels, the 'fine-structure' information, may in addition be the key for restoring music reception beyond gross features, and for a renewed enjoyment of music, with implants and electric stimulation only. Some fine-structure information may be conveyed in the low-frequency range with combined EAS, and this may underlie in large part the success of the approach.

A strategy to provide a closer mimicking of normal auditory processing is described in Wilson et al. (2003a), and preliminary data are presented in two recent reports (Schatzer et al., 2003; Wilson et al., 2003b). Issues associated with providing potentially useful representations of fine-structure information are described and discussed in Wilson et al. (2004). With the possible exception of combined EAS, present processing strategies for implants convey only a small amount of this information at best to their users. Fundamentally new approaches under development may change that (e.g. Stickney et al., 2002; Litvak et al., 2003; Rubinstein and Hong, 2003; Zeng et al., 2003; Wilson et al., 2004; Zeng, 2004a, 2004b).

These are just some among the many possibilities for the further development of cochlear implants. Recent papers on future directions for implants include those by Clark (2001), Clopton and Spelman (2003), Wilson et al. (2003a), Dorman and Wilson (2004), and Zeng (2004b).

## Concluding remarks

All present processing strategies for cochlear implants use a 'filterbank' or 'waveform' approach. Explicit extraction and representation of specific features of speech was abandoned in the early 1990s. All but one of the present strategies use biphasic pulses as stimuli. With the exception of the PPS strategy, the pulses are presented in a non-simultaneous sequence across electrodes. In the PPS strategy, pairs of widely separated electrodes are stimulated simultaneously, and each pair is stimulated in a non-simultaneous sequence. The SAS strategy presents 'analog' or continuous waveforms as stimuli simultaneously to all (utilized) electrodes. This and the PPS strategy produce good results for some patients but now have been largely supplanted along with the prior implementation of CIS by the HiRes strategy for recipients of the Clarion CII and HiRes 90K implant devices. HiRes is a variation of CIS that uses relatively high rates and a relatively high number of stimulus sites, as supported with improved current sources in the Clarion CII and HiRes 90K receiver/stimulator. Implementations of CIS and ACE in other implant systems also use high rates and up to 12 or more stimulus sites. The performance of those systems and strategies is comparable to that of HiRes.

The design of processing strategies is evolving rapidly, with the advent of bilateral implants and combined EAS, and with many possibilities for further improvements. Although much progress has been made, especially during the past 15 years or so, much remains to be done. Patients with the best results still do not hear as well as listeners with normal hearing, particularly in demanding situations such as speech presented in competition with noise at typical S/Ns, e.g. +5 dB. Implant recipients do not have much access to music and other sounds that are more complex than speech. Even the 'star' performers report a need for great concentration in attaining their high scores in speech-reception tests. Such a cognitive load must separate implant listeners from their normal-hearing peers. Most importantly, though, is the fact that scores are widely distributed across patients with any of the present processing strategies and associated implant systems. Whereas most patients achieve relatively high scores, others do not. A key question in current research on implants is 'why?' The answer may lead to substantial improvements for patients presently at the low end of the performance spectrum.

## Terminology and glossary

Commonly used terms and abbreviations in referencing aspects of cochlear implants include the following:

**ACE**: acronym for *Advanced Combination Encoder*, a processing strategy for cochlear implants.

**AGC**: abbreviation for *Automatic Gain Control*.

**BM**: abbreviation for *Basilar Membrane*, a highly specialized structure that divides the cochlea along its length and acts as a type of frequency analyser, by vibrating or responding maximally near the basal end of the cochlea in response to high-frequency sounds, and by vibrating or responding maximally closer to the apical end of the cochlea for lower frequencies.

**BTE**: abbreviation for *Behind The Ear*, as in a BTE housing for the microphone and electronics for a hearing aid or cochlear implant.

**CA**: abbreviation for *Compressed Analog*, a processing strategy for cochlear implants.

**Channel or channels**: this can reference a channel of processing, stimulation, or reception. A channel of processing is usually associated with a restricted range of frequencies, as determined by a bandpass filter for the channel. A channel of stimulation refers to a site of stimulation in the cochlea, and a channel of reception refers to a perceptually independent source of information that can be utilized as such by the patient. Closely spaced sites of stimulation may not produce independent channels of reception due to overlapping electric fields and other factors. Thus, the number of perceptual channels may be lower or far lower than the number of stimulus or processing channels.

**CIS:** abbreviation for *C*ontinuous *I*nterleaved *S*ampling, a processing strategy for cochlear implants.

**Conditioner pulses:** a train of uniform and rapidly presented pulses designed to produce stochastic patterns of discharge within and among auditory neurons, much like the patterns of 'spontaneous activity' in normal hearing. The conditioner pulses are presented in conjunction with the stimuli determined with standard processing strategies for implants. The spontaneous-like activity imparted by the conditioner pulses is expected to 'condition' the neurons to be more receptive (e.g. with a greater dynamic range of responses) to the deterministic stimuli.

**Current steering:** a term used to reference the construction of virtual channels, see *Electrode coupling configuration* and *Virtual channel* below.

**DSP:** abbreviation for *D*igital *S*ignal *P*rocessing, as in a DSP chip or integrated circuit, or as in a DSP algorithm.

**EAS:** this refers to combined *E*lectric and *A*coustic *S*timulation of the auditory system, for persons with some residual (low-frequency) hearing either ipsilateral or contralateral to a cochlear implant. (In some contexts, EAS refers only to the combination of the two modes of stimulation in the same ear, i.e. acoustic stimulation ipsilateral to the implant.)

**Electrode:** a generic term that can reference a particular electrode among multiple electrodes in a cochlear implant or a particular site of stimulation produced by (1) a single electrode in the cochlea in combination with a remote 'return' electrode outside the cochlea or (2) a combination of electrodes within the cochlea, to produce bipolar pairs of closely spaced electrodes or more complicated combinations involving more than two intracochlear electrodes. (These arrangements are described further in *Electrode coupling configuration* below.)

**Electrode array:** the set of intracochlear electrodes, usually held in place with a silastic carrier. The array is inserted into the scala tympani at surgery, usually through a fenestration made by the surgeon (a cochleostomy) near the basal end and round window membrane of the cochlea. In some implant designs, additional structures or procedures are used to position the array close to the inner or modiolar wall of the ST to bring the electrodes closer to the spiral ganglion, the putative site of neural excitation for implants.

**Electrode coupling configuration:** this refers to the arrangement of electrodes for stimulation with an implant. The configurations include *monopolar stimulation*, in which a single electrode within the cochlea is stimulated with reference to a return electrode outside the cochlea for each site of stimulation, *bipolar stimulation*, in which one intracochlear electrode is stimulated with reference to a nearby electrode also within the cochlea, *tripolar* or *quadrupolar stimulation*, in which three or more electrodes are stimulated together in a 'beamforming' arrangement to produce restricted fields of excitation, and *virtual channel stimulation*, in which pairs of electrodes are stimulated simultaneously or in rapid succession to produce effective sites of stimulation between the electrodes.

**Emulation mode:** the fitting software for the Clarion CII implant system includes an emulation mode that supports implementations of the CIS, PPS and SAS processing strategies previously used in conjunction with the Clarion 1.2 implant system. These implementations in the Clarion CII system do not reproduce exactly the implementations in the Clarion 1.2 system due to differences in hardware for the two systems, e.g. different current sources and electrode designs. (The newer HiRes 90K implant system also includes an emulation mode for its fitting software that supports implementations of CIS and PPS strategies.)

**HiRes:** acronym for *H*igh *R*esolution, a processing strategy for cochlear implants.

**IHC:** abbreviation for *I*nner *H*air *C*ell, the sensory hair cells in the cochlea that transduce motions of the basilar membrane into excitatory chemical stimuli for adjacent neurons in the auditory nerve.

**MPS:** abbreviation for *M*ultiple *P*ulsatile *S*ampler, a processing strategy for cochlear implants. *MPS* is another (newer) name for *PPS*, an identical strategy.

**Modiolus**:      the inner core of the cochlea that contains the auditory nerve.

**$n$-of-$m$**:      a processing strategy for cochlear implants in which $n$ channels and associated electrodes are selected from among $m$ channels and electrodes for each cycle of stimulation. The $n$-of-$m$ strategy was the progenitor of the *SPEAK* and *ACE* strategies. Present implementations of the $n$-of-$m$ and *ACE* strategies are essentially identical.

**OHC**:      abbreviation for *Outer Hair Cell*, the sensory hair cells in cochlea involved in an active feedback loop that 'sharpens' the longitudinal or spatial response of the *BM* to low- and mid-intensity sounds and that increases the sensitivity of the *BM* to faint sounds.

**PPS**:      abbreviation for *Paired Pulsatile Sampler*, a processing strategy for cochlear implants. The name *MPS* also has been used for this strategy; see above.

**Receiver/stimulator**:      a hermetically sealed package of electronics implanted beneath the skin above and posterior to the pinna and seated in the skull. The electronics receive signals from an external transmitting coil held in place with attracting magnets, one in the center of the coil (or headpiece) and the other in the receiver/stimulator package. The received signals are decoded to specify stimuli for the electrode array (see definition above). In addition, the signals are rectified and integrated (with a lowpass filter) to provide power for the implanted electronics. The stimuli are conveyed from the receiver/stimulator to the array via a multi-wire cable. Feedthroughs for the cable also are hermetically sealed to prevent damage to the electronics by corrosive body fluids and to prevent damage to tissue by toxic materials or voltages in the electronics.

**SAS**:      acronym for *Simultaneous Analog Stimulation*, a processing strategy for cochlear implants.

**S/N**:      abbreviation for *Signal-to-Noise* ratio, usually expressed in decibels (dB).

**SPEAK**:      acronym for the *Spectral Peak* processing strategy for cochlear implants.

**ST**:      acronym for *Scala Tympani*, one of three chambers in the cochlea, into which the electrode array for all present-day implants is inserted. The other chambers are the scala media and scala

| | vestibuli. These chambers divide the cross section of the cochlea and continue along its length. |
|---|---|
| **Virtual channel:** | a site of stimulation formed between two electrodes, see *Electrode coupling configuration* above. Recently, the term *current steering* has also been used to reference the concept of virtual channels. The two terms may be used interchangeably. |
| **Vocoder:** | acronym for *Voice Coder*, an analysis-synthesis system used to extract essential parameters from speech in the analysis stage, then transmit those parameters over a distance through a phone line or other link, and finally to reconstruct a speech signal at the receiving end in the coding stage. Some designs of cochlear implants are based on the analysis stages of various vocoder systems, or on knowledge obtained in vocoder studies about parts of the speech signal that must be preserved or transmitted to maintain intelligibility. |

# Acknowledgments

Preparation of this chapter was supported by NIH project N01-DC-2-1002. Portions of text in the chapter were updated or adapted from prior publications (Wilson et al., 2003a; Wilson, 2004).

# References

Abbas PJ, Miller CA (2004) Biophysics and physiology. In: F-G Zeng, AN Popper, RR Fay (eds), Cochlear Implants: Auditory prostheses and electric hearing. New York: Springer-Verlag, pp. 149–212.

Arndt P, Staller S, Arcaroli J et al. (1999) Within-subjects comparison of advanced coding strategies in the Nucleus 24 cochlear implant. Technical Report, Englewood, CO: Cochlear Corporation.

Arnold W, Bredberg G, Gstoettner W et al. (2002) Meningitis following cochlear implantation: pathomechanisms, clinical symptoms, conservative and surgical treatments. ORL J Otorhinolaryngol Relat Spec 64: 382–9.

Badi AN, Kertesz TR, Gurgel RK et al. (2003) Development of a novel eighth-nerve intraneural auditory neuroprosthesis. Laryngoscope 113: 833–42.

Balkany TJ, Eshraghi AA, Yang N (2002) Modiolar proximity of three perimodiolar cochlear implant electrodes. Acta Otolaryngol 122: 363–9.

Battmer RD, Zilberman Y, Haake P et al. (1999) Simultaneous Analog Stimulation (SAS) – Continuous Interleaved Sampler (CIS) pilot comparison study in Europe. Ann Otol Rhinol Laryngol 108(suppl. 177): 69–73.

Battmer RD, Büchner A, Frohne-Büchner C et al. (2002) The Clarion CII high resolution mode: Experience after 6 months. Presented at the 7th International Cochlear Implant Conference, Manchester, UK.

Bierer JA, Middlebrooks JC (2004) Cortical responses to cochlear implant stimulation: Channel interactions. J Assoc Res Otolaryngol 5: 32–48.

Boëx C, Pelizzone M, Montandon P (1996) Speech recognition with a CIS strategy for the Ineraid multichannel cochlear implant. Am J Otol 17: 61–8.

Boëx C, de Balthasar C, Kos MI et al. (2003) Electrical field interactions in different cochlear implant systems. J Acoust Soc Am 114: 2049–57.

Brill S, Hochmair I, Hochmair ES (1998) The importance of stimulation rate in pulsatile stimulation strategies in cochlear implants. Presented at the XXIV International Congress of Audiology, Buenos Aires, Argentina.

Brown CJ, Geers A, Herrmann B et al. (Working Group on Cochlear Implants) (in press) Cochlear implants. Technical Report, American Speech-Language-Hearing Association. ASHA suppl. 24.

Büchner A, Frohne C, Battmer R-D et al. (2003) Investigation of stimulation rates between 800 and 5000 pps with the Clarion CII implant. Presented at the 2003 Conference on Implantable Auditory Prostheses, Pacific Grove, CA, p. 116 in the book of Abstracts.

Büchner A, Frohne-Büchner C, Battmer R-D et al. (2004) Two years of experience using high stimulation rates with the Clarion CII device. Presented at the Eighth International Cochlear Implant Conference, Indianapolis, IN, p. 46 in the book of Abstracts.

Busby PA, Tong YC, Clark GM (1993) The perception of temporal modulations by cochlear implant patients. J Acoust Soc Am 94: 124–31.

Clark GM (2000) The cochlear implant: A search for answers. Cochlear Implants Int 1: 1–15.

Clark GM (2001) Cochlear implants: Climbing new mountains. Cochlear Implants Int 2: 75–97.

Clopton BM, Spelman FA (2003) Technology and the future of cochlear implants. Ann Otol Rhinol Laryngol 112(suppl. 191): 26–32.

Cohen LT, Saunders E, Clark GM (2001) Psychophysics of a prototype peri-modiolar cochlear implant electrode array. Hear Res 155: 63–81.

Crosby PA, Daly CN, Money DK et al. (1985) Cochlear implant system for an auditory prosthesis. US patent 4532930.

David EE, Ostroff JM, Shipp D et al. (2003) Speech coding strategies and revised cochlear implant candidacy: An analysis of post-implant performance. Otol Neurotol 24: 228–33.

de Balthasar C, Boëx C, Cosendai G et al. (2003) Channel interactions with high-rate biphasic electrical stimulation in cochlear implant subjects. Hear Res 182: 77–87.

Dorman MF, Loizou PC (1997) Changes in speech intelligibility as a function of time and signal processing strategy for an Ineraid patient fitted with continuous interleaved sampling (CIS) processors. Ear Hear 18: 147–55.

Dorman MF, Wilson BS (2004) The design and function of cochlear implants. Am Scientist 92: 436–45.

Dorman MF, Smith L, Parkin JL (1993) Loudness balance between acoustic and electric stimulation by a patient with a multichannel cochlear implant. Ear Hear 14: 290–2.

Dorman MF, Loizou PC, Fitzke J et al. (1998) The recognition of sentences in noise by normal-hearing listeners using simulations of cochlear-implant signal processors with 6–20 channels. J Acoust Soc Am 104: 3583–5.

Dorman MF, Loizou PC, Spahr AJ et al. (2002) A comparison of the speech understanding provided by acoustic models of fixed-channel and channel-picking signal processors for cochlear implants. J Speech Lang Hear Res 45: 783–8.

Eddington DK (1980) Speech discrimination in deaf subjects with cochlear implants. J Acoust Soc Am 68: 885–91.

Eddington DK, Dobelle WH, Brackman DE et al. (1978) Auditory prosthesis research with multiple channel intracochlear stimulation in man. Ann Otol Rhinol Laryngol 87(suppl. 53): 1–39.

Favre E, Pelizzone M (1993) Channel interactions in patients using the Ineraid multichannel cochlear implant. Hear Res 66: 150–6.

Firszt JB (2004) HiResolution sound processing. Technical Report, Advanced Bionics Corporation, Sylmar, CA. (This report is available at the Advanced Bionics website; the present direct link is http://www.cochlearimplant.com/printables/HiRes-WhtPpr.pdf.)

Fishman KE, Shannon RV, Slattery WH (1997) Speech recognition as a function of the number of electrodes used in the SPEAK cochlear implant speech processor. J Speech Lang Hear Res 40: 1201–15.

Flanagan JL (1972) Speech Analysis, Synthesis and Perception, 2nd edn. Berlin, Heidelberg, New York: Springer-Verlag, pp. 330–1.

Friesen LM, Shannon RV, Baskent D et al. (2001) Speech recognition in noise as a function of the number of spectral channels: comparison of acoustic hearing and cochlear implants. J Acoust Soc Am 110: 1150–63.

Frijns JH, Briaire JJ, Grote JJ (2001) The importance of human cochlear anatomy for the results with modiolus-hugging multichannel cochlear implants. Otol Neurotol 22: 340–9.

Frijns JH, Briaire JJ, de Laat JA et al. (2002) Initial evaluation of the Clarion CII cochlear implant: speech perception and neural response imaging. Ear Hear 23: 184–97.

Frijns JH, Klop WM, Bonnet RM et al. (2003) Optimizing the number of electrodes with high-rate stimulation of the Clarion CII cochlear implant. Acta Otolaryngol 123: 138–42.

Frohne-Büchner C, Battmer R-D, Büchner A et al. (2003) The Clarion CII high resolution mode: paired or sequential stimulation paradigm? Presented at the 2003 Conference on Implantable Auditory Prostheses, Pacific Grove, CA, p. 117 in the book of Abstracts.

Fu Q-J, Shannon RV (2000) Effect of stimulation rate on phoneme recognition by Nucleus 22 cochlear implant listeners. J Acoust Soc Am 107: 589–97.

Garnham C, O'Driscoll M, Ramsden R et al. (2002) Speech understanding in noise with a Med-El COMBI 40+ cochlear implant using reduced channel sets. Ear Hear 23: 540–52.

Glasberg BR, Moore BCJ (1990) Derivation of auditory filter shapes from notched-noise data. Hear Res 47: 103–38.

Greenwood DD (1990) A cochlear frequency-position function for several species: 29 years later. J Acoust Soc Am 87: 2592–605.

Gstoettner WK, Hamzavi J, Baumgartner WD (1998) Speech discrimination scores of postlingually deaf adults implanted with the Combi 40 cochlear implant. Acta Otolaryngol 118: 640–5.

Gstoettner WK, Adunka O, Franz P et al. (2001) Perimodiolar electrodes in cochlear implant surgery. Acta Otolaryngol 121: 216–19.

Hamzavi J, Baumgartner W-D, Pok SM et al. (2003) Variables affecting speech perception in postlingually deaf adults following cochlear implantation. Acta Otolaryngol 13: 493–8.

Helms J, Müller J, Schön F et al. (1997) Evaluation of performance with the COMBI 40 cochlear implant in adults: A multicentric clinical study. ORL J Otorhinolaryngol Relat Spec 59: 23–35.

Helms J, Müller J, Schön F et al. (2001) Comparison of the TEMPO+ ear-level speech processor and the CIS pro+ body-worn processor in adult Med-El cochlear implant users. ORL J Otorhinolaryngol Relat Spec 63: 31–40.

Hillman T, Badi AN, Normann RA et al. (2003) Cochlear nerve stimulation with a 3-dimensional penetrating electrode array. Otol Neurotol 24: 764–8.

Hinojosa R, Marion M (1983) Histopathology of profound sensorineural deafness. Ann N Y Acad Sci 405: 459–84.

Hochmair-Desoyer IJ, Hochmair ES, Burian K et al. (1983) Percepts from the Vienna cochlear prosthesis. Ann N Y Acad Sci 405: 295–306.

Kasturi K, Loizou PC, Dorman M et al. (2002) The intelligibility of speech with 'holes' in the spectrum. J Acoust Soc Am 112: 1102–11.

Kessler DK (1999) The Clarion multi-strategy cochlear implant. Ann Otol Rhinol Laryngol 108(suppl. 177): 8–16.

Kiefer J, von Ilberg C, Hubner-Egener J et al. (2000) Optimized speech understanding with the continuous interleaved sampling speech coding strategy in cochlear implants: Effect of variations in stimulation rate and number of channels. Ann Otol Rhinol Laryngol 109: 1009–20.

Kiefer J, Hohl S, Sturzebecher E et al. (2001) Comparison of speech recognition with different speech coding strategies (SPEAK, CIS, and ACE) and their relationship to telemetric measures of compound action potentials in the nucleus CI24M cochlear implant system. Audiology 40: 32–42.

Koch DB, Osberger MJ, Segel P et al. (2004) HiResolution and conventional sound processing in the HiResolution Bionic Ear: using appropriate outcome measures to assess speech-recognition ability. Audiol Neurootol 9: 214–23.

Lawson DT, Wilson BS, Zerbi M et al. (1996) Speech processors for auditory prostheses: 22 electrode percutaneous study – Results for the first five subjects. Third Quarterly Progress Report, NIH project N01-DC-5-2103, Neural Prosthesis Program, National Institutes of Health, Bethesda, MD. (This report is available at http://www.rti.org/capr/caprqprs.htm.)

Leake PA, Rebscher SJ (2004) Anatomical considerations and long-term effects of electrical stimulation. In: F-G Zeng, AN Popper, RR Fay (eds), Cochlear Implants: Auditory prostheses and electric hearing. New York: Springer-Verlag, pp. 101–48.

Litvak LM, Delgutte B, Eddington DK (2003) Improved neural representation of vowels in electric stimulation using desynchronizing pulse trains. J Acoust Soc Am 114: 2099–111.

Loeb GE, Byers CL, Rebscher SJ et al. (1983) Design and fabrication of an experimental cochlear prosthesis. Med Biol Eng Comput 21: 241–54.

Loizou PC (1998) Mimicking the human ear: an overview of signal processing strategies for cochlear prostheses. IEEE Sig Proc Mag 15: 101–30.

Loizou PC (1999) Signal-processing techniques for cochlear implants. IEEE Eng Med Biol Mag 18: 34–46.

Loizou PC, Poroy O, Dorman M (2000) The effect of parametric variations of cochlear implant processors on speech understanding. J Acoust Soc Am 108: 790–802.

Loizou PC, Stickney G, Mishra L et al. (2003) Comparison of speech processing strategies used in the Clarion implant processor. Ear Hear 24: 12–19.

McDermott HJ, McKay CM, Vandali AE (1992) A new portable sound processor for the University of Melbourne/Nucleus Limited multielectrode cochlear implant. J Acoust Soc Am 91: 3367–91.

McDermott HJ, Vandali AE (1997) Spectral maxima sound processor. US patent 5597380.

McKay CM, McDermott HJ, Clark GM (1994) Pitch percepts associated with amplitude-modulated current pulse trains in cochlear implantees. J Acoust Soc Am 96: 2664–73.

Merzenich MM (1985) UCSF cochlear implant device. In: RA Schindler, MM Merzenich (eds), Cochlear Implants. New York: Raven Press, pp. 121–30.

Merzenich MM, Rebscher SJ, Loeb GE et al. (1984) The UCSF cochlear implant project. Adv Audiol 2: 119–44.

Miura M, Sando I, Hirsch BE et al. (2002) Analysis of spiral ganglion cell populations in children with normal and pathological ears. Ann Otol Rhinol Laryngol 111: 1059–65.

Moore BCJ, Glasberg BR (1983) Suggested formulae for calculating auditory-filter bandwidths and excitation patterns. J Acoust Soc Am 74: 750–3.

Müller J, Schön F, Helms J (2002) Speech understanding in quiet and noise in bilateral users of the Med-El COMBI 40/40+ cochlear implant system. Ear Hear 23: 198–206.

Osberger MJ, Fisher L (2000) New directions in speech processing: Patient performance with simultaneous analog stimulation. Ann Otol Rhinol Laryngol 109(suppl. 185): 70–3.

Pasanisi E, Bacciu A, Vincenti V et al. (2002) Comparison of speech perception benefits with SPEAK and ACE coding strategies in pediatric Nucleus CI24M cochlear implant recipients. Int J Pediatr Otorhinolaryngol 64: 159–63.

Patrick JF, Seligman PM, Clark GM (1997) Engineering. In: GM Clark, RSC Cowan, RC Dowell (eds), Cochlear Implantation for Infants and Children: Advances. San Diego, CA: Singular Publishing Group, pp. 125–45.

Pelizzone M, Tinembart J, François J et al. (1998) Very high stimulation rates for cochlear implants. Presented at the 4th European Symposium on Paediatric Cochlear Implantation. Hertogenbosch, The Netherlands, Abstract 61 in the book of Abstracts.

Pelizzone M, Cosendai G, Tinembart J (1999) Within-patient longitudinal speech reception measures with continuous interleaved sampling processors for Ineraid implanted subjects. Ear Hear 20: 228–37.

Rabiner LR, Shafer RW (1978) Digital Processing of Speech Signals. Englewood Cliffs, NJ: Prentice-Hall, pp. 24–6.

Rubinstein JT, Hong R (2003) Signal coding in cochlear implants: exploiting stochastic effects of electrical stimulation. Ann Otol Rhinol Laryngol 112(suppl. 191): 14–19.

Schatzer R, Wilson BS, Wolford RD et al. (2003) Speech processors for auditory prostheses: Signal processing strategy for a closer mimicking of normal auditory functions. Sixth Quarterly Progress Report, NIH project N01-DC-2-1002,

Neural Prosthesis Program, National Institutes of Health, Bethesda, MD. (This report is available at http://www.rti.org/capr/caprqprs.htm.)

Seligman P, McDermott H (1995) Architecture of the Spectra 22 speech processor. Ann Otol Rhinol Laryngol 104 (suppl. 166): 139–41.

Shannon RV (1983) Multichannel electrical stimulation of the auditory nerve in man. I. Basic psychophysics. Hear Res 11: 157–89.

Shannon RV, Adams DD, Ferrel RL et al. (1990) A computer interface for psychophysical and speech research with the Nucleus cochlear implant. J Acoust Soc Am 87: 905–7.

Shannon RV, Galvin JJ 3rd, Baskent D (2002) Holes in hearing. J Assoc Res Otolaryngol 3: 185–99.

Skinner MW, Clark GM, Whitford LA et al. (1994) Evaluation of a new spectral peak (SPEAK) coding strategy for the Nucleus 22 channel cochlear implant system. Am J Otol 15 (suppl. 2): 15–27.

Skinner MW, Arndt PL, Staller S (2002a) Nucleus 24 advanced encoder conversion study: Performance versus preference. Ear Hear 2002 23 (suppl. 1): 2–17.

Skinner MW, Holden LK, Whitford LA et al. (2002b) Speech recognition with the Nucleus 24 SPEAK, ACE, and CIS speech coding strategies in newly implanted adults. Ear Hear 23: 207–23.

Smith ZM, Delgutte B, Oxenham AJ (2002) Chimaeric sounds reveal dichotomies in auditory perception. Nature 416: 87–90.

Stickney GS, Loizou PC, Assmann PF et al. (2001) Electrode interaction and speech intelligibility in multichannel cochlear implants. Presented at the 2001 Conference on Implantable Auditory Prostheses, Pacific Grove, CA, p. 156 in the book of Abstracts.

Stickney GS, Nie K, Zeng F-G (2002) Realistic listening improved by adding fine structure. J Acoust Soc Am 112(Pt. 2): 2355.

Stollwerck LE, Goodrum-Clarke K, Lynch C et al. (2001) Speech processing strategy preferences among 55 European Clarion cochlear implant users. Scand Audiol(suppl. 2001): 36–8.

Tong YC, Blamey PJ, Dowell RC et al. (1983) Psychophysical studies evaluating the feasibility of a speech processing strategy for a multiple-channel cochlear implant. J Acoust Soc Am 74: 73–80.

Townshend B, Cotter N, Van Compernolle D et al. (1987) Pitch perception by cochlear implant subjects. J Acoust Soc Am 82: 106–15.

Tyler RS, Parkinson A, Wilson BS et al. (2000) Evaluation of different choices of $n$ in an $n$-of-$m$ processor for cochlear implants. Adv Oto-Rhino-Laryngol 57: 311–15.

Vandali AE, Whitford LA, Plant KL et al. (2000) Speech perception as a function of electrical stimulation rate: using the Nucleus 24 cochlear implant system. Ear Hear 21: 608–24.

White MW (1986) Compression systems for hearing aids and cochlear prostheses. J Rehabil Res Dev 23: 25–39.

White MW, Merzenich MM, Gardi JN (1984) Multichannel cochlear implants: Channel interactions and processor design. Arch Otolaryngol 110: 493–501.

Wilson BS (1997) The future of cochlear implants. Brit J Audiol 31: 205–25.

Wilson BS (2000a) Strategies for representing speech information with cochlear implants. In: JK Niparko, KI Kirk, NK Mellon et al. (eds), Cochlear Implants: Principles and Practices. Philadelphia, PA: Lippincott, Williams and Wilkins, pp. 129–70.

Wilson BS (2000b) New directions in implant design. In: SB Waltzman, N Cohen (eds), Cochlear Implants. New York: Thieme Medical and Scientific Publishers, pp. 43–56.

Wilson BS (2004) Engineering design of cochlear implant systems. In: F-G Zeng, AN Popper, RR Fay (eds), Cochlear Implants: Auditory prostheses and electric hearing. New York: Springer-Verlag, pp. 14–52.

Wilson BS, Finley CC, Farmer JC Jr et al. (1988) Comparative studies of speech processing strategies for cochlear implants. Laryngoscope 98: 1069–77.

Wilson BS, Finley CC, Lawson DT et al. (1991) Better speech recognition with cochlear implants. Nature 352: 236–8.

Wilson BS, Lawson DT, Zerbi M et al. (1992) Speech processors for auditory prostheses: Virtual channel interleaved sampling (VCIS) processors. First Quarterly Progress Report, NIH project N01-DC-2-2401, Neural Prosthesis Program, National Institutes of Health, Bethesda, MD. (This report is available at http://www.rti.org/capr/caprqprs.htm.)

Wilson BS, Finley CC, Zerbi M et al. (1994a) Speech processors for auditory prostheses: Temporal representations with cochlear implants – Modeling, psychophysical, and electrophysiological studies. Seventh Quarterly Progress Report, NIH project N01-DC-2-2401, Neural Prosthesis Program, National Institutes of Health, Bethesda, MD. (This report is available at http://www.rti.org/capr/caprqprs.htm.)

Wilson BS, Lawson DT, Zerbi M et al. (1994b) Recent developments with the CIS strategies. In: IJ Hochmair-Desoyer, ES Hochmair (eds), Advances in Cochlear Implants. Vienna: Manz, pp. 103–12.

Wilson BS, Zerbi M, Finley CC et al. (1997) Speech processors for auditory prostheses: relationships between temporal patterns of nerve activity and pitch judgments for cochlear implant patients. Eighth Quarterly Progress Report, NIH project N01-DC-5-2103, Neural Prosthesis Program, National Institutes of Health, Bethesda, MD. (This report is available at http://www.rti.org/capr/caprqprs.htm.)

Wilson BS, Wolford RD, Lawson DT (2000) Speech processors for auditory prostheses: effects of changes in stimulus rate and envelope cut-off frequency for CIS processors. Sixth Quarterly Progress Report, NIH project N01-DC-8-2105, Neural Prosthesis Program, National Institutes of Health, Bethesda, MD. (This report is available at http://www.rti.org/capr/caprqprs.htm.)

Wilson BS, Lawson DT, Müller JM et al. (2003a) Cochlear implants: Some likely next steps. Annu Rev Biomed Eng 5: 207–49.

Wilson BS, Wolford RD, Schatzer R et al. (2003b) Speech processors for auditory prostheses: combined use of dual-resonance nonlinear (DRNL) filters and virtual channels. Seventh Quarterly Progress Report, NIH project N01-DC-2-1002. Neural Prosthesis Program, National Institutes of Health, Bethesda, MD. (This report is available at http://www.rti.org/capr/caprqprs.htm.)

Wilson BS, Sun X, Schatzer R et al. (2004) Representation of fine-structure or fine-frequency information with cochlear implants. Int Cong. Ser. 1273: 3–6.

Wouters J, Geurts L, Peeters S et al. (1998) Developments in speech processing for cochlear implants. Acta Otorhinolaryngol Belg 52: 129–32.

Zeng F-G (2002) Temporal pitch in electric hearing. Hear Res 174: 101–6.

Zeng F-G (2004a) Trends in cochlear implants. Trends Amplification 8: 1–34.

Zeng F-G (2004b) Auditory prostheses: past, present, and future. In F-G Zeng, AN Popper, RR Fay (eds), Cochlear Implants: Auditory prostheses and electric hearing. New York: Springer-Verlag, pp. 1–13.

Zeng F-G, Shannon RV (1992) Loudness balance between acoustic and electric stimulation. Hear Res 60: 231–5.

Zeng F-G, Nie K, Stickney G et al. (2003) Using fine structure to improve cochlear implant performance. Presented at the 2003 Conference on Implantable Auditory Prostheses, Pacific Grove, CA, p. 39 in the book of Abstracts.

Zierhofer CM (2003) Electrical nerve stimulation based on channel specific sampling sequences. US Patent 6594525.

Ziese M, Stutzel A, von Specht H et al. (2000) Speech understanding with the CIS and the n-of-m strategy in the Med-El COMBI 40+ system. ORL J Otorhinolaryngol Relat Spec 62: 321–9.

Zimmerman-Philips S, Murad C (1999) Programming features of the Clarion multistrategy cochlear implant. Ann Otol Rhinol Laryngol 108(suppl. 177): 17–21.

Zwicker E, Fastl H (1990) Psychoacoustics: Facts and Models. Berlin, Heidelberg, New York: Springer-Verlag, pp. 103–5.

Zwolan T, Kileny PR, Smith S et al. (2001) Adult cochlear implant patient performance with evolving electrode technology. Otol Neurotol 22: 844–9.

# CHAPTER 3
# The cochlear implant team

DAVID W. PROOPS

The cochlear implant team is one of the most successful multi/inter-disciplinary collaborations in the healthcare systems of the modern world. To understand the form, function and development of cochlear implant teams requires a basic understanding of the theories of teams, the roles assumed and required within them and the input necessary to sustain them. As a child emerges from infancy, it first establishes a sense of self as it grows in its family. Learning how to become part of a team instead of an isolated individual is an essential part of the process of socialization that occurs as a child matures into adulthood. The dictionary definition of a team is 'two or more persons working together'. Membership of a team can be a highly valued experience, and the importance of teams has been known since earliest human history; one could argue that man would not have survived as a species, let alone have achieved our complex civilization, without the ability to co-operate with others in teamwork. However, until the modern age, most teams, apart from family or tribal units, were segregated by gender. Even industrialization did not change this until recent times; of course, teams comprising a mixture of both genders are now commonplace and undoubtedly strengthened by this.

In order to integrate clinical care, professionals often prefer disease-specific teams, such as in diabetes or hypertensive teams. The rehabilitation of the profoundly hearing-impaired is a specific clinical area, and the cochlear implant team is one such specific group, with a common aim of offering specialist care.

Such teams can offer a co-ordinated range of skills, expertise and clinical experience in a setting with inter-professional support. Teams may adopt several formats: multi-disciplinary, inter-disciplinary and transdisciplinary. In multi-disciplinary teams, the different professions work individually to set goals and meet to discuss their progress. In inter-disciplinary teams, goals are first agreed by the team, whose members then co-ordinate their input to the common treatment plan.

In trans-disciplinary teams, not only goals but skills are shared. Teamwork allows the co-ordination of input and the sharing of skills and experiences in solving complex clinical problems. Greater flexibility and integration of work makes the best use of resources. These teams act as an educational resource and stimulate awareness of the condition and should undertake clinical research to strengthen their practice and demonstrate their effectiveness.

## Aspects of multi-disciplinary teamworking

Within health care, teamworking is regarded as an essential prerequisite of modern clinical care. However, for most of medical history the roles were very separate. The assumption made in this model was of medical leadership although there was often little formal co-ordination. The explosion of professions allied to medicine led to the concept of multi-disciplinary teams, that is, bringing various professionals together to understand a particular problem, in this sense affording different perspectives on specific clinical issues at hand.

Issues of territory and professional boundaries impact on multi-disciplinary working, which does not guarantee the development of shared understanding. The concept of inter-disciplinary care has emerged, which, although not denying the importance of specific skills, seeks to blur the professional boundaries and requires trust, tolerance and a willingness to share responsibility.

An effective team will show:

* purpose and values – for example, evidence of well-defined values, standards, functions and responsibilities, and strategic direction;
* performance – which will involve evidence of leadership, competent management, good systems, good performance records and effective internal performance monitoring and feedback;
* consistency – including evidence of thoroughness and a systematic approach to providing patient care;
* effectiveness and efficiency – evidence that, amongst other things, they are assessing the care they provide and its clinical results;
* a chain of responsibility – demonstrating that responsibilities are well defined and understood;
* openness – for example, willingness to let others see in, and evidence of performance presented in ways that people outside the team can understand;
* overall acceptability – including evidence that the performance and results achieved by the team inspire the trust and confidence of patients, employers and professional colleagues.

# Team dynamics

Good team dynamics achieve more than would be possible from the sum of the work of its individual team members. To achieve this, individual team members must have a knowledge of their functions, clear achievable goals, work in a well-co-ordinated fashion, give and receive support to other team members and, finally, feel a valued member of that team.

Dr Meredith Belbin has written extensively on team roles which are defined as 'a tendency to behave, contribute and interrelate with others in a particular way' (Belbin, 1993).

A team is not just a group of people with different job titles but a congregation of individuals, each of whom has a role understood by the other members. Members of a team have clearly defined professional roles but may also seek out certain additional/secondary roles and they perform most effectively in the one that is most natural to them.

Belbin has described a number of identifiable team roles which can be adopted naturally by various personality types found amongst people working together in a team. The accurate delineation of these team roles is critical in the understanding of the dynamics of any team.

# Team roles

Belbin identified successful clusters of behaviour and nine roles emerged within three subgroups as follows:

## Action-orientated roles

1. shaper
2. implementer
3. completer, finisher

## People-orientated roles

1. co-ordinator
2. teamworker
3. resource investigator

## Cerebral roles

1. plant
2. monitor evaluator
3. specialist

The characteristics of each type, in terms of their contribution to the team and 'allowable weaknesses', that is their negative qualities, are shown in Table 3.1

**Table 3.1** Team roles described by Belbin

| Belbin Team Role Type | Contribution | Allowable Weaknesses |
|---|---|---|
| Plant | Creative, imaginative, unorthodox, solves difficult problems | Ignores incidentals, too preoccupied to communicate effectively |
| Co-ordinator | Mature, confident, a good chairperson, clarifies goals, promotes decision making, delegates well | Can often be seen as manipulative, offloads personal work |
| Monitor, evaluator | Sober, strategic, discerning, sees all options, judges accuracy | Lacks drive and ability to Inspire others |
| Implementer | Disciplined, reliable, conservative, efficient, turns ideas into practical actions | Somewhat inflexible, slow to respond to new possibilities |
| Completer, finisher | Painstaking, conscientious, anxious, searches out errors and omissions, delivers on time | Inclined to worry unduly and reluctant to delegate |
| Resource investigator | Extrovert, enthusiastic, communicates and explains opportunities, develops contacts | Over-optimistic, loses interest once individual enthusiasm has passed |
| Shaper | Challenging, dynamic, thrives on pressure, drive and courage to overcome obstacles | Prone to provocation, offends people's feelings |
| Team worker | Co-operative, mild, perceptive and diplomatic, listens, builds, averts friction | Indecisive in crunch situations |
| Specialist | Single-minded, self-starting, dedicated, provides knowledge and skills in rare supply | Contributes only on a narrow field, dwells on technicalities |

Not all teams contain all these types and certain teams may be loaded with more than one subtype than another. The representation of sub-types within a team will affect not only team dynamics but also the success of the team in achieving its goals.

# Cochlear implant teams

Cochlear implant teams are frequently divided between adult and paediatric services, and although many skills are transferable between these schemes there are distinct differences in their composition and roles and goals.

There is an essential difference between the habilitation of children who have no previous experience of sound and restoring hearing to deafened adults. Adult teams are primarily concerned with the rehabilitation of individuals who have had some experience of hearing, although some congenitally deaf adults are being implanted more frequently as confidence about their potential to benefit grows. Rehabilitation tends to focus on improvement of the communication skills that enable patients to access the world of hearing.

Paediatric teams are usually working with young children and under-16-year-olds, and the work focuses on helping them develop the skills to use their newly acquired hearing to develop speech and language. There is a huge educational role both at the pre-school and school stages, as well as, most vitally, the family. This area is covered in greater detail in Chapter 14 in this book.

Eventually, all patients will inevitably be managed by an adult cochlear implant team, although it must be recognized that the needs of those implanted as young children when they become adult may be very different from those of older adults who have had their ability to perceive sound restored.

The transition between childhood and adulthood is known to be a difficult one for us all, and the concept of an adolescent programme to facilitate this transition is a model that has been increasingly adopted by many cochlear implant teams. Given that the very large numbers of those receiving cochlear implants in the world are children, the adolescent group is growing rapidly and so the need for specialist services designed to cater for the needs of this population is increasing.

A paediatric cochlear implant team is typically composed of a surgeon, audiologist, nurse, teacher of the deaf, speech and language therapist, psychologist and administrator.

An adult cochlear implant team is composed of a surgeon, audiologist, nurse, hearing therapist (although this profession does not exist outside the UK, the skills provided by them are essential), speech and language therapist, clinical psychologist and administrator. Ideally, there is a close working relationship between these teams and in some instances the same roles can be occupied on both teams by the same individual.

# Roles of the individual team members

## Surgeon

Most usually an ENT surgeon who has specialized in otology is required, with an understanding and empathy for the hearing-impaired. They obviously must be competent to perform advanced ear surgery. They must be prepared to run separate clinics for cochlear implantation and attend a separate business meeting. They must have an understanding and interest in the whole process and become involved in decision making. They are usually the point of referral and must involve all the team in the decision on selection. They are vitally involved in the medical assessment of the patient, totally responsible for the surgery and the medical follow-up and they must be involved in outcome by undertaking regular audit. Most important of all, they must be accessible both to the rest of the team and to their patients. Of all the team members the surgeon over a life time will see the patient least as the great bulk of professional interaction post- and pre-implant surgery is with the other team members. Further details concerning the role of the ENT surgeon are to be found in Chapters 8 and 10 in this book.

## Audiologist

These individuals will be senior, experienced audiologists with great experience of hearing aid fitting and managing patients with significant hearing loss. They should therefore have significant experience of working with severely or profoundly deaf individuals and be very confident at electrophysiological as well as behavioural testing. In-depth knowledge of cochlear implant programming and troubleshooting is essential. The audiologists usually have most of the patient contact long term as they are responsible for maintaining the patient and with the present technology there is a requirement for the repeated 'tuning' of the device. Further details of the role of the audiologist and device programming are discussed in Chapters 4 and 12.

## Hearing therapist

Hearing therapists are usually members of the adult team and are skilled in understanding communication problems. They investigate issues concerning the patient's domestic, work and emotional needs and understand clearly the family dynamics, especially where there is a deafened member. They very often need to play the part of the patient's advocate and are able to help patients through early disappointments when they need to be motivated and be able to cope with the stresses and strains of depression that can affect adults with profound hearing loss.

## Psychologist

Not all teams have a psychologist, but access to psychological services is invaluable. A psychologist can assess the patient's emotional and psychological status and thus can offer insight to the team in terms of patient selection and potential difficulties in rehabilitation or habilitation. Implantation can change family dynamics, and all members of the team should be aware of this.

## Nurse

A nurse is vital to a complete implant team, as it is well recognized that patients talk to nurses more than any other medical worker. Patients and their families will ask nurses questions that they feel are too minor or trivial for the supposedly busy medical staff. The nurse should have a full knowledge of the process and in an ideal world be able to visit the patient at home and be the contact point for all non-technical problems. Even if home visits are not possible, a link nurse from the team can perform routine health checks prior to admission, be on hand at clinics to administer meningitis vaccines and provide continuity between out- and in-patient care.

## Teacher of the deaf

Teachers of the deaf have a well-defined role in the educational system and are vital to the working of a paediatric cochlear implant team. They can work with the family to assess a child's educational needs and, because of their knowledge of the educational services that are available in different areas, they can assist parents in making appropriate choices of educational environments for each child. Also, early intervention via pre-school home visits ensures parents maximize opportunities for speech and language development in young deaf children.

## Speech and language therapist (SLT)

Specialist SLTs have essential roles to play on both paediatric and adult programmes, as disorders of speech and language are so prevalent in the severe to profoundly deaf population. They can offer the parents, teachers and other professionals involved with the deaf child advice and information on how best to normalize their communication skills. Individual therapy programmes may be offered or advice given to local therapists and parents on how to facilitate speech and language development in children. Adult therapy programmes may focus on language skills and also on specific speech work, pre- and post-implantation. SLTs may also have a role in supporting children as they transit through adolescence into an adult programme. Further discussion about the role of the SLT is found in Chapter 4 on the assessment of adult patients.

## The co-ordinator

The role of the co-ordinator is to ensure that the patient makes a smooth process through the referral, evaluation, selection, implantation and rehabilitation phases. They must have a thorough understanding of the roles of other members of the team and facilitate clear lines of communication between all the professionals on the team. The co-ordinator is the first point of contact on the team and must liaise with fellow professionals, patients and their families, outside agencies, cochlear implant manufacturers, contracts and finance departments and referrers. Co-ordinators may be from any of the professional groups represented on the team, and, although models of line management vary between teams, they must ensure that clinical practice is in line with published quality standards.

## Administrative support

Good communication between all members of the team, the patients, the patient's family and the general practitioner, educational system and external agencies is essential. The administrator and co-ordinator work closely together to ensure patients progress smoothly along the patient pathway and that the programme is adequately resourced in terms of funding for patient care and also stock and equipment.

# Challenges to implementing inter-professional teamwork

Professionals from different backgrounds have differing pay scales, management structures, cultures, technical languages and expectations. All of these may cause difficulties and offer challenges to the team.

The practical issues must be addressed by a management structure that is acceptable to all by having as near equitable pay and access to support and professional development from within each team member's own professional area. This is being implemented to a certain extent via the new measures in the modernization of the National Health Service pay structure, 'Agenda for Change'.

Management of patients' records, data, budgets and ultimate responsibility for clinical care must be identified and this is best done by the co-ordinator. As previously discussed, models of management vary between teams, and the co-ordinator may have substantial managerial duties including professional management on some teams but not on others. However, as the team leader, the following requirements must be fulfilled:

- listening to team members;
- valuing individual contributions;
- respecting individual differences;

- communicating effectively;
- having clear objectives and clarity about roles within the team;
- involving all staff in decisions;
- showing appreciation of jobs well done;
- allocating time for team development;
- encouraging individual development within the team.

## Hierarchy vs. democracy

Most societies acknowledge an inevitable hierarchy. In the military, this is at its most obvious and a strict adherence to its vertical command structure is expected. Moreover, intense loyalty to regiment and intense affection between soldiers (comradeship) is strongly fostered and this will reinforce the hierarchical structure further.

In contrast, the cochlear implant programme is an inter-disciplinary team of professionals working in a more democratic structure, where no one professional group dominates and where members share a high level of specialism and expertise. Within this peer structure, the general principles of teamwork still apply. This includes a belief that all opinions are valid on all topics, that relevant topics are discussed and the disparate views given equivalent weight, no matter the experience of that individual in that field.

A true democracy is, of course, highly unlikely and the more probable model which gives the best opportunity of giving the right decision involving all members is 'representative' democracy. Here the relevant experts will write a report incorporated into a corpus to be discussed at team meetings. To ensure all evaluations and assessments have been covered for all patients, a checklist may be used. In Birmingham we use the AIP (Adult Implant Profile), shown in Figure 3.1 and the CHIP (Children's Implant Profile). Each aspect of the assessment, such as audiology, medical and radiology, are listed and ticks are made in columns headed 'no concern', 'moderate concern' and 'great concern'. If there are no concerns regarding any aspect of the assessment, there is little to discuss and the decision as to the suitability of implantation for that individual is self-evident. If, on the other hand, there are significant concerns, this has to be resolved through a group discussion where specialist opinions are sought. The decision must be agreed by all to offer collective responsibility. These forms, the AIP and the CHIP, signed off by those who contributed to them, are the basis of the report on each candidate and therefore confirm and legitimize the selection process.

While this method may be more time-consuming, it gives the team confidence that all members have had the opportunity to express their views. There is a paper record of the process, so any future review of the decision-making process can be undertaken without bias using contemporaneous documentation.

Patient's name:

| Factors important to use of cochlear implant | No concern | Moderate concern | Great concern | Comments |
|---|---|---|---|---|
| Audiological | | | | |
| Functional hearing | | | | |
| Duration of profound deafness | | | | |
| Additional special needs | | | | |
| Communication skills | | | | |
| Support:<br>a) home<br>b) work | | | | |
| Environment | | | | |
| Expectations:<br>a) patient<br>b) family and friends | | | | |
| Motivation and commitment | | | | |
| Medical | | | | |
| Other (please specify) | | | | |

Completed by:                          Date:

**Figure 3.1** Adult Implant Profile (AIP).

Those working on cochlear implant teams recognize the benefits of team membership. These are the intellectual stimulation of working and collaborating with colleagues from other professional groups, the opportunities for new developments and scientific research and, most importantly, the satisfaction of delivering a high-quality clinical service.

# Reference

Belbin RM (1993) Team Roles at Work. Oxford: Butterworth-Heinemann.

# CHAPTER 4

# Assessment of adult patients

CLAIRE A. FIELDEN

## Introduction

Cochlear implantation has been an established form of treatment for profoundly deaf adults for more than a decade. It is a high-cost, low-volume speciality, with only 23 active providers of the service in the UK. There are an estimated 400 new cases to a population of 58 million in the UK a year (Summerfield and Barton, 2001), a number that is likely to increase with the introduction of more-relaxed selection criteria.

Outcomes from cochlear implantation in both adults and children are widely documented, often showing dramatically enhanced speech discrimination ability, both with and without other speech cues. Improvements in communication ability and sound detection lead to greater patient safety and the opportunity to lead a more independent life. Along with improved listening comes a greatly improved quality of life. An implantee once reported,

> Losing my hearing was like being locked in a room all alone, and only when I received my implant did it feel as though someone had opened the door.

However, an implant is not the most appropriate form of treatment for every individual with hearing impairment. It is therefore necessary to conduct a detailed assessment procedure to establish which adults are most likely to benefit from implantation.

## Cochlear implant candidacy

### Changing criteria

In the early-to-mid-1980s, implantation was restricted to those with total or profound hearing loss, and as such derived no benefit from an acoustic hearing aid. In more recent years, and with increasing confidence in cochlear implant systems and outcomes, criteria have relaxed. Several landmark reports have advocated the use of cochlear implants as a treatment for severe deafness, i.e. for those with considerably more aidable hearing than was traditionally the case. The UK study 'Predicting Outcomes from Cochlear Implantation in Adults', or POCIA (results outlined in UKCISG, 2004a) acknowledged the benefits of implanting cochlear implant candidates who were 'marginal hearing aid users'. That is, candidates who presented with aidable residual hearing and with minimal open-set speech discrimination scores with their hearing aids. Implant centres around the world are constantly re-evaluating criteria for selection, leading to the relaxation of existing constraints as the potential benefits of implantation become more evident.

In 1995, the NIH published a document recommending that cochlear implantation be extended to adults with open-set speech discrimination of less than or equal to 30% in the best-aided condition, a recommendation corroborated by the US FDA. In the UK, this is the figure that is still most closely adhered to. The UKCISG (2004a) argue that to make an intervention cost-effective, implantation should occur in ears that have at least an 80% chance of showing an improvement. These probabilities can also be used as a tool for selecting the more appropriate ear for implantation by calculating the odds for each ear separately. In Melbourne, a recent audit of results led to the suggested criterion of 70% open-set speech discrimination in the best-aided condition, and up to 40% in the ear-to-be-implanted (Dowell et al., 2004). This criterion level would give the candidate a 75% probability of achieving a post-operative speech score higher than their pre-operative score. Rubinstein et al. (1999) suggest that the expected performance and confidence intervals in cases of short duration of auditory deprivation of ten years or less could justify a further expansion in selection criteria due to the anticipated preservation of spiral ganglion cells, with the UKCISG (2004a) also demonstrating superior performance in candidates with shorter durations of profound deafness. With highly successful outcomes, it seems reasonable that selection criteria should be altered so more people could benefit from the intervention. A full review of this topic is to be found in Chapter 6.

Another group of candidates for whom implantation has become a very real possibility is the group with a severely sloping high-frequency hearing loss. These candidates would not normally have been considered for implantation, owing to the preserved residual low-frequency hearing. However, it is now thought that implantation may be a viable option, either with a full electrode array or very recently a short electrode array (Gantz and Turner, 2003), with the possibility of a combination of acoustic and electronic information in the same ear.

These relaxations in criteria raised a further issue for consideration: the increased risk for the candidate. Surgery is likely to destroy the residual

hearing in the implanted ear, with no reliable method of predicting outcomes or any guarantee of a higher speech discrimination score
post-operatively. Today, as the majority of adults referred for consideration of a cochlear implant in the clinic have some degree of residual
hearing in the ear to be implanted, the risk of hearing deterioration following unsuccessful implantation/habilitation becomes a very real
possibility. It is therefore imperative that a carefully planned assessment
procedure be conducted. It is essential that the right candidates be selected for implantation so that the wrong candidates do not undergo a
potentially harmful and irreversible surgical procedure.

## Current assessment procedure

The FDA published initial recommendations for pre-implant assessment
protocol in 1990. Such guidelines included:

- complete medical examination and radiological evaluation;
- audiological test battery including sound field auditory assessment;
- speech discrimination and recognition;
- patient counselling;
- evaluation of communication ability;
- psychological evaluation.

With the change from traditional to marginal candidates came changes in
the assessment requirements. Specifically, these are to ascertain the exact
amount of functional hearing and aided benefit to minimize the risks
associated with the operation.

### History taking

As with all other clinical procedures, the importance of a full and extensive
patient history cannot be over-emphasized. An initial referral letter can only
provide minimal information about the patient, so it is important to establish information both from the patient and other family members about
issues relevant to the assessment, implant procedure and subsequent outcome and rehabilitation. The clinician must obtain subjective information
about key issues such as age of onset and duration of existing hearing level,
aetiology and current benefit obtained from hearing aids. Information on
whether there may be a hereditary component to the hearing loss, the
development of the hearing loss and whether the candidate has tinnitus or
balance disturbance is also useful to ascertain. The candidate's ability to
communicate with the current level of hearing loss may give important
clues as to how well they are able to process limited auditory information.
It is also important to establish whether there may be any factors that might
preclude cochlear implantation, such as retrocochlear pathology.

## Aetiology

In the UK, the report provided by the Medical Research Council evaluating cochlear implantation between 1990 and 1994 stated that in half the patients suitable for unilateral implantation the underlying aetiology was not identified (Summerfield and Marshall, 1995). Aetiology in itself has not been found to provide a useful guide to candidate selection (Lehnhardt and Aschendorff, 1993) except in instances where a retrocochlear abnormality is suspected. However, certain aetiologies can have an effect on performance outcome or decision to implant if unidentified. The ossification within the cochlea that occurs as a result of meningitis can hinder successful implantation, so in such cases it is essential to consider implantation as soon as possible following recovery from the disease (Dodds et al., 1997). The continual bone formation that occurs as a result of otosclerosis can lead to undesirable outcomes including facial nerve stimulation (Ruckenstein et al., 2001); therefore, if treatment to halt the progression of the disease is unsuccessful, the candidate must receive adequate counselling with realistic expectations. Candidates with Usher's syndrome or other visual impairment should receive special consideration, as such individuals may be restricted in the amount of visual information they have post-operatively. Candidates with cochlear abnormality, such as that seen in Mondini dysplasia, should also receive counselling about potential difficulties post-operatively in areas such as programming (Turrini et al., 1997), although outcomes with this condition can be favourable (Munro et al., 1996). The age of the adult when assessed is not an important consideration *per se* for implant suitability, as the older adult (aged 65 years or over) has been shown to perform no worse than the younger adult (e.g. Pasanisi et al., 2003; Labadie et al., 2000).

## Duration of deafness

Many studies have claimed that duration of profound deafness is correlated to post-implant speech recognition (e.g. Geier et al., 1999; van Dijk et al., 1999). The more recently deafened ear is frequently considered to be the optimum choice for implantation due to the presumed better survival of spiral ganglion cells in an ear that has been more recently stimulated. It seems that the effectiveness of cochlear implants commonly declines as the duration of profound deafness increases (e.g. UKCISG, 2004a). A recent onset of deafness, i.e. under ten years, gives the best chance of a successful outcome while a long duration of more than thirty years gives the poorest prognosis of success. The middle years are slightly less predictable as many other variables are known to contribute to outcomes.

Research by Friedland et al. (2003) showed that, although duration of deafness seems to be one of the most key predictive factors in post-operative outcomes, it may not necessarily be ear-specific and may refer to the overall auditory receptivity of the individual. However, most research has looked at outcomes from individual ears, with the suggestion that, when subjects who receive benefit from an acoustic hearing aid then go on to receive an implant in an ear that has been profoundly deaf for over thirty years, effectiveness may be limited (e.g. UKCISG, 2004a). The assumption is that the duration of deafness in the implanted ear is one of the key factors in the prediction of outcomes: the more recently deafened the ear, the greater the likelihood of a successful outcome. Careful questioning during history taking is therefore essential.

# The role of the audiologist

## Hearing assessment

The procedure for hearing assessment in the UK is outlined by British Society of Audiology recommendations (1981) and should be followed exactly. This is the only way to ensure that test-retest variability and inter-tester biases are reduced to a minimum. However, it is worth mentioning that in the population of patients seen by Cochlear Implant Programmes, i.e. people with severe–profound hearing impairments, there is a high prevalence of tinnitus (Tyler, 1995; Miyamoto et al., 1997) which may have an adverse affect on hearing-threshold measurement. The subject will often report being unable to hear the very quiet pure tones above the intense level of his/her own tinnitus. In such cases, it may be necessary to test on more than one occasion to get a more accurate portrayal of the hearing levels or to use a more alerting stimulus, such as an interrupted tone.

Otoscopy and immittance measures should also be routinely conducted to establish the condition of the outer and middle ear, and to look for signs of active infection requiring treatment before the implant surgery.

## Optimizing current aiding

In spite of the widely documented benefits of cochlear implantation, it would be unethical to offer a candidate an invasive treatment procedure unless all non-invasive options had been explored and exhausted in advance. As part of the implant assessment procedure, it is necessary to examine current hearing aid provision, optimizing wherever possible. The aim of this hearing aid re-evaluation should be to improve one or more of the following:

- signal detection;
- signal discrimination;
- signal localization;
- speech discrimination in quiet;
- speech discrimination in noise.

In theory, the use of binaural aids will be more successful in improving performance on these tasks than monaural fitting alone, so the patient should be given the opportunity to try binaural aiding wherever possible. There may be contraindications to binaural aiding, such as binaural interference, increased costs, cosmetic concerns, decreased manipulation skills and additional hearing aid management issues, particularly in the elderly (Holmes, 2003), but it is recommended that binaural aiding should be attempted in each assessment. Routine bilateral fitting may help to minimize the effects of auditory deprivation and promote spiral ganglion cell survival.

Monaural hearing aid fitting in cases of bilateral hearing loss may result in a reduced ability to recognize speech in the unaided ear, which has been termed the late-onset auditory deprivation effect (e.g. Silman et al., 1984). This is a functional decline in speech recognition ability, not necessarily reversible following aiding of a previously unaided ear (see Arlinger, 2003, for a review) and may be crucial in deciding which is the more appropriate ear to receive an implant. Ponton et al. (2001) have demonstrated gradual but measurable changes in cortical activity following hearing loss in candidates with profound unilateral adult-onset hearing loss. Other theoretical benefits of binaural aiding would include head shadow benefit, loudness summation and improved sound quality (Feston and Plomp, 1986). An additional aim would be to fit an ear with a hearing aid that can be worn post-operatively, contralaterally to the implant. Recent research has reported additional benefits of bimodal hearing when compared to implant use alone (see Chapter 15).

Another important consideration in hearing aid provision, often underestimated, is earmould optimization. Implant candidates have traditionally needed extremely powerful aiding with maximum gain, and although criteria for referrals are relaxing to include patients with more residual hearing, this is still true in many cases. To achieve optimum amplification, careful consideration should be given to earmould requirements. The most obvious parameter is to seal the ear canal as effectively as possible to minimize sound leakage and acoustic feedback, which can be problematic in patients with severe–profound deafness, particularly in the high-frequency range (Dyrlund and Lundh, 1990). To create a good seal the impression should adequately fill the canal, concha and helix, with good depth into the canal (i.e. the second bend of the ear canal should be visible on the impression). A soft, hypoallergenic material filling the entire concha is recommended for the earmould to maximize patient comfort, and minimize feedback. An open-jaw impression can be useful to minimize the feedback resulting from movements of the jaw (see Mueller and Hall, 1998, for a review of open-jaw impressions). In the case of the patient with profound high-frequency sensori-neural hearing loss (SNHL), perhaps with suspected dead regions of the cochlea (Moore et al., 2000), it may be sensible to reduce high-frequency gain from the instrument. This would allow a more comfortable vented earmould, which may increase the usability of the aid without compromising too much in the way of benefit.

The ultimate goal of the audiologist should be to ensure the most appropriate aids are provided to the patient with the most optimal settings, to ensure maximum speech discrimination pre-operatively. It is recommended that the highest-quality and most-appropriate digital hearing aids be fitted, as the intention should be to try the very best options before considering the more expensive and invasive procedure of cochlear implantation. If the patient still falls within the selection criteria, even following optimum hearing aid trials, the audiologist can be confident that an implant is the most logical next step for the patient.

## Aided threshold measurement

Aided threshold testing is a method of hearing aid evaluation based on behavioural threshold measurement in the sound field. The measured difference between unaided and aided threshold levels is the amount of functional gain attributed to the hearing aid. Aided thresholds are measured using warble tones presented at octave and half-octave frequencies, between 250 Hz and 4000 Hz inclusive. Thresholds can be averaged over the five frequencies to produce a measure of sound sensitivity with aiding. It may be useful as a direct measure of comparison between hearing aids, although it is important to remember sound field calibration issues. According to Hawkins et al. (1987), in order to account for calibration difficulties inherent in free field testing there needs to be a difference of at least 15 dBA between two hearing aids on sound field threshold measurements in order for them to be considered significantly different. Even a slight alteration in head position within the sound field can affect results considerably (Northern, 1992). There are similar difficulties in using speech-based measurement to select the best-performing hearing aid for fitting: calibration difficulties inherent in free-field speech testing may mean that the variability of the speech materials themselves is greater than that of the aids being evaluated (Jerger 1987; Mueller and Grimes, 1983).

## Probe microphone measurement

Probe microphone measurement has become a routine method of hearing aid fitting and verification within the audiology clinic and makes a previously unscientific method of selecting appropriate amplification more scientific. Acoustic measurements are performed close to the tympanic membrane in the individual ear canal, producing clear recordings of the changes attributable to the hearing device and earmould, also taking into account the natural resonance of the ear canal. A target gain can be calculated using one of several published prescription formulae. There has been a considerable amount of work examining the most appropriate methods of calculating optimum gain in patients with severe or profound

hearing impairments. The National Acoustic Laboratories (NAL) procedure is frequently used (Byrne and Dillon, 1986), although Byrne et al.
(1990) note that this category of patient tends to prefer on average 10 dB
more gain than prescribed by the NAL formula, particularly at the low frequencies. This extra gain requirement is incorporated into the NAL-RP
formula. More recently, the NAL-NL formula and DSL (Desired Sensation
Level) method (Seewald and Scollie, 2003) have gained widespread use.
These formulae provide targets for different input levels, thus enabling
the verification of non-linear hearing aid outputs.

The use of probe microphone insertion gain methods to verify hearing
aid fittings rather than the traditional functional gain measurement can
have several advantages. For instance, the measurement can be made
across all frequencies rather than at a few discrete frequencies. It does not
require a behavioural response and avoids the many sound field calibration issues. When conducted accurately, the amount of functional gain
measured in the sound field should be the same as insertion gain measurements when using a probe microphone (McCandless, 1994).

With equipment readily available for clinicians, real ear measurements
can be conducted on every patient to ensure that prescribed targets are
met. Earmould modifications, alterations to aid settings and even earmould tubing variability could be used to achieve the closest possible
match to the prescribed target (Swan and Gatehouse, 1995). The routine
use of real ear insertion gain in all hearing aid fittings would result in
many patients having a more accurately fitted hearing aid.

## Subjective hearing aid benefit

Once the hearing aid has been selected, fitted and verified, it is then necessary to allow the patient sufficient opportunity for a hearing aid trial in
different listening environments: at home, at work, with family members,
listening to the radio, using the telephone or other challenging auditory
scenarios. After a trial period of around six weeks, the candidate should
return to the implant centre for further testing and evaluation of benefit,
as it takes at least six weeks for the process of perceptual acclimatization
to occur (Gatehouse, 1992). There are several methods of assessing disability and handicap resulting from a hearing loss. One method is the
Abbreviated Profile of Hearing Aid Benefit (APHAB, Cox and Alexander,
1995). This questionnaire uses everyday scenarios to evaluate the degree
of benefit offered by the hearing aids. This questionnaire can also be used
to compare one hearing aid to another, so it may be useful to complete
section A (original aiding) when they first attend the clinic, and section B
(optimized aiding) when they have completed their hearing aid trial. This
will give the clinician a better idea of the situations in which the hearing
aids are/are not useful, because the overall performance of an aid will vary
depending upon the physical and acoustical environment. Another
questionnaire useful to determine hearing aid benefit is the Glasgow

Hearing Aid Benefit Profile (GHABP, Gatehouse, 1999). This evaluates initial disability, handicap, use, benefit, residual disability and satisfaction before and after hearing aid provision, based on the principle that the best hearing aid is the one that the patient finds the most beneficial. It has been reported that demonstrating audibility of sound, for instance free-field warble tones, is not sufficient to predict speech discrimination ability particularly in severe–profound hearing losses (Ching et al., 1998). It may therefore be sensible to identify several hearing aids offering appropriate amplification and then allow the patient to decide upon the most beneficial hearing aid for them as an individual.

Questionnaires can be valuable in assessing subjective benefit from different amplification systems, but should be used carefully as there can be order effects and other biases if the questionnaires are used to evaluate benefit from several different hearing aid trials. It might be most beneficial if it were completed on just one occasion, after selection and verification methods indicate the optimal aided condition for one hearing aid trial.

In individuals with impaired cochlear function, performance with an aid cannot always be accurately predicted, even when the most precise fitting methods are used. As audibility does not necessarily mean intelligibility, the implant audiologist may see patients with good aided threshold levels but with very poor speech discrimination ability and vice versa. Pre-operative residual speech recognition acts as a 'trophic factor', protecting spiral ganglion cells and/or central auditory pathways from degeneration (Gomaa et al., 2003). If a candidate is making extremely good use of limited remaining hearing and obtains reasonable speech scores in spite of this, it suggests they are likely to be successful implant users.

## Speech discrimination ability

In assessment for cochlear implant candidacy, there has to be a pre-implant baseline speech discrimination measurement, which the audiologist can use both to advise whether the individual would be a suitable candidate for implantation and also to counsel the candidate on post-implant expectations. This assessment should be completed only after the hearing aid trial, as described above.

In the UK, many of the implant centres contributed data to the POCIA study in the 1990s (results documented in UKCISG 2004a, 2004b, 2004c). Many of the tests used for that study are still used today, including questionnaires examining hearing handicap, quality of life, depression levels and expectations about cochlear implantation. The battery includes standardized measures of speech perception, both with and without lipreading cues, and single-word and phoneme discrimination. Sentence test lists are all pre-recorded and used in addition to the live voice testing conducted by the hearing therapist. The three main sentence tests used are:

- CUNY (City University New York), using high-fidelity audio-visual recording (Aleksy and Boyle, 1994);
- BKB: Bench–Kowal–Bamford (Bench et al., 1979);
- IHR: Institute of Hearing Research (MacLeod and Summerfield, 1987). IHR sentences were modelled on the BKB sentences lists, containing similar syntax and vocabulary.

Monosyllabic word lists and vowel/consonant recognition tests are also used.

The purpose of the sentence lists is to evaluate:

- lipreading skills without sound using a high-fidelity video laser disc;
- speech discrimination using lipreading with sound using an audio-visual image as above;
- open-set speech discrimination using sound alone.

This procedure is used to test speech understanding in each individual ear and binaurally where appropriate to find the best aided condition. Sentence scores can be measured both in quiet and in noise conditions. Open-set speech in quiet is the most widely used method of assessing speech discrimination ability in cochlear implant candidates within the UK. Many UK centres recommend implants for patients obtaining open-set speech discrimination scores of 30% or less in the best aided condition, but criteria are currently being evaluated.

### Candidates with non-organic hearing loss

Non-organic hearing loss (NOHL) may be defined as 'any hearing loss that cannot be accounted for by an organic cause' (Aplin and Rowson, 1990). There have been several reported occurrences of candidates with non-organic hearing loss presenting for implant assessment (e.g. Spraggs et al., 1994), and analysis suggests that the incidence may be increasing (Lynch et al., 2001). It is therefore an issue that the implant team needs to consider during the assessment process. Inappropriate cochlear implantation of a candidate with NOHL would have a detrimental effect in that it would create or exacerbate a hearing impairment with medico-legal implications, and is a waste of time and resources. NOHL may present itself as a total hearing loss where hearing levels are in fact normal, or a partial hearing loss with a non-organic overlay. Recent research suggests that a model of two extremes, conscious malingering for personal gain versus a subconscious conversion indicative of psychological problems, is inadequate. Austen and Lynch propose a model of NOHL in which there exists a continuum between the two extremes, with a third diagnostic category which they refer to as 'factitious loss', in which the patient is not entirely conscious or unconscious of their actions (Austen and Lynch, 2004). Assessment in such cases must account for the complex relationship between conscious and unconscious behaviours and the underlying motivation. The capacity to refer to a clinical psychologist is invaluable and the assessment is not complete without this expertise.

There are accepted objective test procedures the audiologist can use to confirm the presence of a non-organic element to the hearing loss. The Auditory Brainstem Response Test (ABR) is an objective method of threshold estimation using either a click stimulus, which evaluates hearing status in the range of 2000–4000 Hz, or tone bursts at specific frequencies. It is a non-invasive method of confirming a profound hearing impairment or detecting a non-organic overlay, and should be conducted on all potential implant candidates. However, the fact that the click ABR primarily provides information regarding high-frequency hearing levels seriously limits its usefulness in providing a complete objective measure of the hearing status. Developed in the 1980s at the University of Melbourne, a new category of auditory evoked potentials may provide objective frequency-specific hearing assessment. The auditory steady-state response (ASSR), also called the steady-state evoked potential (SSEP), can be reliably evoked by frequency-specific tonal stimuli. Research indicates that thresholds correlate well with behavioural audiogram thresholds (e.g. Stueve and O'Rourke, 2003; Swanepoel et al., 2004a). The Tone-Burst ABR is a more frequency-specific method of threshold estimation than the click ABR, and recent research on normal listeners has compared it favourably to the dichotic ASSR except that it was not as time-efficient (Swanepoel et al., 2004b). It also remains dependent upon subjective evaluation of waveforms, whereas the ASSR can be conducted objectively.

The primary advantage of the ASSR over the standard evoked potential test seems to be the ability to differentiate between severe and profound hearing loss as well as distinguishing between levels of profound hearing losses, e.g. the difference between a 90 dB and a 110 dB hearing loss (e.g. Firszt et al., 2004; Roberson et al., 2003). This ability is crucial in instances where a cochlear implant is being considered as well as to fit amplification accurately, particularly but not exclusively in the paediatric population. Continued research is needed to obtain a clearer understanding of the ASSR, in particular to establish the reliability of threshold estimates, which will assist in the refinement of guidelines for clinical application (Firszt et al., 2004).

Otoacoustic emissions (OAEs) are an objective measure of outer hair cell (OHC) function in the cochlea, the premise being that preserved cochlear function is reflective of normal hearing. OAEs are usually not recordable in ears with a hearing loss greater than around 30 dB or if there is any middle ear effusion. The absence of a recordable OAE response does not provide an estimate of hearing thresholds but merely suggests the existence of a hearing loss. The fundamental difficulty with OAEs is that they measure the response only up to OHC level and no further along the auditory pathway. In the case of VIII Nerve pathology such as acoustic neuroma, OAEs may or may not remain measurable, with the influencing factor most likely to be an indirectly mediated compromise of the organ of Corti's vascular supply by the growing tumour (Telischi et al., 1995).

There are documented cases of profound hearing loss with absent ABRs but with measurable OAEs, and such cases will have passed an OAE hearing screening test. This has been called 'auditory neuropathy'. One research paper looked at a group of infants who were at risk of hearing impairment and examined the number of cases of auditory neuropathy in their group. They quote a prevalence figure of 0.23%, which may be higher than previously thought (Rance et. al., 1999), illustrating that perhaps auditory neuropathy may be of some concern in neonatal hearing screening programmes, where any negative effect on screening sensitivity has yet to be quantified. However, children with profound deafness resulting from auditory neuropathy have been successfully implanted (e.g. Peterson et al., 2003; Mason et al., 2003; Shallop et al., 2001). This suggests that 'neuropathy' is a misnomer, reflecting not a true neuropathy but perhaps a malfunction of another as yet unconfirmed part of the auditory pathway.

# The role of the hearing therapist

In the UK, responsibility for aural rehabilitation is frequently shared between the audiologist, hearing therapist (HT) and speech and language therapist. The HT in an adult cochlear implant team uses a holistic approach to evaluating and assessing cochlear implant candidates. For instance, s/he not only evaluates the amount of disability, impairment and handicap presented by the hearing loss but also examines effects on every aspect of the patient's life: in relationships, in work situations and others, in the past, present and future.

In an initial assessment of the candidate, the HT will take a thorough history to establish the extent of difficulties that arise from the hearing loss, encouraging contributions from both the patient and other family members. The HT might typically ask the patient to identify three aspects of their life where they have been experiencing difficulty and where they would like to see improvement following cochlear implantation, if found to be suitable. The patient's communication skills with the family and the clinician will be informally assessed at this point. The HT may opt to use any of a number of available questionnaires, for example quality-of-life or hearing handicap measures, tinnitus or dizziness evaluation. The outcomes can then be used to prepare an assessment tailored to the individual needs of the client. The HT will use rehabilitative methods where appropriate to ensure that the needs of the candidate cannot be met without consideration of an implant. Advice on assistive listening devices, such as amplified telephones, loop systems and visual alarm systems, is provided to the patient as appropriate. Lipreading ability is assessed, and the candidate is offered lipreading classes to allow all cues to be accessible to the patient. Tinnitus counselling is frequently required due to the high prevalence of tinnitus in implant candidates (Mo et al., 2002), as is vestibular rehabilitation and advice on hearing tactics to make life easier for the patient and the family.

Following hearing aid optimization by the audiologist, the HT will typically examine the amount of functional hearing using live voice testing, maintaining a constant voice level of 70 dBA. Verbal materials with varying levels of redundancy are used, from continuous discourse tracking to everyday sentences to single words, both with and without lipreading, to obtain a measurement of functional hearing ability in the candidate. Performance on a live voice test is usually superior to performance using pre-recorded materials. It is therefore necessary to complete the HT assessment before a final team decision can be made as to the suitability of the candidate, as it provides important additional information about the 'real-life' communication abilities of the candidate, which complements the more formal testing performed with recorded speech materials.

Should the patient fall within the criteria for cochlear implantation, the HT will assess expectations and counsel appropriately. The HT will arrange for the candidate to meet with an existing implant user, matched in as many ways as possible to the candidate, particularly in the duration of deafness in the implanted ear. The HT will encourage the candidate to find out as much about the procedure and outcomes as possible from someone who has been through it. S/he will then ensure that the candidate is comfortable about the surgical procedure and demonstrate all the

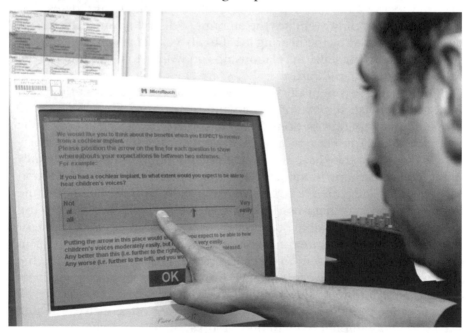

**Figure 4.1** Patient under assessment completing questionnaire via computer touch screen.

implant equipment, including a choice of implant devices as appropriate so that the recipient can go through the procedure as smoothly as possible. The HT spends extensive time with each candidate to establish whether an implant is the appropriate method of treatment for the individual. If at any time there is any concern, then the HT will refer, appropriately, to a psychologist or other agency.

# The role of the speech and language therapist

There is often significant overlap between the roles performed by hearing therapists and speech and language therapists (SLTs) on an adult cochlear implant team. For example, both professions will work with the candidate and their family to assess and optimize listening and communication skills. They will also help the candidate develop complete understanding of the assessment and rehabilitative process, thereby forming appropriate expectations in order to make an informed decision should a cochlear implant be offered. Team working between the two professions allows for individually tailored assessment and rehabilitation packages, which draws on the expertise of both the HT and SLT, in both individual and group therapy.

The role of the SLT in adult cochlear implant assessment is very different from the role in paediatric assessment. The paediatric SLT is very often helping the child with a cochlear implant acquire speech and language skills from the outset, whereas the vast majority of adults on assessment are those who have already acquired speech and language.

Ideally, all candidates referred for implantation should have a complete voice, speech, language and communication assessment conducted by an SLT. This would include an evaluation of the client's speech perception abilities, understanding and use of spoken language, written and signed language as appropriate, voice skills, speech production and overall intelligibility, preferred method of communication and any communication tactics used (RCSLT, 1996). The results of this assessment will give an indication of how well the client has used their hearing abilities over the years, which, when combined with the audiologist's results and a full history, is essential in ascertaining whether the candidate would benefit from an implant. However, a full, detailed assessment for every candidate is not always possible and therefore the SLT may use a screening assessment for all candidates, or other members of the team may request involvement when necessary (RCSLT, 1996).

While postlingually deafened adults typically do not require help with the acquisition of speech and language, some require assistance with the maintenance of voice skills due to hearing loss and the re-acquisition of speech sounds lost through a long history of reduced auditory input and feedback. The SLT will also judge where expectations for improvements in voice and/or speech are realistic, and counsel the patient appropriately.

Non-typical adult candidates are now becoming an increasing cohort of successful implant users, for instance those with:

- congenital or long-term deafness;
- acquired deafness due to or in addition to acquired or progressive neurological disorders (e.g. traumatic brain injury, cerebellar vascular incident, Parkinson's disease, meningitis);
- varying degrees of learning difficulty;
- identified syndromes associated with deafness or communication difficulties (e.g. Treacher-Collins);
- other complex requirements.

These candidates should receive particular attention from the SLT, to evaluate whether a cochlear implant would be an appropriate option, and the extent to which the candidate would be likely to benefit.

A final group of candidates who particularly benefit from speech and language therapy evaluation are those young people still in education who have been referred directly into adult cochlear implant services. The evaluation of speech, language and listening skills and close liaison with local educational support services provides a useful insight into how the young person is coping with their hearing loss, often at the most demanding time of their academic career.

# The role of the clinical psychologist

As implant programmes are identifying more patient-related factors that can affect post-implant outcomes, the role of the clinical psychologist becomes more apparent. There is surprisingly little research to date on the psychological evaluation of implant candidates, but it may add valuable information in assessing candidacy (Aplin, 1993) and is recommended by the FDA report (1990). A thorough evaluation of psychological aspects of cochlear implantation can be found in Chapter 7.

The NIH (1995) suggests that candidates with severe psychiatric disorders be excluded from implantation; however, such individuals are often difficult to identify. Ideally, all candidates should undergo psychological assessment prior to implantation, but, if that is not achievable, clinicians should refer for a psychological opinion any candidate in whom they recognize issues that they feel may affect the outcome of a cochlear implant, remembering that people with an acquired severe–profound hearing loss are likely to exhibit some degree of emotional disturbance. Austen (2004) makes some suggestions for appropriate referrals, for instance candidates with learning disability or multiple handicaps in whom the ability to understand procedures and give informed consent is questionable. Candidates with a confirmed non-organic element to their hearing loss should also be referred. She also recommends the implant team fully explores motives for implantation: are they predominantly psychological, for example to improve confidence, rather than audiological? Is the candidate attending for personal reasons or to please other family members? There has been no consensus as to whether psychometric screening tests have any predictive value in audiological outcomes, for instance IQ or personality inventories, but such measures may be useful in selecting appropriate candidates for psychological assessment. Clinical depression, which may have a negative effect on motivation to succeed with a cochlear implant, should also be considered carefully and subjective depression ratings can be ascertained by questionnaire, for example the Beck Depression Inventory (Beck et al., 1961).

It is recommended that all implant teams have access to psychological input. However, a psychological issue may not necessarily be a contraindication to implantation as it may result from the isolation caused by deafness, the alleviation of which can lead to improved psychological outcomes (Knutson et al., 1998).

## Optional assessment tools

### Promontory Stimulation Testing and Round Window Stimulation Testing

Techniques using electrical stimulation are available to assess neural pathway activity in profoundly deaf patients being considered for cochlear implantation. There are two widely accepted methods: the Promontory Stimulation Test (PST) and the Round Window Stimulation Test (RWST). The PST is conducted with the use of a trans-tympanic needle electrode. The needle is fed through the tympanic membrane by the surgeon and is placed onto the promontory along the medial wall of the tympanic cavity. Small electric pulses are delivered relative to a reference electrode, which is normally located on the mastoid process. The resulting current stimulates the VIII nerve and may be perceived as sound. The tympanic membrane heals very quickly and the test can be performed under local anaesthetic.

The RWST is more invasive, where a flap of tympanic membrane is opened to allow a ball electrode to pass through, to be positioned directly within the round window niche with a reference electrode again placed outside the ear. As the electrode is positioned closer to the neural fibres than a promontory electrode, it is thought to be a more sensitive test (Aso and Gibson, 1994); however, it is more invasive and requires a greater degree of anaesthesia. In adult subjects a response is usually measured subjectively, i.e. whether the subject is able to perceive the stimulus as sound. In less co-operative populations such as children or in subjects with little previous experience of sound such as prelingually deafened adults, it is possible to record an electrically evoked auditory brainstem response (EABR) from the stimulation of the auditory nerve, using a general anaesthetic if required.

In the early days of implantation, when only 'traditional' profoundly or totally deaf candidates were considered for implantation, PST and RWST had a greater role in the selection process. It was advisable to ascertain the quality or quantity of the surviving neural population prior to implantation where no hearing information could be derived, and to help determine the site of lesion. Today, however, the candidate with no measurable behavioural hearing threshold levels is amongst the minority of referrals to the implant programme. In the main, adult candidates have some degree of residual hearing in at least one ear, which negates the urgent need for PST and RWST. However, in cases of head injury or skull fracture, it may still be a useful addition to the test battery.

There is not much evidence to support the use of one procedure in favour of the other. Sauvaget et al. (2002) successfully recorded evoked potentials in 93% of ears using the PST and 79% using the RWST, suggesting that PST may be a better choice, particularly as the recording procedure is less invasive.

As to whether the tests are useful in predicting outcomes from cochlear implantation, results have been inconclusive (Ito et al., 1994; Albu and Babighian 1997; Nikolopoulos et al., 2000). Schmidt et al. (2003) used functional Magnetic Resonance Imaging (f-MRI) to measure activation in the auditory cortex following promontory stimulation. They demonstrated cortical activation in 85% of patients who had reported perceiving a sound, and lack of cortical stimulation in 75% of patients who had reported not hearing a sound, which suggests that a negative test result does not necessarily indicate a non-functioning auditory pathway. It is therefore suggested that such procedures remain optional assessment tools, until any further potential becomes apparent.

**Vestibular investigation**

Traditionally, the vestibular test battery, consisting of electronystagmography and caloric irrigation, was used to establish the status of the vestibular apparatus prior to every implant surgery, theoretically to predict post-operative vestibular disturbance. The tests were found to have low predictive value in our clinic and were therefore discontinued from routine pre-implant assessment. In spite of this, vestibular investigation may still assist in counselling regarding the possibility of dizziness postoperatively. The risk of post-operative vertigo may be greater in patients with a recordable response on caloric testing than those in which there is no evidence of peripheral vestibular function pre-operatively. Therefore, vestibular testing may assist in selecting the ear for implantation. If there is a known case of vestibular disorder in an implant candidate, it may be worth ascertaining the amount of measurable residual vestibular function in each ear. If caloric investigation suggests that there is unilateral vestibular hypofunction, perhaps the surgeon would consider implanting that ear, rather than risk the ear with the remaining measurable function.

Inadvertent destruction of remaining function might lead to problems associated with bilateral hypofunction, for example oscillopsia post-operatively (Chen et al., 2001).

Vestibular test results should be interpreted with some caution, as the caloric test only measures a specified part of the balance system, so should be used as a tool in conjunction with other tests in the assessment battery.

## Genetic investigation

In our clinics we see many adults and children with probable or confirmed hereditary hearing losses and it is sometimes the case that more than one blood relative will go on to receive an implant in any one family. As the number of genes identified as being responsible for hearing loss increases, it may become possible to identify likely genetic causes for the large population of referrals with unknown aetiologies, which may even hold implications for post-operative outcomes. Appropriate counselling and advice could then be offered as part of the wider service.

## Typical patient pathway through the system

Figure 4.2 demonstrates the stages of the typical patient pathway through the system, from referral through to implantation or permanent discharge from the service if an implant will never be an appropriate treatment for the patient. In Birmingham, those patients who are found to be outside the current criteria for cochlear implantation remain under the overall care of the programme. These patients are reviewed annually until such time as they become suitable candidates for implantation, either because of deterioration in their hearing or because selection criteria have expanded enough to include them.

## Selection of ear

Current practice of unilateral cochlear implantation presents the assessment team with a dilemma: which ear is likely to give the better listening performance post-operatively? The two main prognostic factors have traditionally been a shorter duration of deafness in the ear-to-be-implanted and greater residual speech discrimination ability pre-operatively (e.g. Rubinstein et al., 1999; Dowell et al., 2002; Gomaa et al., 2003). The supposition in both instances relates to a presumably higher proportion of spiral ganglion cells likely to be preserved, therefore ear selection should be made using one or both factors. However, the decision is not always straightforward. A clinical trial of simultaneous bilateral cochlear implantation by the Iowa team could not isolate any factor pre-operatively in their small group of ten that was able to predict post-operative speech discrimination performance in any one ear (Gantz et al., 2002). The UKCISG (2004a) was unable to demonstrate conclusively that implanting a candidate in a zero-scoring ear results in a worse outcome than a candidate

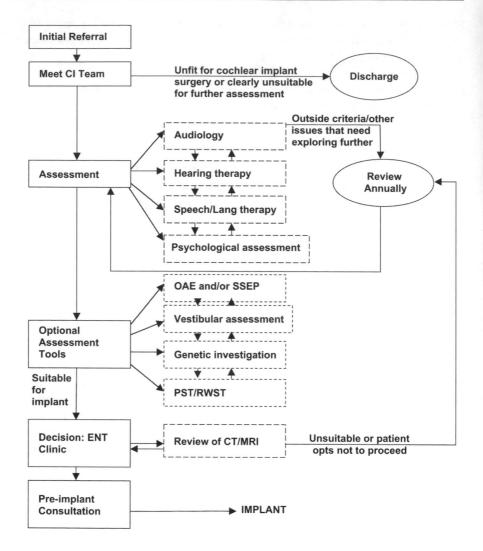

**Figure 4.2** Typical patient pathway through the Cochlear Implant Assessment Process.

with a small amount of residual speech discrimination pre-operatively, providing duration of deafness was not a factor. Stark et al. (2004) present a single case of a bilateral implantee with a difference between the ears in duration of deafness. They demonstrate better post-operative speech discrimination scores in the ear which had the longer duration of deafness, of more than 25 years.

In the case of the bilateral hearing aid user with equal speech discrimination and duration of deafness in each ear, and nothing to choose between them on the basis of the scan, decisions about ear selection may be discussed with the candidate and based upon other factors (which are discussed in greater detail in Chapter 15). In the case of a unilateral hearing aid user the decision becomes more difficult. Some candidates use a single hearing aid, perhaps due to a lack of success in aiding the opposite ear, implying that the aided ear (the better performing and more recently used ear) is the better choice for implantation. However, it is a much greater risk for this group of candidates in that the operation would potentially destroy the residual hearing that they have relied upon. A similar dilemma occurs when the clinician is presented with a bilateral hearing aid user with a definite 'better' and 'poorer' ear. Should the better performing ear be implanted or should this be retained for the continuation of hearing aid use?

Many recent studies, aimed particularly towards paediatric teams, have stressed the importance of continuing hearing aid use in the contralateral ear post-implantation, to allow 'bimodal' hearing. Tyler and his colleagues examined speech perception and localization ability in a small group of implantees using an implant and a contralateral hearing aid (Tyler et al., 2002). They were able to observe some binaural advantage to both elements, but do stress that their numbers were small. Armstrong et al. (1997) also report binaural benefits, as do Waltzman et al. (1992). It is important to remember that when continuing contralateral hearing aid use following implantation, it needs to be optimized in terms of loudness and frequency response to provide the best match to the implant, and guidance on how this may be achieved can be obtained from cochlear implant manufacturers. This seems to offer the best chance of binaural integration between the electric and acoustic stimulation, allowing subsequent binaural benefits (Blamey et al., 2000; Ching et al., 2001). Ching and her colleagues also report that in their group there were no apparent auditory disadvantages to wearing a contralateral aid, such as picking up extra interfering noise that would not have been detected using an implant alone. Bimodal fitting provides continual stimulation and this may contribute to the preservation of spiral ganglion cells in the non-implanted ear.

There are strong arguments in favour of bimodal fitting wherever possible, and expanding criteria may lead to routine bimodal fitting in most cases. However, it requires a compromise over whether the best side to implant would be the side with the most residual hearing to maximize potential with the implant ear alone or whether to implant the poorer ear with a view to increasing the potential binaural benefits following implantation. Should cochlear implant benefit be measured in terms of binaural outcome? It is a question not easily answered and is confounded by other factors such as speech discrimination ability as opposed to hearing threshold levels and whether the poorer ear has been without stimulation for many years, leading to questionable neural survival.

Each case should be evaluated on an individual basis, looking at durations of deafness and residual speech discrimination in the better and poorer ears. This is a good reason for adopting a whole team approach, to discuss each case individually and reach a team decision as to the best way forward, including the candidate being involved in the decision wherever possible.

**Counselling of risks and expectations**

It is the responsibility of the clinician to outline all potential risks and benefits to the implantee prior to surgery. Many risks are outlined in the FDA (1990) report, for example post-operative dizziness or tinnitus and facial nerve disturbance. (Medical risks are outlined in Chapter 8.) One of the greatest risks is that all residual hearing may be lost in the implanted ear following surgery. As audiological criteria are relaxed, this risk becomes more significant. The implantee should understand the risk that they would no longer be able to revert to using their hearing aid in the implanted ear should they decide not to use the implant, or in those rare cases of device failure.

The assessment indicates whether the implant would be an improvement on the current aiding provision and the team can therefore counsel the patient as to what they should expect. Using information such as duration of deafness and current speech discrimination scores in the ear to be implanted, the clinician can counsel on the probability that the patient will achieve open-set speech understanding post-operatively, although it remains impossible to predict exactly how an implantee will perform.

Many complications can be successfully treated, and most are rare. However, all known risks should be outlined to candidates pre-operatively, allowing them to make an informed decision as to whether they feel the expected potential benefits outweigh the potential risks. Implant centres also have a responsibility to record any such occurrences as part of their clinical audit procedures so that the incidence of problems can be monitored.

# Future directions

The field of cochlear implants benefits from widespread research, and as such is constantly developing. Such developments are crucial in the assessment of new candidates. The overwhelming trend in current implant research seems to be to make implantation available to more people. As outcomes from adult implantation steadily improve, more relaxed selection criteria are indicated. As electrode array technology and surgical techniques become more sophisticated, with the aim of maximum preservation of residual hearing, implantation becomes a viable form of treatment for more people with lesser degrees of deafness.

The majority of adult cochlear implant recipients have had acquired postlingual deafness. However, many centres have implanted prelingually deaf adults in recent years, with an increasing knowledge of the results that may be anticipated. With such knowledge and appropriate counselling, there is evidence to suggest that these candidates, particularly those who have been consistently aided and integrated into the hearing community, may be able to attain worthwhile benefits from an implant (e.g. Kaplan et al., 2003).

# Conclusion

Cochlear implantation remains a highly successful treatment for severe and profound hearing losses. However, as there are still many risks associated with implantation, it is vital that clinicians carefully select only the candidates who are likely to obtain additional benefits. There are a number of assessment tools available to cochlear implant teams which can be used to obtain a full and detailed picture of each candidate's suitability. Further advances will require alterations to the assessment and selection processes, and the increasing knowledge and experience of potential outcomes should be used to provide specific information and counselling in each case.

### Acknowledgements

Grateful thanks to Tracy Wright, Hearing Therapist, Kate Hanvey, Speech and Language Therapist and Sally Austen, Clinical Psychologist, for their assistance in the writing of this chapter.

# References

Albu S, Babighian G (1997) Predictive factors in cochlear implants. Acta Otorhinolaryngologica Belg. 51(1): 11–16.

Aleksy W, Boyle P (1994) An audio-visual recording of the CUNY sentence lists on laser disc. Cochlear Implant Programme, internal report. University College Hospital, London.

Aplin DY (1993) Psychological assessment of multi-channel cochlear implant patients. Journal of Laryngology and Otology 107(4): 298–304.

Aplin DY, Rowson VJ (1990) Psychological characteristics of children with functional hearing loss. British Journal of Audiology 24: 77–87.

Arlinger S (2003) Negative consequences of uncorrected hearing loss – a review. International Journal of Audiology 42(suppl. 2): 2S17–20.

Armstrong M, Pegg P, James C et al. (1997) Speech perception in noise with implant and hearing aid. American Journal of Otology 18(suppl. 6): S140–1

Aso S, Gibson WP (1994) Electrocochleography in profoundly deaf children: comparison of promontory and round window techniques. American Journal of Otology 15(3): 376–9.

Austen S (2004) Cochlear Implants in adults: the role of the psychologist. In S Austen, S Crocker (eds), Deafness In Mind: Working Psychologically with Deaf People across the Lifespan. London: Whurr.

Austen S, Lynch C (2004) Non-organic hearing loss redefined: understanding, categorizing and managing non-organic behaviour. International Journal of Audiology 43(8): 449–57.

Beck A, Ward C, Mendelson M et al. (1961) An inventory for measuring depression. Arch. Gen. Psychiatr. 4: 561–71.

Bench J, Kowal A, Bamford J (1979) The BKB (Bench–Kowal–Bamford) sentence lists for partially hearing children. British Journal of Audiology 13(3): 108–12.

Blamey PJ, Dooley GJ, James CJ et al. (2000) Monaural and binaural loudness measures in cochlear implant users with contralateral residual hearing. Ear and Hearing 21(1): 6–17.

British Society of Audiology recommended procedures for pure-tone audiometry using a manually operated instrument (1981). British Journal of Audiology 15(3): 213–16.

Byrne D, Dillon H (1986) The National Acoustic Laboratories' (NAL) new procedure for selecting the gain and frequency response of a hearing aid. Ear and Hearing 7(4): 257–65.

Byrne D, Parkinson A, Newall P (1990) Hearing aid gain and frequency response requirements for the severely/profoundly hearing impaired. Ear and Hearing 11(1): 40–9.

Chen JM, Shipp D, Al-Abidi A et al. (2001) Does choosing the 'worse' ear for cochlear implantation affect outcome? Otology Neurology 22(3): 335–9.

Ching TY, Dillon H, Byrne D (1998) Speech recognition of hearing impaired listeners: predictions from audibility and the limited role of high-frequency amplification. Journal of the Acoustical Society of America 103(2): 1128–40.

Ching TY, Psarros C, Hill M et al. (2001) Should children who use cochlear implants wear hearing aids in the opposite ear? Ear and Hearing 22(5): 365–80.

Cox RM, Alexander GC (1995) The abbreviated profile of hearing aid benefit. Ear and Hearing 16: 176–86.

Dodds A, Tyszkiewicz E, Ramsden R (1997) Cochlear implantation after bacterial meningitis: the dangers of delay. Archives of Disease in Childhood 76(2): 139–40.

Dowell RC, Hollow R, Winton E et al. (2002) Outcomes for adults using cochlear implants: re-thinking selection criteria. Paper presented at the 7th International Cochlear Implant Conference. Manchester, UK: 4–6 September.

Dowell RC, Hollow R, Winton E (2004) Outcomes for cochlear implant users with significant residual hearing: implications for selection criteria in children. Archives of Otolaryngology: Head and Neck Surgery 130(5): 575–81.

Dyrlund O, Lundh P (1990) Gain and feedback problems when fitting behind-the-ear hearing aids to profoundly hearing-impaired children. Scandinavian Audiology 19(2): 89–95.

Feston J, Plomp R (1986) Speech reception threshold in noise with one and two hearing aids. Journal of the Acoustical Society of America 79: 465–71.

Firszt JB, Gaggl W, Runge-Samuelson CL et al. (2004) Auditory sensitivity in children using the auditory steady-state response. Archives of Otolaryngology: Head and Neck Surgery 130(5): 536–40.

FDA (Food and Drug Administration, US) (1990) Guideline for the arrangement and content of a premarket approval (PMA) application for a cochlear implant in adults of at least 18 years. US Department of Health and Human Services.

Friedland DR, Venick HS, Niparko JK (2003) Choice of ear for cochlear implantation: the effect of history and residual hearing on predicted post-operative performance. Otology Neurotology 24(4): 582–9.

Gantz BJ, Turner C (2003) Combining acoustic and electrical hearing. Laryngoscope 113(10): 1726–30.

Gantz BJ, Tyler RS, Rubinstein JT et al. (2002) Binaural cochlear implants placed during the same operation. Otology Neurotology 23(2): 169–80.

Gatehouse S (1999) A self-report outcome measure for the evaluation of hearing aid fittings and services. Health Bulletin (Edinburgh) 57(6): 424–36.

Gatehouse S (1992) The time course and magnitude of perceptual acclimatization to frequency responses: evidence of monaural fitting of hearing aids. Journal of the Acoustical Society of America 92(3): 1258–68.

Geier L, Barker M, Fisher L et al. (1999) The effect of long-term deafness on speech recognition in postlingually deafened adult Clarion cochlear implant users. Annals of Otology, Rhinology and Laryngology(suppl. 177): 80–3.

Gomaa NA, Rubinstein JT, Lowder MW et al. (2003) Residual speech perception and cochlear implant performance in postlingually deafened adults. Ear and Hearing 24(6): 539–44.

Hawkins D, Montgomery A, Prosek R et al. (1987) Examination of two issues concerning functional gain measurements. Journal of Speech and Hearing Disorders 52: 56–63.

Holmes AE (2003) Bilateral amplification for the elderly: are two aids better than one? International Journal of Audiology 42(suppl. 2): 63–7.

Ito J, Tsuji J, Sakakihara J (1994) Reliability of the promontory stimulation test for the preoperative evaluation of cochlear implants: a comparison with the round window stimulation test. Auris Nasus Larynx 21(1): 13–16.

Jerger J (1987) On the evaluation of hearing aid performance. ASHA 29: 49–51.

Kaplan DM, Shipp DB, Chen JM et al. (2003) Early deafened adult cochlear implant users: assessment of outcomes. Journal of Otolaryngology 32(4): 245–9.

Knutson JF, Murray KT, Husarek S et al. (1998) Psychological change over 54 months of cochlear implant use. Ear and Hearing 19(3): 191–201.

Labadie RF, Carrasco VN, Gilmer CH et al. (2000) Cochlear implant performance in senior citizens. Journal of Otolaryngology: Head and Neck Surgery 123(4): 419–24.

Lenhardt E, Aschendorff A (1993) Prognostic factors in 187 adults provided with the Nucleus Cochlear Mini-System 22. In: B Fraysse, O Deguine (eds), Cochlear Implants: New Perspectives, Advances in Otorhinolaryngology, Vol. 48. Basel: Karger, pp. 146–52.

Lynch CA, Wintersgill S, Meerton LJ et al. (2001) Non-organic behaviour during cochlear implant assessment. Paper presented at British Cochlear Implant Group Meeting.

McCandless G (1994) Overview and rationale of threshold-based hearing aid selection procedures. In: M Valente (ed), Strategies for Selecting and Verifying Hearing Aid Fittings. New York: Thieme Medical.

Macleod A, Summerfield Q (1987) Quantifying the contribution of vision to speech perception in noise. British Journal of Audiology 21(2): 131–41.

Mason JC, De Michele A, Stevens C et al. (2003) Cochlear implantation in patients with auditory neuropathy of varied etiologies. Laryngoscope 113(1): 45–9.

Miyamoto RT, Wynne MK, McKnight C et al. (1997) Electrical suppression of tinnitus via cochlear implants. International Tinnitus Journal 3(1): 35–8.

Mo B, Harris S, Lindback M (2002) Tinnitus in cochlear implant patients – a comparison with other hearing-impaired patients. International Journal of Audiology 41(8): 527–34.

Moore BC, Huss M, Vickers DA et al. (2000) A test for the diagnosis of dead regions in the cochlea. British Journal of Audiology 34(4): 205–24.

Mueller H, Grimes A (1983) Speech audiometry for hearing aid selection. Seminars in Hearing 4(3): 255–72.

Mueller H, Hall J (1998) Audiologist's Desk Reference. Vol. 2: Audiologic Management, Rehabilitation and Terminology. San Diego: Singular Publishing.

Munro KJ, George CR, Haacke NP (1996) Audiological findings after multichannel cochlear implantation in patients with Mondini dysplasia. British Journal of Audiology 30(6): 369–79.

NIH (National Institute of Health) (1995) Cochlear Implants in Adults and Children. National Institute of Health Consensus Statements 13(2): 1–30. Washington DC.

Nikolopoulos TP, Mason SM, Gibbin KP et al. (2000) The prognostic value of promontory electric auditory brainstem response in paediatric cochlear implantation. Ear and Hearing 21(3): 236–41.

Northern JL (1992) Introduction to computerized probe-microphone real-ear measurements in hearing aid evaluation procedures. In HG Mueller, DB Hawkins, Northern JL (eds), Probe Microphone Measurements: Hearing Aid Selection and Assessment. London: Singular Publishing, pp. 1–19.

Pasanisi E, Bacciu A, Vincenti V et al. (2003) Speech recognition in elderly cochlear implant recipients. Clinical Otolaryngology 28(2): 154–7.

Peterson A, Shallop J, Driscoll C et al. (2003) Outcomes of cochlear implantation in children with auditory neuropathy. Journal of the American Academy of Audiology 14(4): 188–201.

Ponton CW, Vasama JP, Tremblay K et al. (2001) Plasticity in the adult human central auditory system: evidence from late-onset profound unilateral deafness. Hearing Research 154(1–2): 32–44.

Rance G, Beer DE, Cone-Wesson B et al. (1999) Clinical findings for a group of infants and young children with auditory neuropathy. Ear and Hearing 20(3): 238–52.

Roberson JB Jr, O'Rourke C, Stidham KR (2003) Auditory steady-state response testing in children: evaluation of a new technology. Archives of Otolaryngology: Head and Neck Surgery 129(1): 107–13.

Royal College of Speech and Language Therapists (RCSLT) (1996) Communicating Quality 2. Professional Standards for Speech and Language Therapists. London: RCSLT.

Rubinstein JT, Parkinson WS, Tyler RS et al. (1999) Residual speech recognition and cochlear implant performance: effects of implant criteria. American Journal of Otology 20(4): 445–52.

Ruckenstein MJ, Raftyer KO, Montes M et al. (2001) Management of far advanced otosclerosis in the era of cochlear implantation. Otology Neurotology 22(4): 471–4.

Sauvaget E, Pereon Y, Nguyen The Tich S et al. (2002) Electrically evoked auditory potentials: comparison between transtympanic promontory and round-window stimulations. Neurophysiologie Clinique 32(4): 269–74.

Schmidt AM, Weber BP, Zacharias R et al. (2003) Functional MR imaging of the auditory cortex with electrical stimulation of the promontory in 35 deaf patients before cochlear implantation. American Journal of Neuroradiology 24(2): 201–7.

Seewald RC, Scollie SD (2003) An approach for ensuring accuracy in pediatric hearing instrument fitting. Trends in Amplification 7(1): 29–40.

Shallop JK, Peterson A, Facer GW et al. (2001) Cochlear implants in five cases of auditory neuropathy: postoperative findings and progress. Laryngoscope 111(4–1): 555–62.

Silman S, Gelfand SA, Silverman CA (1984) Late-onset auditory deprivation: effects of monaural versus binaural hearing aids. Journal of the Acoustical Society of America 76: 1357–62.

Spraggs PD, Burton MJ, Graham JM (1994) Nonorganic hearing loss in cochlear implant candidates. American Journal of Otology 15(5): 652–7.

Stark T, Engel A, Borkowski G (2004) Bilateral cochlear implantation in varying duration of deafness. (German). Laryngorhinotologie 83(1): 20–2.

Stueve MP, O'Rourke C (2003) Estimation of hearing loss in children: comparison of auditory steady-state response, auditory brainstem response, and behavioral test methods. American Journal of Audiology 12(2): 125–36.

Summerfield AQ, Marshall DH (1995) Cochlear Implantation in the UK 1990–1994: Report by the MRC Institute of Hearing Research on the Evaluation of the National Cochlear Implant Programme. London: HMSO Publications.

Summerfield AQ, Barton GR (2001) Alternative Approaches to Commissioning Cochlear Implantation in England: Discussion Document. Medical Research Council Institute of Hearing Research. Nottingham.

Swan IR, Gatehouse S (1995) The value of routine in-the-ear measurement of hearing aid gain. British Journal of Audiology 29(5): 271–17.

Swanepoel D, Hugo R, Roode R (2004a) Auditory steady-state responses for children with severe to profound hearing loss. Archives of Otolaryngology: Head and Neck Surgery 130(5): 531–5.

Swanepoel D, Schmulian D, Hugo R (2004b) Establishing normal hearing with the dichotic multiple-frequency auditory steady-state response compared to an auditory brainstem response protocol. Acta Otolaryngologica 124(1): 62–8.

Telischi FF, Roth J, Stagner BB et al. (1995) Patterns of evoked otoacoustic emissions associated with acoustic neuromas. Laryngoscope 105(7 pt. 1): 675–82

Turrini M, Orzan E, Gabana M et al. (1997) Cochlear implantation in bilateral Mondini dysplasia. Scandinavian Audiology (suppl. 46): 78–81.

Tyler RS (1995) Tinnitus in the profoundly hearing impaired and the effects of cochlear implants. Annals of Otology, Rhinology and Laryngology (suppl. 165): 25–30.

Tyler RS, Parkinson AJ, Wilson BS et al. (2002) Patients utilizing a hearing aid and a cochlear implant: speech perception and localization. Ear and Hearing 23(2): 98–105.

UKCISG (UK Cochlear Implant Study Group) (2004a) Criteria of candidature for unilateral cochlear implantation in post-lingually deafened adults I: Theory and measures of effectiveness. Ear and Hearing 25(4): 310–35.

UKCISG (UK Cochlear Implant Study Group) (2004b) Criteria of candidature for unilateral cochlear implantation in post-lingually deafened adults II: Cost effectiveness analysis. Ear and Hearing 25(4): 336–60.

UKCISG (UK Cochlear Implant Study Group) (2004c) Criteria of candidature for unilateral cochlear implantation in post-lingually deafened adults III: Prospective evaluation of an actuarial approach to defining a criterion. Ear and Hearing 25(4): 361–74.

van Dijk JE, van Olphen AF, Langereis MC et al. (1999) Predictors of cochlear implant performance. Audiology 38(2): 109–16.

Waltzman SB, Cohen NL, Shapiro WH (1992). Sensory aids in conjunction with cochlear implants. American Journal of Otology 13(4): 308–12.

# Chapter 5

# Assessment of children

Mary Joe Osberger, Amy McConkey Robbins
and Patricia G. Trautwein

## Introduction

Cochlear implants are accepted as an effective treatment for profound deafness. Many profoundly deaf children acquire spoken language with these devices, an accomplishment realized by few deaf children who use conventional acoustic amplification. Children with cochlear implants often function as well as children with less severe hearing impairments (Boothroyd and Eran, 1994; Meyer et al., 1998), allowing them to acquire spoken language through incidental learning (Robbins, 2000). The impact of implants on deaf children's oral language acquisition is evidenced in improved reading abilities and other linguistic skills required for academic success (Spencer et al., 1999; Spencer et al., 2003). Consequently, deaf children with implants are educated in less restrictive environments and may require fewer educational special support services than their peers with hearing aids (Francis et al., 1999).

The need to determine cochlear implant candidacy and post-implant benefit led to the development of procedures that now are commonly used in pediatric assessments. Pre-operatively, the typical evaluation battery consists of audiological tests to establish the degree and type of hearing loss and measures of auditory skill development or speech recognition to determine functional hearing aid benefit. The pre-operative results also serve as a baseline for later comparison with post-implant. Post-operative assessment of cochlear implant performance serves to document device benefit, track progress over time, and assist with development of intervention goals and educational needs. Because hearing loss also impacts speech and language skills, assessment in these areas also occurs. Many cochlear implant programs employ a team approach consisting of an audiologist, speech-language pathologist, educator of the hearing impaired, and psychologist (in addition to medical personnel described elsewhere in this book). This allows input from a wide range of professionals with different perspectives on the child's performance and needs.

Since the inception of cochlear implants, technological advances have resulted in incremental improvements in performance (Sehgal et al., 1998; Geers et al., 2003a) that have led to expanded selection criteria and modifications in evaluation procedures. During the early days of cochlear implants, candidacy was limited to older children who clearly demonstrated a plateau in the development of auditory skills and whose performance could be reliably assessed with traditional audiological procedures (Berliner and Eisenberg, 1985; Miyamoto et al., 1995). These children did not even demonstrate sound awareness with conventional hearing aids. Gradually, criteria were expanded to include younger children and those with more residual hearing (Zwolan et al., 1997; Waltzman and Cohen, 1998; Osberger et al., 2002). It is now common practice to implant children between 12 and 18 months of age, with an emerging trend to implant children younger than one year. The younger age at implant is motivated by numerous research findings that show substantial differences in device benefit as a function of age at implant (Tye-Murray and Kirk; 1993; Fryauf-Bertschy et al., 1997; Connor et al., 2000), even in children implanted between one and three years of age (Robbins et al., 2004).

Older children continue to be cochlear implant candidates even though the trend is to implant children at younger ages (Osberger et al., 2002). These children form two distinct groups. The first group consists of children with severe-to-profound hearing loss who did not meet the selection criteria when they were younger because they had too much hearing. They use oral communication and tend to be mainstreamed in regular schools. With advances in technology, these children now obtain more benefit from a cochlear implant than from hearing aids. After implantation, many of these children use a hearing aid in the contralateral ear (Ching et al., 2003). The other group is older children who use total communication. Advances in technology, improved benefit, and greater acceptance of cochlear implants presumably accounts for increased referrals for children from total communication programs. Although numerous studies have shown that children who use oral education attain higher scores on post-implant measures of speech perception, speech production, and language than children who use total communication, children from total communication programs, nevertheless, derive more benefit from cochlear implants than hearing aids (Meyer et al., 1998; Osberger et al., 1998; Geers et al., 2003a; Geers et al., 2003b; Tobey et al., 2003).

The focus of this chapter is on children younger than age five because they pose the greatest assessment challenges. Procedures for older children are well documented in previous publications (e.g. Tyler, 1993; Robbins and Kirk, 1996; Kirk, 2000). The first section addresses audiological procedures to determine degree and type of hearing loss with objective and behavioral measures. Next, assessment of auditory, speech, language, and communication skills is presented for infants and toddlers (children younger than 2–3 years of age) and young children (children 3–5 years of age). This classification is used as a framework for the chapter and does not reflect strict categorization by chronological age. In addition, specific candidacy criteria will not be discussed, because of the evolutionary nature of this information. Rather, clinicians can employ the measures described in the chapter and current selection criteria can be applied as appropriate.

## Audiological evaluation

The audiological evaluation determines or reconfirms the degree of hearing loss and appropriate fitting of hearing aids. Accurate audiological data are critical to determine if a child will receive greater long-term benefit from a cochlear implant or conventional amplification. Children present a unique set of challenges for audiological assessment including more limited language skills and experience with audition as well as shorter attention spans than adults. These challenges are addressed with an audiological test battery that includes both pediatric behavioral and objective assessments in aided and unaided conditions. Audiological data are used in conjunction with speech perception testing to determine a child's candidacy for cochlear implantation. The reader is referred to Eisenberg (2003) for a review of clinical procedures and research with infants and toddlers.

The increasing popularity and mandating of newborn screening has led to early identification of hearing loss through the use of an objective measures test battery. Most newborns who fail the screening are referred for a comprehensive diagnostic evaluation. A clinician evaluating a child for a cochlear implant should review previous results and minimally re-administer unaided and aided behavioral tests. Objective measures should be repeated if inconsistencies between behavioral and objective data are noted or if there is a question about the reliability of previous findings.

### Objective measures

#### Auditory brainstem response

Auditory evoked potentials (AEP) are very small electrical voltage potentials originating from the auditory pathway typically recorded using small, non-invasive electrodes placed on the scalp. Auditory brainstem response (ABR) audiometry is the most common clinical application of an AEP. The reader is referred to Jacobson (1994) or Hall (1992) for a detailed description of clinical set-up for AEP recording. ABR wave V is the component used most often as an objective correlate to audiometric threshold. For infants and young children, the ABR can be used in the initial fitting of amplification when behavioral thresholds are unreliable (Winter and Eisenberg, 1999; Sininger, 2003) or can assist in the early cochlear implant counseling process. Therefore, it is imperative that the most accurate estimation of audiometric configuration and degree of hearing loss be deduced from ABR audiometry. Although click stimuli can be used to elicit an ABR (and rule out auditory neuropathy, as discussed later in this chapter), tone burst stimuli are preferred because of the better estimation of the behavioral audiogram across the speech spectrum (Stapells and Oates, 1997; Sininger, 2003). The addition of notched-noise masking may further improve the accuracy of the estimated audiogram, especially in cases of steeply sloping hearing loss (Stapells et al., 1995).

*Steady state evoked responses*

Research has shown that tone-burst ABR, using current clinical equipment, does not distinguish severe-to-profound hearing losses in the range of 85–95 dB HL from those greater than 100 dB HL (Rance et al., 1998; Vander Werff et al., 2002). Determining the degree of residual hearing, especially if thresholds are in the profound range of impairment, is critical for hearing aid fitting as well as for the determination of cochlear implant candidacy.

The auditory steady state evoked response (SSEP) shows a distinct advantage over ABR testing because recordings have been reliably produced up to 127 dB nHL (Roberson et al., 2003). SSEP is an AEP recorded from the scalp in response to periodic modulations of the amplitude and/or frequency of a continuous tone (Picton et al., 2003). A frequency-based analysis and algorithm are applied to the evoked potential to determine a threshold response from background EEG. Research has shown that SSEP can be used clinically to estimate behavioral threshold (Cone-Wesson et al., 2002; Dimitrijevic et al., 2002; Rance and Rickards, 2002). Moreover, studies have reported the improved sensitivity of SSEP-estimated frequency-specific audiograms for distinguishing between the presence or absence of residual hearing in children with profound hearing loss compared to ABR (Vander Werff et al., 2002). Many cochlear implant centers, therefore, have incorporated SSEP into the audiological evaluation of cochlear implant candidates.

*Tympanometry*

Tympanometry is used to assess middle ear function and determine if a conductive component to the hearing loss is present. For children under four months of age, multi-frequency immittance testing may be more informative, although normative data are limited (Sprague et al., 1985; Holte et al., 1991). Multi-frequency reflex testing can also be performed to verify the degree of hearing loss indicated via objective or behavioral measures (Margolis, 1993).

## Otoacoustic emissions

Otoacoustic emissions (OAEs) are sounds of cochlear origin caused by the motion of the sensory hair cells in response to auditory stimulation (Kemp, 2002). OAEs have been proven to be clinically valuable in the differential diagnosis of sensorineural hearing loss and in the screening of cochlear function in infants and other difficult-to-test patients (Ohlms et al., 1990). OAEs are present in persons with normal inner ear function, but are absent in persons with a hearing loss of 30 dB or greater (Zorowka, 1993). OAEs cannot be used for determining the hearing threshold. Children being evaluated for a cochlear implant should have hearing thresholds in the severe-to-profound range and therefore will not have OAEs. However, OAEs are typically incorporated into the audiological test battery to rule out auditory neuropathy (see later section on auditory neuropathy).

## Behavioral procedures

While the objective measures provide information regarding auditory function and hearing sensitivity, they are not a substitute for the behavioral hearing evaluation. Both behavioral and objective measures should be used whenever possible. Pure tone audiometry is routinely used for the determination of hearing sensitivity across the speech spectrum to assist in hearing aid fitting and determine cochlear implant candidacy. The behavioral method varies based on the child's age and developmental level, which is described briefly below. The reader is referred to Northern and Downs (1991) for a detailed description of the methodology. These methods can be used to determine the degree of hearing loss, verify the hearing aid fitting, and to program appropriate stimulation levels of the cochlear implant.

## Behavioral observation audiometry

Behavioral observation audiometry (BOA) assesses hearing with unconditioned, reflexive responses to sound. BOA is not used to determine thresholds, but rather is used to assess supra-threshold response to sound. It is most commonly used with children under five or six months of age. BOA is typically conducted in the sound field, but insert earphones can also be used. BOA should be used as a cross check to objective measures in very young children. For example, a child with profound hearing thresholds on objective AEPs should not have a startle response observed to speech at 75 dB HL.

## Visual reinforcement audiometry

With visual reinforcement audiometry (VRA), the child is conditioned to provide a specific response, typically a head turn, to an acoustic stimulus. Correct responses are reinforced visually using animated and/or lighted toys. This method is most appropriate with children from five to six months to approximately two-and-half years of age. Once the child is conditioned, VRA can be used to accurately determine hearing threshold (Wilson and Thompson, 1984; Diefendorf, 1988).

## Conditioned play audiometry

With conditioned play audiometry (CPA), the child is conditioned to perform a play activity (i.e. dropping a block in a bucket) whenever a sound is heard. Once the child is conditioned, the threshold of hearing can be determined by decreasing signal intensity. Games are selected to engage children from two-and-a-half to approximately five years of age. Some children can be evaluated by age two with CPA but the probability of success increases as the child approaches age three and older (Thompson and Weber, 1974). Children over the age of five can generally follow standard audiometric procedures in which the hand is raised in response to hearing a sound in either ear.

For both VRA and CPA, insert earphones are generally recommended to provide ear-specific information. Sound-field testing is typically used for the verification of appropriately fitted amplification.

## Hearing aid evaluation

The goal of a cochlear implant pre-evaluation is to determine if a child will gain more benefit from a cochlear implant than from hearing aids. With the exception of special cases where cochlear patency is at risk, such as deafness secondary to meningitis, a hearing aid trial is recommended prior to implantation. With the change in cochlear implant candidacy over the past three decades to include individuals with more residual hearing, it is even more important to evaluate the appropriateness of the hearing aid fitting, potential long-term benefit with hearing aids, and the possibility of continued hearing aid use in the non-implanted ear.

The combined use of objective measures, specifically tone burst ABR or SSEP, and age-appropriate behavioral measures, provide the clinician with an accurate estimation of frequency threshold information to fit amplification even in very young children. Prescriptive formulas have become increasingly popular, especially with advanced hearing aid technology. Many formulas require loudness growth measures that can be reliably obtained in adults but not in children. For children, prescriptive formulas based on threshold are most appropriate.

The performance of a hearing aid can be tested in a 2-cc coupler to compare the aid to the manufacturer's specifications. Real-ear measures obtained with a probe-tube microphone system should be used to evaluate the function of the hearing aid in the child's ear. These measures take into account the individual differences of a child's ear canal size relative to the 2-cc coupler to better match the target gain of the prescriptive formula with the aid in situ. Hearing aids that are set to match target gain in a 2-cc coupler will often provide excessive gain in situ due to the reduced ear canal volume. Measuring or using an estimated Real Ear to Coupler Difference (RECD) can assist with fitting verification in children. The Desired Sensation Level (DSL) is a threshold-based prescriptive hearing aid formula frequently used for fitting acoustic amplification in children (Seewald, 1992). DSL converts thresholds in dB HL to thresholds in dB SPL and then corrects with measured RECD or age-specific estimated RECDs when necessary (Seewald et al., 1999; Bagatto et al., 2002).

Aided threshold data, obtained with the age-appropriate behavioral procedure, provide insight into audibility of sound with acoustic input. However, clinical measures routinely used to assess performance with linear analog amplification are not as well suited for advanced technology that employs compression and noise suppression found in digital hearing aids and cochlear implant sound processors (Boymans et al., 1999). Therefore, multi-channel compression technology is often fit with narrow band noise or speech signals (Moore et al., 1998). Sound-field testing with narrow band noise or speech signals should be used in conjunction with supra-threshold speech perception measures (described later in the chapter) to verify the hearing aid fitting.

## Auditory neuropathy

Auditory neuropathy is a recently classified hearing disorder that presents with a grossly abnormal or absent neural response measured with AEPs in the presence of normal cochlear function as measured with OAEs (Doyle et al., 1998; Berlin et al., 2003). Rehabilitation for auditory neuropathy cases is challenging due to the uncertain etiology and pathophysiology coupled with the heterogeneity of the audiological and neurological findings in this population of patients. One pervasive finding with auditory neuropathy is poor speech discrimination in relation to the degree of hearing loss. OAEs should be used in conjunction with click-evoked ABR to assess the potential for auditory neuropathy in patients being evaluated for a cochlear implant. Case studies have reported benefit following cochlear implantation in patients with auditory neuropathy (Mason et al., 2003; Peterson et al., 2003). While the results of these studies are promising, a diagnosis of auditory neuropathy is not considered an immediate indicator for cochlear implant referral. Some infants and children diagnosed with auditory neuropathy showed fluctuating auditory responses and significant benefit with conventional amplification (Rance et al., 1999). Therefore, a limited trial period with amplification and monitoring of the stability of audiological thresholds is recommended before cochlear implantation. At this time, the post-implant benefits in these children are encouraging and, therefore, an implant should be considered after appropriate hearing aid use and parent counseling.

# Assessment of auditory, speech, and language skills

**Table 5.1** Summary of measures to assess auditory, speech, and language skills in infants and toddlers and young children with cochlear implants

### Infants and Toddlers

| Auditory | Speech | Language |
|---|---|---|
| Infant–Toddler-Meaningful Auditory Integration Scale (IT-MAIS) | Production Infant Scale Evaluation (PRISE) | Communication and Symbolic Behavior Scales (CSBS) |
| | | MacArthur Communicative Development Inventory (CDI): Words and Gestures and Words and Sentences |
| | | Reynell Developmental Language Scales (RDLS) |
| | | Preschool Language Scale (PLS) |

### Young Children

| Auditory | Speech | Language |
|---|---|---|
| Meaningful Auditory Integration Scale (MAIS) | Goldman–Fristoe Test of Articulation | Reynell Developmental Language Scales (RDLS) |
| Auditory Behavior in Everyday Life (ABEL) | Identifying Early Phonological Needs in Children with Hearing Impairment (IEPN) | Preschool Language Scale (PLS) |
| Categories of Auditory Performance (CAP) | Speech Intelligibility Rating (SIR) | Peabody Picture Vocabulary Test |
| Early Speech Perception Test (ESP) | Sound inventories | Analysis of spontaneous language sample |
| Lexical Neighborhood Test (LNT) | | |
| Multisyllabic Lexical Neighborhood Test (MLNT) | | |

## A practical approach

The procedures that are used to assess pre- and post-implant performance in children should be ones that are appropriate for the resources of each center. The staff need to select instruments that can be administered and scored within a reasonable amount of time, an issue that becomes even more important as the implant population grows at a center. It also is recommended that a common set of procedures be administered to all children who fall within a pre-determined age or developmental category. This will allow a comparison of a single child's performance over time as well as comparisons across children. Ideally, a clinical database should be maintained at each center to derive an index of 'average' performance on each measure. The examination of a child's history might identify factors that account for performance that is below or above the average (e.g. hearing loss history, familial factors, educational issues). If this is not feasible, clinicians will still develop performance expectations if they administer a standard set of tests to common groups of children. Tests outside the core battery can be administered to obtain additional diagnostic information on a given child. The measures that are described in the following sections are ones that are practical to use clinically and do not include those that are more appropriate in a research or laboratory setting.

## Assessment methodology

Until the advent of cochlear implants, auditory skills in young children were traditionally assessed with simple detection tasks because there was no great need to assess speech understanding in these children. Once a sensorineural hearing loss was identified, the course of intervention was clear – hearing aid amplification. The greatest challenge was the appropriate fitting of acoustic amplification that led to the development of prescriptive hearing aid procedures for children (Seewald et al., 1985; Moodie et al., 1994). The assessment of speech recognition in young children became important when professionals were confronted with recommending a cochlear implant or continued use of conventional hearing aids for their pediatric patients.

Assessing functional auditory and speech recognition skills in children under age three is challenging because the tasks that provide the most straightforward information (i.e. object/picture pointing, word repetition) are developmentally inappropriate for these young children. Consequently, techniques employed in other disciplines to obtain developmental information from young children are routinely used to assess auditory skill acquisition in children pre- and post-implant. Notably, parental report measures and other types of questionnaires and rating scales are now components of test batteries with young cochlear implant candidates, and there is a growing trend to apply such measures with young children who use hearing aids (Purdy et al., 2002). Measures of this nature are also employed with older children and adults to quantify everyday listening experiences that cannot be gleaned from traditional speech perception tests administered in a clinical setting (Cox and Alexander, 1995). The use of questionnaires and rating scales also may be more time-efficient for the assessment of speech and language skills than more traditional, standardized tests. In addition, some of these measures can be administered by an audiologist if the implant center does not have the resources to support a speech-language pathologist or educator on the team. Thus, the proposed assessment procedures include parental report/questionnaire measures as well as more traditional measures of speech perception.

## Assessment of auditory skills

### Infants and toddlers

There are significant challenges in assessing implant benefit in infants and toddlers because of their very young age (Robbins, 2003). Nonetheless, numerous studies have documented the auditory benefits that these young children derive from cochlear implants compared to their pre-implant performance with hearing aids (e.g. Kirk, 2000; Zimmerman-Phillips et al., 2000; Robbins et al., 2004).

The tool that has been used most often to document auditory-skill development in young children is the Infant–Toddler-Meaningful Auditory Integration Scale (IT-MAIS) (Zimmerman-Phillips et al., 2001). The IT-MAIS is a criteria-referenced measure that employs a structured parent interview to assess the frequency of occurrence of targeted auditory behaviors in everyday situations. It is a modification of the Meaningful Auditory Integration Scale (MAIS) (Robbins et al., 1991), a measure originally designed to capture the benefit of early cochlear implant technology in everyday listening situations in school-age children. Research has shown that the MAIS has high inter-rater reliability (Robbins et al., 1991) and is significantly correlated ($r = .70$) with post-operative open-set word scores on the PB-K test (Robbins et al., 1998).

To create the IT-MAIS, items and criteria-response behaviors on the MAIS were modified to be more appropriate for infants and toddlers. Like the MAIS, the IT-MAIS consists of ten probes or questions that assess three domains of auditory behavior. Questions 1 and 2 capture changes in vocalizations associated with device use, Questions 3–6 assess spontaneous alerting to sounds in everyday environments, and Questions 7–10 assess auditory recognition (i.e. deriving meaning from sound). Using information provided by the parent during the interview, the examiner scores each question based upon the frequency of occurrence of the target behavior in everyday situations using the following scoring system: 0 = never demonstrates the target behavior, 1 = rarely, 2 = occasionally, 3 = frequently, and 4 = always demonstrates the target behavior. Strict scoring criteria have been developed to ensure uniformity among examiners in scoring the parent's responses.

One of the advantages of the IT-MAIS is that it taps auditory behaviors that are universal and independent of a child's native language.

Consequently, the IT-MAIS has been translated into many languages. Normative data have been collected by Kishon-Rabin and colleagues (2001) for 109 normal-hearing children, ranging in age from two weeks to 36 months (mean age = 12.5 months). Parents were administered a translated version of the IT-MAIS in Hebrew or Arabic. Each child's total IT-MAIS score was converted to a percentage and plotted as a function of his or her chronological age at the time of testing. Figure 5.1 shows the developmental pattern reported by Kishon-Rabin et al. (2001) for the infants with normal hearing. The IT-MAIS data indicate that normal-hearing children show rapid progress in auditory skill acquisition, attaining a score of 80% by approximately 12 months of age.

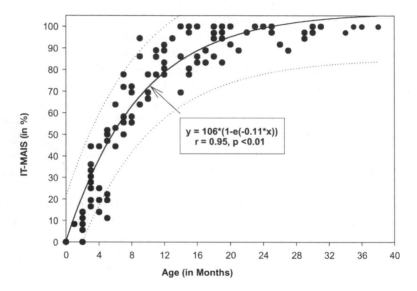

**Figure 5.1** Individual IT-MAIS scores by age for children with normal hearing. Solid line is best-fit exponential function. Dashed line is $-/+2$ standard errors. (From Kishon-Rabin et al., 2001, with permission.)

A study by Robbins et al. (2004) compared the pre- and post-implant IT-MAIS of children implanted under age three to the normative data reported by Kishon-Rabin et al. (2001). The children with cochlear implants were divided into three groups based on age at time of implant: 12–18 months (n = 45), 19–23 months (n = 23), and 24–36 months (n = 30). Over half of the children in the youngest age group achieved auditory milestones approximating those of hearing peers after only six months of device use. For the children implanted between 19 and 23 months, only about one-quarter of them attained scores within the broad normal range after six months of device use. Only a handful of children implanted between 24 and 36 months achieved scores comparable to their peers with normal hearing at the six-month follow-up visit. In sum, while all children benefited from their implants, the youngest children achieved auditory milestones at ages close to those of their peers with normal hearing.

Research indicates that the IT-MAIS is a clinically useful tool that is sensitive to auditory skill development in young children. Moreover, performance on the measure is consistent with developmental trends in children with normal hearing and results can be compared between children who use different native languages. In addition to the IT-MAIS, the reader is referred to the Nottingham Early Assessment Package (NEAP) (2003), which also describes procedures for assessing auditory perception, speech production, and communication and language development in children under two years of age.

## Young children

Auditory development of children in the three-to-five-year age range can be assessed with either the IT-MAIS or MAIS, depending on the child's skill level. A measure that is useful after the IT-MAIS or MAIS is no longer sensitive to skill development is the Auditory Behavior in Everyday Life (ABEL) (Purdy et al., 2002). The ABEL also employs parental report of children's auditory skills in everyday situations but it covers a wider range of auditory behaviors than the IT-MAIS and MAIS and, thus, it is appropriate for hard of hearing children who use conventional hearing aids, as well as severely and profoundly hearing impaired children with cochlear implants. Unlike the IT-MAIS and MAIS, the ABEL is completed by the parent. Research with the ABEL resulted in a 24-item instrument with three groups of items: auditory-oral (e.g. says a person's name to gain their attention, initiates spoken conversations with familiar people, etc.); auditory-awareness (e.g. answers telephone appropriately, responds to own name, etc.), and social-conversational skills (e.g. initiates spoken conversations with unfamiliar people, takes turns in conversations, etc.). Initial findings from a small group of children with cochlear implants indicate that this tool can be used to assess pre- to post-implant benefit.

**Table 5.2** Criteria to categorize children's performance on the Categories of Auditory Performance scale

| Category | Description of behaviour |
|----------|--------------------------|
| 7 | Use of telephone with known listener. |
| 6 | Understanding of conversation without lipreading. |
| 5 | Understanding of common phrases without lipreading. |
| 4 | Discrimination of some speech sounds without lipreading. |
| 3 | Identification of environmental sounds. |
| 2 | Response to speech sounds (e.g. 'go'). |
| 1 | Awareness of environmental sounds. |
| 0 | No awareness of environmental sounds. |

Source: Archbold et al., 1995.

The Categories of Auditory Performance (CAP) is a rating scale used to describe speech perception abilities of children with implants (Archbold et al., 1995; Archbold et al., 1998). It is a hierarchical scale of auditory skills, ranging from no sound awareness to telephone use with a known speaker (Table 5.2). Research has shown that significantly more children implanted below the age of five reach the highest categories after four years of implant use compared to those children implanted over age five (McCormick and Archbold, 2003). The measure is a good tool for a quick evaluation of listening progress with a cochlear implant.

Tests that employ a more traditional format – picture pointing or object identification – may be appropriate for some young children, especially if they have residual hearing or received an implant at a young age. Recorded versions of the tests can be employed if appropriate.

The Early Speech Perception (ESP) test battery was developed to assess speech perception abilities of profoundly hearing impaired children (Moog and Geers, 1990). There are two versions of the measure – one for younger children with limited vocabulary and language skills (Low Verbal version) and one for older children (Standard version). The two versions differ with respect to response format (object identification for Low Verbal version; picture identification for Standard version) and number of items (12 on each subtest of Low Verbal version; 24 on each subtest of Standard version). Each version consists of three subtests. The Pattern Perception subtest contains words that differ in syllable number or stress pattern. A response to any word in the same stress category as the target word is counted as correct. The Spondee Identification subtest evaluates the child's identification of two-syllable words with the same stress pattern with a closed-set response task. The Monosyllable Identification task evaluates identification of one-syllable words that differ from one another primarily in the vowel sound in a closed-set response format. Performance is scored on the basis of the percentage of words correctly identified.

The Lexical Neighborhood Test (LNT) is an open-set measure that can be administered to hearing impaired children as young as three years of age (Johnson and Winter, 2003). The LNT was designed to assess speech recognition in children, controlling for lexical properties of the stimulus words (Kirk et al., 1995). Previous measures of speech recognition did not equate words for the number of phonemes shared by other words or for the frequency of occurrence of the words. For example, the word 'cat' is considered to have many 'lexical neighbors' (words that rhyme with it, e.g. hat, bat, mat, etc.). It is also a high-frequency word. The word 'computer' has few lexical neighbors but may be considered somewhat high in frequency. There are two subtests with 25 items that measure word recognition as a function of lexically 'easy' words (high-frequency words with few neighbors) or lexically 'hard' words (low-frequency words with many neighbors). The Multisyllabic Lexical Neighborhood Test (MLNT) is similar to the LNT except that the multi-syllabic words are used and there are

12 items per list of easy and hard words. Performance is scored as percentage correct recognition for hard and easy words, and the test as a whole. Responses can also be scored for percentage of phonemes correctly identified.

## Assessment of speech skills

### Infants and toddlers

Research has shown the positive effect of cochlear implant use on the development of speech skills, which should be monitored as an important indicator of device benefit in infants and toddlers. Studies have shown improved production of segmental and supra-segmental features of speech and overall speech intelligibility (Tobey et al., 1994; Robbins et al., 1995; Tobey et al., 2003). Dramatic improvements in speech production are often apparent after only several months of device use, even in very young children (Zimmerman et al., 2000). Because changes occur so rapidly in very early implanted children, re-evaluation of skills at three-month intervals is appropriate.

A tool similar to the IT-MAIS has been developed to assess vocal development in infants with cochlear implants (Kishon-Rabin et al., 2003). The Production Infant Scale Evaluation (PRISE) assesses vocal development in infants with implants based on the developmental stages of infants with normal hearing (Oller, 1980). Like the IT-MAIS, the PRISE also employs a structured parent interview to obtain information on the frequency of occurrence of targeted behaviors that the clinician rates on a scale of 0 (the child never demonstrates the behavior) to 4 (the child always demonstrates the behavior). The PRISE contains 11 probes that assess voice quality and stages of vocal development, including the emergence of canonical babbling and first-word use.

Analysis of early productions in implanted babies is warranted because these productions are associated with auditory feedback capability. Canonical babbling involves the baby's use of both a consonant and vowel unit that conform to mature language restrictions, such as 'ada'. A subcategory of canonical babbling is reduplicated babbling where the baby produces a series of consonant/vowel syllables (e.g. 'babababababa' or 'dudududu') (Oller, 1980). Canonical babbling typically emerges in children with normal hearing between seven and ten months of age. It is considered an important landmark in pre-linguistic development both because it is more complex than earlier vocalizations and because its emergence is almost always severely delayed in profoundly deaf children. Kishon-Rabin et al. (2003) found that the developmental pattern on the PRISE in infants with normal hearing is monotonic, reaching first-word use (90% on the test) at approximately 13 months of age. Results obtained from a small sample of children with cochlear implants revealed that at

the pre-implant stage hearing impaired infants (regardless of age) performed similar to six-month-old babies with normal hearing. Post-
implant, the use of PRISE revealed changes in vocal development that was
attributed to cochlear implant use.

Previous research has shown a significant correlation between parent
report data and speech intelligibility as measured by listener judgments.
Robbins et al. (1998) report a significant correlation (r = .60) between
speech intelligibility scores and parent report results on the Meaningful
Use of Speech Scale (MUSS) for 29 children with multichannel implants.
An even higher correlation (r = .75) was found when the analysis
included only children implanted before age six. These results suggest
that information from the MUSS could be used to provide a reasonable
measure of speech intelligibility for children who cannot or will not perform on one of the more traditional clinical speech intelligibility
measures.

## Young children

The clinical assessment of speech in young deaf children is challenging,
particularly at pre-implant intervals when children's speech may contain
articulatory behaviors and utterances that cannot be described using traditional phonetic transcription. The evaluation of speech production in
young children may be carried out using three types of tools: articulation
tests, sound inventories, and ratings of speech intelligibility. Each of these
three tools is described below.

### Articulation tests

Standardized articulation tests typically require the child to name pictured items that contain target phonemes. The examiner transcribes the
child's productions and compares the child's use to correct adult models.
Often, a percentage correct score is generated. Because the stimuli are
highly controlled, articulation tests have the advantage of eliciting a wide
number of consonants and vowels in a short period of time. In addition,
the examiner knows the intended target word and, thus, what substitution or omission has occurred in the child's speech. (In spontaneous
speech samples, the child's intended target may be unknown, complicat-
ing attempts to correspond the child's phonology to that of adult
models.) Finally, most articulation tests have been normed on a sample of
hearing children, allowing comparison of the deaf child's performance to
that of age-matched peers. Some disadvantages of articulation tests
include evaluation of elicited, rather than spontaneous, productions, and
productions are limited to single words. Test results, therefore, may not
accurately reflect the intelligibility of a child's connected spoken language. An articulation test commonly used with children wearing
implants is the Goldman–Fristoe Test of Articulation (Goldman and
Fristoe, 2000), appropriate for children as young as two years.

Paden and Brown (1990) designed a clinical tool to assess early phonological processes. Identifying Early Phonological Needs in Children with Hearing Impairment (IEPN) samples broad categories of speech rather than every phoneme. Twenty-five pictured items serve as the stimuli, and scores are calculated for word patterns, syllable number and stress, presence of initial and final consonants, and vowel height and place accuracy. Results from a study of 24 implanted children suggested that the IEPN was a useful tool in describing changes in speech production in the early stages of implant use (Brown and McDowall, 1999).

## Sound inventories

This method of speech analysis involves constructing an accurate representation of the individual speech sounds used by the child. Typically, this is done by recording a sample of the child's spontaneous utterances, often during a play session, and creating a systematic inventory of vowels and consonants heard during the session. Osberger and colleagues (1991) used such a system to analyze frequency of occurrence for consonant feature acquisition over time in children with implants. The results suggested that sound inventories were sensitive to changes in speech production associated with sensory aid use over time. For clinical purposes, this can be a very useful method for documenting small improvements in a child's speech that may not be measurable using other tools, particularly in children with limited spoken language. However, inventories are generally more time-consuming than other speech production methods and yield only intra-subject comparisons, as normative data are not available from groups of implanted children.

## Rating scales

A third speech assessment tool for young children is the use of a rating

**Table 5.3** Criteria used to categorize children's performance on the Speech Intelligibility Rating (SIR)

| Category | Description of behaviour |
| --- | --- |
| 5 | Connected speech is intelligible to all listeners. Child is understood easily in everyday contexts. |
| 4 | Connected speech is intelligible to a listener who has a little experience of a deaf person's speech. |
| 3 | Connected speech is intelligible to a listener who concentrates and lipreads. |
| 2 | Connected speech is unintelligible. Intelligible speech is developing in single words when context and lipreading cues are available. |
| 1 | Connected speech is unintelligible. Pre-recognizable words in spoken language; primary mode of communication may be manual. |

Source: Allen et al., 1998.

scale that classifies children's speech production according to one of several hierarchical categories. One useful tool is the Speech Intelligibility Rating (SIR) (Allen, et al., 1998), a 5-point scale designed to evaluate the intelligibility of children wearing cochlear implants (Table 5.3). Wilkinson and Brinton (2003) report good inter-rater reliability for the SIR, and a strong relationship has been reported between post-implant performance on the SIR and CAP rating scales (O'Donoghue et al., 1999). Rating scales have the advantage of being less time-consuming than methods such as sound inventories. On the other hand, because there are only a few points on most rating scales, they may not be sensitive to small improvements in a young child's speech production, particularly for children with limited intelligibility. Rating scales are most appropriate for children whose spoken language is characterized by connected phrases and sentences.

## Assessment of language skills

### Infants and toddlers

In addition to auditory perceptual and speech production benefits, children with cochlear implants show significant improvement in their receptive and expressive language development (see Robbins, 2000). Improvements in the use of communication strategies and conversational skills have also been reported (Tait, 1993; Nicholas, 1994) and more children with implants demonstrate higher levels of reading achievement than reported for their peers with hearing aids (Spencer et al., 1999). Nonetheless, even with marked improvements in performance, children with cochlear implants remain delayed in linguistic development compared to children with normal hearing of the same chronological age. However, children with cochlear implants do not continue to fall further behind in their language performance as has been reported for their profoundly hearing impaired peers with hearing aids. As deaf children are implanted at younger ages, the gap will be smaller between their skills and those of their age-matched peers with normal hearing.

As much as possible, language assessment in children with implants should be separate from auditory skill assessment. For measuring underlying language, children should be assessed in their preferred modality, meaning an oral-aural test presentation to children who use oral communication and combined speech and sign presentation to children who use total communication. Of course, it is also helpful to assess the language of total communication children in the oral-aural mode if one wishes to evaluate these children's language ability without sign support. Such an evaluation, however, would likely underestimate the child's communicative competence. As children are implanted at younger ages, the dichotomy between oral and total communication is disappearing. In many cases, young children who use total communication prior to implantation gradually become oral communicators, especially if appropriate aural-oral training is provided. In any case, the most appropriate language assessment tools for implanted children are those that do not penalize the child for poor auditory ability.

The Communication and Symbolic Behavior Scales or CSBS (Wetherby and Prizant, 1993) evaluate important prelinguistic skills such as communicative functions, social-affective abilities, use of gestures, turn-taking, and eye contact. It has been standardized on normally developing children from birth to age four. Pre-linguistic communication is rated in 22 scales measuring parameters of communicative competence and aspects of symbolic development. A structured play session is videotaped and the child's behaviors are analyzed to assess communicative function, noting gestural means, vocalizations, verbalizations, reciprocity, social-affective signaling and symbolic expressions in play. This measure yields information that can be useful in identifying children who might have cognitive impairment in addition to a hearing loss. Such identification becomes critically important as age at implantation decreases, particularly as a means of parent counseling and establishing realistic expectations. Kane (2004) correlated pre-implant CSBS scores with post-implant Reynell scores in a group of early implanted children. Results suggested that very low performance on the CSBS pre-implant was a red flag for low Reynell scores after two years of device use. These preliminary observations suggest that if children lack appropriate pre-linguistic behaviors, the development of age-appropriate formal language may be at risk.

MacArthur Communicative Development Inventory (CDI): Words and Gestures is designed for use with eight- to 16-month normally developing infants (Fenson et al., 1994). The instrument is completed by the parent and queries such skills as the use of representational gestures, games and play routines, and appropriate use of objects. A major portion of the inventory is an extensive vocabulary checklist organized into 19 semantic categories. Parents indicate whether their child shows comprehension and/or spontaneous use of these specific vocabulary items. The MacArthur CDI is a valuable tool in the assessment of communication changes in early implanted children because it assesses very early pre-linguistic behaviors, does not require the child's compliance to complete, and is based upon the child's natural use of language in the home.

The MacArthur Communicative Development Inventory: Words and Sentences is used with children between 16 and 30 months of age. It, like the CDI: Words and Gestures, contains an extensive vocabulary checklist and also assesses later-developing morphological and syntactic structures, including bound morphemes. This version of the CDI also surveys the child's use of references to the past, future, and absent objects and events. Such references are highly illustrative of a child's language development because they are viewed as an important index of the child's emerging ability to represent the world (Ingram, 1981). In normal-hearing children, these references begin to occur late in the single-word period of language development.

Both versions of the MCDI are normed on hearing children and yield percentile rankings based upon the age and gender of the child.

The Reynell Developmental Language Scale (RDLS) (Reynell and Gruber, 1990) is an assessment tool that has been used extensively with deaf children. The test format of the RDLS involves object manipulation and description based on questions that vary in length and complexity. This format reflects real-world communication to a greater degree than do many other language tests. The test evaluates receptive and expressive language independently, yielding age-equivalent and standard scores that compare the child's performance to that of hearing children of the same age. Separate norms are available for British and American children. The Reynell is normed on children aged 12 months to six years, 11 months. As with most tests, the instrument is most sensitive if used with children in the mid-age range of the normative sample, and less sensitive for children at the very lower or upper age ranges.

The Preschool Language Scale, Fourth Edition (PLS) (Zimmerman et al., 2002) is another measure that also evaluates receptive and expressive communication independently. It is normed on hearing children ages birth through six years, 11 months, and therefore is applicable to children a year younger than the Reynell. Caution should be used in interpreting results from deaf children, particularly pre-implant, on the receptive section (called Auditory Comprehension section) because it contains a large number of items that can only be achieved through hearing. Nevertheless, the PLS is a useful clinical tool because it spans a broad age range and uses objects and formats that are motivating to young children.

## Young children

For children in the three- to five-year range, language testing should include measures of single-word vocabulary, grammatical skills, and connected language. A measure of single-word vocabulary comprehension should always be included in an assessment battery but should not be used as the only measure of language ability. Single-word tests may under-estimate a deaf child's communicative competence because of the nature of the task. That is, in these picture selection tasks, redundancy has been restricted and only one lexical selection is correct. Conversely, a single-word test may overestimate a deaf child's communicative competence. This occurs in children who have a broad base of single-word vocabulary but are deficient in processing longer, complex sentence-level material. The results of a vocabulary test should always be interpreted in light of results obtained from other language measures. The most widely used vocabulary test is the Peabody Picture Vocabulary Test-III (PPVT) (Dunn and Dunn, 1997). As the PPVT is normed on hearing individuals ages two years, six months to 90 years of age, it may be used throughout the lifespan of deaf children.

Comprehension and use of connected language may be assessed in young children using the RDLS or PLS, described above. The most accurate measure for assessing a child's proficiency in linguistic structure (syntax and morphology) is a spontaneous language sample. A spontaneous sample reflects a less structured, more natural language milieu and is an indication of how well children can 'put it all together' to express themselves. Typically, a sample of at least 50 spontaneous, non-imitative utterances is needed in order to complete an analysis. The sample is gathered through natural play interaction with the child. Published methods for analyzing language samples include Lee's Developmental Scoring System (DSS) (Lee, 1974) and the SALT (Miller, 2001). These analyses allow comparison of the implanted child's score to that of hearing children. A spontaneous sample also may be used to calculate mean length of utterance (MLU), a more general indicator of linguistic structure. The PLS-4 provides a supplemental measure to obtain a language sample and compute MLU.

Language structure is an important and sometimes overlooked area of assessment for implanted children. Aspects of grammar, particularly morphology, have been shown to be some of the most fragile subskills of language in children with a variety of communication disorders. Robbins et al. (2000) found that, in a group of children with implants, grammatical skills developed at a slower rate than most other aspects of language. This suggests that implant children may be vulnerable to delays in grammatical development, even when other aspects of language such as vocabulary and concepts improve at a normal-hearing rate. More detailed assessment of language structure in implanted children could help to guide remediation and to increase teacher and parent vigilance in this important aspect of communication acquisition.

# Summary

Cochlear implants have changed the lives of many deaf children and their families. Because of advances in technology and younger age at implant, outcomes are now compared to developmental patterns of children with normal hearing rather than to the performance of severely and profoundly hearing impaired children who use conventional hearing aids. Furthermore, expectations of parents and professionals is for early implanted children to communicate orally and to attend regular schools with support services. Some deaf children with cochlear implants even become fluent orally in more than one language (Waltzman et al., 2003). In addition, children with multiple handicaps, including cognitive deficits, are considered viable candidates for a cochlear implant (Waltzman et al., 2000).

Technological advances will continue. Sound processing has evolved from feature extraction to a more complete representation of the acoustic signal. Emphasis is on delivering high-rate stimulation to induce a more natural (stochastic) response in the auditory system, achieving greater spectral resolution through the use of virtual channels (percepts between electrode contacts), and preserving the temporal fine structure of the original acoustic stimulus (Hong et al., 2003; Koch et al., 2004). Improved processing will impact speech understanding in challenging, real-world situations and music enjoyment (Koch et al., 2004).

Advances in sound processing have important implications for outcomes with bilateral implants. With appropriate signal processing, there is an increased likelihood that the advantages of bilateral versus unilateral implantation can be demonstrated to third-party payors or funding bodies and allow more children access to two devices implanted at the same time. Providing sound to both ears in a young deaf child allows the opportunity for sound to be processed through both sides of the brain. Thus, the right and left auditory cortices can develop in a more natural sequence. Finally, miniaturization will allow many children to use a behind-the-ear speech processor and eventually lead to fully implantable systems. Clearly, the future of cochlear implants and their impact on pediatric recipients is bright.

# References

Allen MC, Nikolopoulos TP, O'Donoghue GM (1998) Speech intelligibility in children after cochlear implantation. American Journal of Otology 19: 742–6.

Archbold S, Lutman M, Marshall DH (1995) Categories of auditory performance. Annals of Otology, Rhinology and Laryngology 104(suppl. 166): 312–14.

Archbold S, Lutman ME, Nikolopoulos TP (1998) Categories of auditory performance: Inter-user reliability. British Journal of Audiology 32: 7–12.

Bagatto MP, Scollie SD, Seewald RC et al. (2002) Real-ear-to-coupler difference predictions as a function of age for two coupling procedures. Journal of the American Academy of Audiology 13: 407–15.

Berlin CI, Hood L, Morlet T et al. (2003) Auditory neuropathy/dys-synchrony: diagnosis and management. Mental Retardation and Developmental Disabilities Research Review 9: 225–31.

Berliner KI, Eisenberg L (1985) Methods and issues in the cochlear implantation of children: an overview. Ear and Hearing 6(suppl.): 6S–13S.

Boothroyd A, Eran O (1994) Auditory speech perception capacity of child implant users expressed as equivalent hearing loss. The Volta Review 96: 151–68.

Boymans M, Dreschler WA, Schoneveld P et al. (1999) Clinical evaluation of a digital-in-the ear hearing instrument. Audiology 38: 99–108.

Brown C, McDowall DW (1999) Speech production results in children implanted with the Clarion implant. Annals of Otology, Rhinology and Laryngology 108: 110–12.

Ching TYC, Psarros C, Incerti P et al. (2003) Management of children using cochlear implants and hearing aids. The Volta Review 103: 39–57.

Cone-Wesson B, Dowell RC, Tomlin D et al. (2002) The auditory steady-state response: comparisons with auditory brainstem response. Journal of the American Academy of Audiology 13: 173–87.

Connor C, Heiber S, Arts H et al. (2000) Speech, vocabulary and the education of children using cochlear implants: oral or total communication. Journal of Speech, Language, and Hearing Research 43: 1185–1204.

Cox RM, Alexander GC (1995) The abbreviated profile of hearing aid benefit. Ear and Hearing 16: 176–86.

Diefendorf A (1988) Pediatric audiology. In: J Lass, L McReynolds, J Northern et al. (eds), Handbook of Speech-Language Pathology and Audiology. Toronto, CA: BC Decker, pp. 1315–38.

Dimitrijevic A, John MS, Van Roon P et al. (2002) Estimating the audiogram using multiple auditory steady state responses. Journal of the American Academy of Audiology 13: 205–24.

Doyle KJ, Sininger YS, Starr A (1998) Auditory neuropathy in childhood. Laryngscope 108: 1374–7.

Dunn LM, Dunn, LM (1997) Peabody Picture Vocabulary Test – 3rd edn. Circle Pines MN: American Guidance Service.

Eisenberg L (ed.) (2003) Assessment of hearing in infants and toddlers. The Volta Review 103.

Fenson L, Dale PS, Reznick JS et al. (1994) MacArthur Communicative Development Inventories. San Diego: Thomson Learning.

Francis HW, Koch ME, Wyatt R et al. (1999) Trends in educational placement and cost-benefit considerations in children with cochlear implants. Archives of Otolaryngology: Head and Neck Surgery 125: 499–505.

Fryauf-Bertschy H, Tyler R, Kelsay D et al. (1997) Cochlear implant use by prelingually deafened children: the influences of age at implant and length of device use. Journal of Speech, Language, and Hearing Research 40: 183–99.

Geers A, Brenner C, Davidson L (2003a) Factors associated with the development of speech perception skills in children implanted by age five. Ear and Hearing 24: 24S–35S.

Geers A, Nicholas J, Sedey AL (2003b) Language skills of children with early cochlear implantation. Ear and Hearing 24: 46S–58S.

Goldman R, Fristoe M (2000) Goldman–Fristoe Test of Articulation. Circle Pines, MN: American Guidance Service.

Hall JW (1992) Handbook of Auditory Evoked Responses. Boston: Allyn & Bacon.

Holte L, Margolis RH, Cavanaugh RM (1991) Developmental changes in multifrequency tympanograms. Audiology 30: 1–24.

Hong RS, Rubinstein JT, Wehner D et al. (2003) Dynamic range enhancement for cochlear implants. Otology and Neurotology 24: 590–5.

Ingram DJ (1981) Procedures for the phonological analyses of children's language. Baltimore: University Park Press.

Jacobson JT (1994) Principles and Applications in Auditory Evoked Potentials. Boston: Allyn & Bacon.

Johnson KC, Winter ME (2003) Audiologic assessment of infants and toddlers. The Volta Review 103: 221–52.

Kane MO, Schopmeyer B, Mellon N, Worg N, Niporko J (2004) Pre-linguistic communication and subsequent language acquisition in children with cochlear implants. Archives of Otolaryngology: Head and Neck Surgery 130: 619–23.

Kemp DT (2002) Otoacoustic emissions, their origin in cochlear function, and use. British Medical Bulletin 63: 223–41.

Kirk KI (2000) Challenges in the clinical investigation of cochlear implant outcomes. In J Niparko (ed.), Cochlear Implants: Principles and Practices. Baltimore: Lippincott, Williams & Wilkins, pp. 225–59.

Kirk KI, Pisoni DB, Osberger MJ (1995) Lexical effects on spoken word recognition by pediatric cochlear implant users. Ear and Hearing 16: 470–1.

Kishon-Rabin L, Taitelbaum R, Elichai O et al. (2001) Developmental aspects of the IT-MAIS in normal-hearing babies. Israeli Journal of Speech and Hearing 23: 12–22.

Kishon-Rabin L, Taitelbaum T, Rotshtein S et al. (2003) Assessing early auditory skills and pre-speech vocalization in normal-hearing and implanted infants. Paper presented at the 9th Symposium on Cochlear Implants in Children. Washington DC, 24–26 April 2003.

Koch DB, Osberger MJ, Segel P et al. (2004) HiResolution and conventional sound processing in the HiResolution Bionic ear: using appropriate outcome measures to assess speech recognition ability. Audiology & Neuro-Otology 9: 214–23.

Lee, LL (1974) Developmental Sentence Analysis. Evanson, IL: Northwestern University Press.

McCormick B, Archbold S (2003) Cochlear implants for young children. London: Whurr.

Margolis RH (1993) Detection of hearing impairment with acoustic stapedius reflex. Ear and Hearing 14: 3–10.

Mason JC, De Michele A, Stevens C et al. (2003) Cochlear implantation in patients with auditory neuropathy of varied etiologies. Laryngoscope 114: 45–9.

Meyer TA, Svirsky MA, Krik KI et al. (1998) Improvements in speech perception by children with profound prelingual hearing loss: effects of device, communication mode, and chronological age. Journal of Speech and Hearing Research 41: 846–58.

Miller J (2001) Systematic Analysis of Language Transcripts (SALT). Madison: University of Wisconsin.

Miyamoto RT, Kirk KI, Todd SL et al. (1995) Speech perception skills of children with multichannel cochlear implants or hearing aids. Annals of Otology, Rhinology and Laryngology 104(suppl. 166): 334–7.

Moodie K, Seewald R, Sinclair S (1994) Procedure for predicting real-ear hearing aid performance in young children. American Journal of Audiology 3: 23–31.

Moog JS, Geers AE (1990) Early Speech Perception Test. St Louis: Central Institute for the Deaf.

Moore BC, Alcantara JI, Glasberg BR (1998) Development and evaluation of a procedure for fitting multi-channel compression hearing aids. British Journal of Audiology 32: 177–95.

Nicholas J (1994) Sensory aid use and development of communicative function. The Volta Review 96: 181–98.

Northern J, Downs M (1991) Hearing in Children. Baltimore: Williams & Wilkins.

Nottingham Early Assessment Package (NEAP) (2003) Nottingham, UK: The Ear Foundation.

O'Donoghue GM, Nikolopoulos TP, Archbold SM et al. (1999) Cochlear implants in young children: the relationship between speech perception and speech intelligibility. Ear and Hearing 20: 419–24.

Ohlms LA, Lonsbury-Martin BL, Martin GK (1990) The clinical application of acoustic distortion products. Archives of Otolaryngology: Head and Neck Surgery 103: 52–9.

Oller K (1980) The emergence of the sounds of speech in infancy. In: GH Yeni-Komshian, JF Kavanagh, CA Ferguson (eds), Child Phonology Volume 1: Production. New York: Academic Press, 93–112.

Osberger MJ, Fisher L, Zimmerman-Phillips S et al. (1998) Speech recognition performance of older children with cochlear implants. American Journal of Otology 19: 152–7.

Osberger MJ, Robbins AM, Berry SW et al. (1991) Analysis of the spontaneous speech samples of children with cochlear implants or tactile aids. American Journal of Otology (suppl. 12): 151–64.

Osberger MJ, Zimmerman-Phillips S, Koch DB (2002) Cochlear implant candidacy and performance trends in children. Annals of Otology, Rhinology, and Laryngology 111(suppl. 189): 61–5.

Paden EP, Brown C (1990) Identifying Early Phonological Needs in Children with Hearing Impairment. Washington: Alexander Graham Bell Association.

Peterson A, Shallop J, Driscoll C et al. (2003) Outcomes of cochlear implantation in children with auditory neuropathy. Journal of the American Academy of Audiology 14: 188–201.

Picton TW, John MS, Dimitrijevic A et al. (2003) Human auditory steady-state response. International Journal of Audiology 42: 177–219.

Purdy SC, Farrinton DR, Chard LL et al. (2002) A parental questionnaire to evaluate children's auditory behavior in everyday life (ABEL). American Journal of Audiology 11: 72–82.

Rance G, Dowell RC, Rickards FW et al. (1998) Steady state evoked potential and behavioral hearing thresholds in a group of children with absent click-evoked auditory brainstem response. Ear and Hearing 19: 48–61.

Rance G, Beer DE, Cone-Wesson B et al. (1999) Clinical findings for a group of infants and young children with auditory neuropathy. Ear and Hearing 20: 238–52.

Rance G, Rickards FW (2002) Prediction of hearing threshold in infants using auditory steady state evoked potentials. Journal of the American Academy of Audiology 13: 236–45.

Reynell JK, Gruber CP (1990) Reynell Developmental Language Scales, US edn. Los Angeles: Western Psychological Services.

Robbins AM (2000) Rehabilitation after cochlear implantation. In J Niparko (ed.), Cochlear Implants: Principles and Practices. Baltimore: Lippincott, Williams & Wilkins, pp. 323–62.

Robbins AM (2003) Communication intervention for infants and toddlers with cochlear implants. Topics in Language Disorders 23: 16–33.

Robbins AM, Kirk KI (1996) Speech perception assessment and performance in pediatric cochlear implant users. Seminars in Hearing 17: 353–69.

Robbins AM, Renshaw JJ, Berry SW (1991) Evaluation of meaningful auditory integration in profoundly hearing-impaired children. American Journal of Otology 12(suppl.): 144–50.

Robbins AM, Kirk KI, Osberger MJ et al. (1995) Speech intelligibility of implanted children. Annals of Otology, Rhinology and Laryngology 104(suppl. 166): 399–401.

Robbins AM, Svirsky M, Osberger MJ et al. (1998) Beyond the audiogram: the role of functional assessments. In FH Bess (ed.), Children with Hearing Impairment: Contemporary Trends. Nashville: Vanderbilt Bill Wilkerson Center Press, pp. 105–24.

Robbins AM, Svirsky MA, Miyamoto RT (2000) Aspects of linguistic development affected by cochlear implantation. In: SB Waltzman, NL Cohen (eds), Cochlear Implants. New York: Thieme Medical, pp. 284–7.

Robbins AM, Koch DB, Osberger MJ et al. (2004) Effect of age at implantation on auditory skill development in infants and toddlers. Archives of Otolaryngology: Head and Neck Surgery 130: 570–74.

Roberson JB Jr, O'Rourke C, Stidham KR (2003) Auditory steady-state response testing in children: evaluation of a new technology. Archives of Otolaryngology: Head and Neck Surgery 129: 107–13.

Seewald RC (1992) The desired sensation level method for fitting children: Version 3.0. Hearing Journal 45: 38–41.

Seewald RC, Ross M, Spiro M (1985) Selecting amplification characteristics for young hearing-impaired children. Ear and Hearing 6: 48–53.

Seewald RC, Moodie KS, Sinclair ST et al. (1999) Predictive validity of a procedure for pediatric hearing instrument fitting. American Journal of Audiology 8: 143–52.

Sehgal ST, Kirk KI, Svirsky MA et al. (1998) The effects of processor strategy on the speech perception performance of pediatric Nucleus multichannel cochlear implant users. Ear and Hearing 19: 149–61.

Sininger YS (2003) Audiological assessment in infants. Current Opinions in Otolaryngology Head and Neck Surgery 11: 378–82.

Spencer LJ, Tomblin JB, Gantz B (1999) Reading skills in children with multi-channel cochlear implant experience. The Volta Review 99: 193–202.

Spencer LJ, Barker BA, Tomblin JB (2003) Exploring the language and literacy outcomes of pediatric cochlear implant users. Ear and Hearing 24: 236–47.

Sprague B, Wiley TL, Goldstein R (1985) Tympanometric and acoustic reflex studies in neonates. Journal of Speech and Hearing Research 28: 265–72.

Stapells DR, Oates P (1997) Estimation of the pure tone audiogram by the auditory brainstem response. Audiology Neurotology 5: 257–80.

Stapells DR, Gravel JS, Martin BA (1995) Thresholds for auditory brainstem responses to tones in notched noise from infants and young children with normal hearing or sensorineural hearing loss. Ear and Hearing 14: 361–71.

Tait M (1993) Video analysis: a method of assessing changes in preverbal and early linguistic communication after cochlear implantation. Ear and Hearing 14: 378–89.

Thompson G, Weber B (1974) Responses of infants and young children to behavior observation audiometry (BOA). Journal of Speech and Hearing Disorders 39: 140–7.

Tobey EA, Geers AE, Brenner C (1994) Speech production results and speech feature acquisition. The Volta Review 96: pp. 109–30.

Tobey EA, Geers AE, Brenner C et al. (2003) Factors associated with development of speech production skills in children implanted by age five. Ear and Hearing 24: 36S–45S.

Tye-Murray N, Kirk KI (1993) Vowel and diphthong production by young users of cochlear implants and the relationship between the phonetic level evaluation and spontaneous speech. Journal of Speech and Hearing Research 36: 488–502.

Tyler RS (1993) Speech perception by children. In RS Tyler (ed.), Cochlear Implants. San Diego: Singular Publishing Group, pp. 191–256.

Vander Werff KR, Brown, CJ, Gienapp BA et al. (2002) Comparison of auditory steady state response and auditory brainstem response thresholds in children. Journal of the American Academy of Audiology 13: 227–35.

Waltzman SB, Cohen NL (1998) Cochlear implantation in children younger than 2 years old. American Journal of Otology 19: 158–62.

Waltzman SB, Scalchunes V, Cohen NL (2000) Performance of multiply handicapped children using cochlear implants. American Journal of Otology 21: 329–35.

Waltzman SB, Robbins AM, Green JE et al. (2003) Second oral language capabilities in children with cochlear implants. Otology and Neurotology 24: 757–63.

Wetherby A, Prizant B (1993) Communication and Symbolic Behavior Scales. Chicago: Riverside Publishing.

Wilkinson AS, Brinton JC (2003) Speech intelligibility rating of cochlear implanted children: inter-rater reliability. Cochlear Implants International 4: 22–30

Wilson WR, Thompson G (1984) Behavioral audiometry. In JJ Jerger (ed.), Pediatric Audiology. San Diego: College-Hill Press, pp. 1–44.

Winter M, Eisenberg L (1999) Amplification for infants: selection and verification. Otolaryngology Clinics of North America 32: 1051–65.

Zimmerman IL, Steiner VG, Pond RE (2002) Preschool Language Scale, 4th edn. San Antonio, TX: Psychological Corporation.

Zimmerman-Phillips S, Robbins AM, Osberger MJ (2000) Assessing cochlear implant benefit in very young children. Annals of Otology, Rhinology and Laryngology 109(suppl. 185): 42–3.

Zimmerman-Phillips S, Robbins AM, Osberger MJ (2001) Infant-Toddler Meaningful Auditory Integration Scale: Sylmar, CA: Advanced Bionics Corporation.

Zorowka PG (1993) Otoacoustic emissions: a new method to diagnose hearing impairment in children. European Journal of Pediatrics 152: 626–34.

Zwolan T, Zimmerman-Phillips S, Ashbaugh CJ et al. (1997) Cochlear implantation of children with minimal open-set speech recognition. Ear and Hearing 18: 240–51.

# CHAPTER 6

# Selection criteria and prediction of outcomes

HUW R. COOPER

## Introduction

Outcomes of cochlear implantation have changed significantly as their widespread application has become established over the last 20 years or so. Around the time of the publication of the first edition of this book, many cochlear implant recipients received single-channel devices, and multi-channel devices were still in a relatively early stage of their development. Over the intervening years technological improvements in design, including refinement of electrode designs and speech processing, have led to steady gains in the performance and benefit that cochlear implant users can expect to receive. Significant improvements in speech reception scores attributable to the implementation of new speech coding strategies over recent years have been well documented (e.g. David et al., 2003).

There remains great variability in outcomes, and most cochlear implant teams are familiar with the unpredictability of results, although much knowledge and insight has been gained with greater experience. There will probably always be a range of outcomes from, at one extreme, only very minimal benefit and awareness of environmental sounds for some to, at the other extreme, fluent open-set speech recognition, telephone use and almost normal hearing abilities. The ability to predict outcomes has been notoriously difficult but understandably desirable for both recipients and implant providers. However, we have learned that a complex range of frequently interacting variables can influence the outcome from an implant, and, although it would be reasonable to state that we now understand much more about the relative importance of all these variables than when cochlear implants were in their infancy, that the precise prediction of an individual's benefit from an implant remains elusive.

Inevitably, the selection criteria commonly used and accepted as standard practice amongst cochlear implant teams have evolved over time as outcomes from implantation have improved. There has also been considerable variation around the world, with some countries maintaining a more conservative approach than others. In some cases this has been the result of differences in the funding systems available, such that, when funding for cochlear implantation is constrained within limited budgets, an inevitable tendency towards giving implants to the most 'obvious' candidates has prevailed.

# Categories of benefit

The benefit that cochlear implant recipients receive from their devices and accompanying rehabilitation falls into various domains. It can be argued that a proportion of the benefit accrued results from the degree of attention and rehabilitative input that ideally precedes and follows the implant surgery itself. For example, increases in confidence and communication ability can certainly be achieved by profoundly deaf adults following intensive rehabilitation from therapists with skills in these areas (methods for this purpose are described extensively in Chapter 13).

However, it is obvious that adults or children who are candidates for cochlear implantation will not be able to gain access to the auditory information required for speech reception, awareness and recognition of environmental sounds and enjoyment of music without the implant itself. The determination of when an implant is more likely to provide this information than optimally fitted hearing aids depends on the careful consideration of each individual and is the basis for selection criteria, as discussed below.

For children, a widely used and very useful way of describing the hierarchy of benefit from an implant has been outlined in the CAP (Categories of Auditory Performance) scale (Archbold et al., 1995). The eight categories used range from 'No awareness of environmental sound' through 'Discriminate some speech sounds without lipreading' up to 'Use telephone with known speaker'. This range of post-implant abilities could equally be applied to adults, although five out of the eight categories relate to speech perception which represents only part of the benefit of being able to hear with an implant. Also, a significant proportion of adult implant users are able to follow conversations with *unknown* speakers on the telephone, which would take their performance beyond the 'top' category of the CAP.

In adults, an open-ended questionnaire can reveal the full range of advantages and disadvantages that implant users actually perceive they obtain from their device, as reported by Tyler (1994). The largest proportion of implant users (86%) reported 'speech reception when speechreading can be used' as an advantage. In decreasing order of the percentage of respondents reporting them, the other advantages listed included:

- environmental sound perception (79%);
- psychological effects (49%);
- speech perception when speechreading cannot be used (56%);
- lifestyle and social effects (40%);
- speech production (14%);
- reduction of tinnitus (7%).

These findings illustrate the wide range of benefits that implant users perceive that they receive. It is possible that the proportion of users reporting the benefit of 'speech perception when speechreading cannot be used' may well be higher today if this survey were repeated with a group of present-day implantees as it is well documented that the performance levels typically achieved now have improved since 1994. However, there is no doubt that the other reported benefits would still emerge as important. There remain a significant number of implant users who, despite enhancements in implant design etc., are unable to obtain open-set speech reception but who would nonetheless report great benefit from their devices in other domains, such as improved confidence when lipreading or reduced tinnitus. This latter benefit will for some implant users be dominant above all others when tinnitus was a major problem pre-operatively. Removal of this most distressing and psychologically disturbing symptom can in itself provide a huge improvement in the quality of life for a proportion of implant users.

The immediate benefit of a correctly inserted and programmed cochlear implant is the detection of environmental sounds. The threshold level of sounds detected tends to vary little between implant listeners. The absolute level of sounds that can be detected depends to a large degree on the setting of the device controls, for example the sensitivity control in the Nucleus system. Most cochlear implant systems do not allow the detection of very quiet sounds at the same levels as in normal listeners, as the input dynamic range is inevitably restricted compared to the normal ear; most implants 'ignore' quiet ambient sounds that could be intrusive and interfere with speech reception. The detection of sounds is of course only the pre-cursor of discrimination, recognition and comprehension of speech and other sounds, and it is at these progressively higher levels of the process of auditory perception that great variability between implant users is observed.

The potential benefits from cochlear implantation include:

- environmental sound awareness;
- speech recognition;
- benefit to lipreading/communication;
- speech and language development;

- reduction of tinnitus;
- enjoyment of music;
- educational achievements;
- improved employment prospects;
- changes in quality of life;
- psychological well-being.

The relative value for each individual implant user of each of these benefits clearly varies and a great deal of the pre-implant assessment process involves exploring the expectations and hopes of the implant candidate. For example, a deafened musician may experience great disappointment, and for them a subjectively poor outcome, if their ability to perceive music through the implant is limited, even if they achieve excellent speech discrimination.

Despite this wide range of potential benefits, outcomes from implantation are very often measured only in terms of the second one in the list, i.e. speech discrimination. Although clearly an important result, which for many implant users may be the key benefit they hope to achieve, it is clear from the length of the list that reception of speech is only one facet of the outcome. Any effort to measure comprehensively the overall benefit from an implant must also include the evaluation of the other areas on the list. A complete outcome evaluation battery that includes these will show the fullest possible picture of implant benefit.

# Variables that could affect outcomes of cochlear implantation

The process of providing useful sound perception to profoundly deaf adults or children is a complex one, with a sequence of events beginning with the picking up of sounds at the speech processor's microphone and ending with the process of auditory perception in the recipient's brain. An analogy might be made to a person listening to an old vinyl record through a hi-fi system. One could have the most expensive needle and amplifier money can buy, but with low-quality speakers the sound heard will be of poor quality. The quality of sound and enjoyment obtained depends on a chain of variables that can each affect the end result, some significantly more than others. Similarly, to obtain the best possible outcome from a cochlear implant a number of factors need to be right, and some will inevitably greatly dominate others in their influence. Any clinician in this field knows that two patients with identical implants, inserted by the same surgeon, with identical insertion depths, programmed using the same processing strategy, can achieve widely different levels of performance; the variables internal to each individual patient may have the greatest influence. Factors that may affect performance include the following:

External to the patient:

• electrode design and insertion;
• speech processing strategy;
• quantity and quality of auditory input.

Internal to the patient:

• physiological factors, i.e. quality/quantity of neural survival;
• central auditory processing;
• cognitive ability;
• motivation;
• emotional state.

The advances in surgical skill and technique, electrode design and speech processing are described sufficiently elsewhere in this book. All have their influence on implant performance, but identifying which *patient* variables really matter is the topic here. The first factor listed above, quantity and quality of auditory neuronal survival, is often thought to be one of the most critical – but is unfortunately difficult to measure directly. The superb scan images to be found in Chapter 8 and Chapter 9 demonstrate the 'state of the art' in current imaging techniques but even the best available imaging can not reliably provide a measure of the quantity of spiral ganglion cells in the cochlea, which are thought to be important for successful electrical stimulation.

Pre-operative trial electrical stimulation has frequently been cited as a viable method for predicting outcomes with varying degrees of success. For example, Kileny et al. (1991) report that pre-operative promontory stimulation thresholds and the slope of the threshold function were 'excellent' predictors of post-operative speech recognition in a group of only 10 implant recipients. Blamey et al. (1992) describe a similar finding with gap-detection thresholds on promontory stimulation. Shipp and Nedzelski (1994) report some significant correlations between detection thresholds and threshold slope functions for round window pre-operative trial stimulation and post-implant open-set speech recognition. More recently, van Dijk et al. (1999) report that the temporal difference of limen in pre-operative round window stimulation was a 'secondary predictor' of post-operative variables after duration of deafness and residual hearing. Despite these previous findings, pre-operative promontory or round window testing is not universally used by many implant teams except in cases where there is some doubt over the integrity of the VIII nerve, in cases of head injury or temporal bone fracture; many clinicians would instead assume that residual hearing thresholds alone provide sufficient evidence of a stimulable auditory nerve and proceed with implantation on that basis.

# Cognitive variables

It is probably true to say that the focus of efforts to understand the variability in cochlear implant outcomes over the years has been on 'hard' physiological factors, as discussed above. However, many implant clinicians would report that there is an elusive 'X factor' that some implant users seem to have in greater abundance than others and which enables them to obtain a really outstanding result. This 'X factor' may relate to central auditory processing and cognitive factors, and has been often neglected or insufficiently understood.

The value of cognitive abilities for implant outcome was explored more by Knutson et al. (1991) and in detail in Chapter 7 of this book. He demonstrated that conventional measures of intelligence such as the WAIS do not correlate with speech reception performance after 18 months of implant use, but more specific tests such as a Visual Monitoring Task and Sequence Learning Task did show significant predictive ability. The conclusion was that the ability to extract and process information from incoming stimuli was highly relevant to success with an implant, and this ability is not related directly to overall intelligence. Clinical experience with large numbers of adult implant users would certainly support this view.

A superb theoretical overview of the roles of perception, learning, memory and information processing in the outcomes of cochlear implants in children is given by Pisoni (2000). In particular, he points to the strong inter-correlation found between open-set speech recognition in implanted children with other language measures such as the Reynell expressive and receptive language scales. This was proposed as evidence of the underlying abilities in information processing, and specifically language processing, that are required for the best use of the information provided by an implant. Tait et al. (2000) report a significant correlation between pre-implant measures of autonomy, as derived from video analysis, and measures of speech identification three years after the implant. They found that the autonomy measures they used explained 27% of the variance in performance on CDT (Connected Discourse Tracking). This is a surprisingly large amount of variance to explain, considering the myriad variables that could influence the results, but the authors may have hit on a key factor that contributes to benefit from an implant in children.

In short, evidence has emerged over recent years that central and cognitive factors have a big influence on the ability of implant users to achieve the best outcomes. Certainly, underlying abilities in the realm of information processing and in particular the ability to extract and process limited information from a reduced signal would appear to be critical and are an area ripe for further research. This topic will be discussed in greater depth in Chapter 7.

# Is it possible to predict outcomes?

Perhaps attempts to answer this question should be preceded by another: why do we need to predict outcomes? There are various reasons why efforts to find ways of predicting the outcomes of cochlear implantation have preoccupied many researchers and clinicians.

Resources available for this expensive treatment are invariably limited, and there has been a natural tendency towards aiming implants at those who can benefit most – hence the ability to predict outcomes has been considered important. In practice, however, many implant teams with no limit on funding recognize the great variability in benefit and would not attempt to 'ration' implantation to those who are likely to be 'star' performers. Provided the assessment process indicates that an individual is likely to benefit to any degree (sometimes with marginal benefit only), the issue of predicting the final outcome becomes more academic than clinically important. When funding is limited, the picture could be different: financial pressure could then lead to those patients expected to gain less benefit being denied the treatment because they did not meet a specified criteria for cost-effectiveness. Luckily, this situation does not arise frequently, at least in western healthcare systems. However, whatever the funding system, there is an ultimate limit to the finances available for cochlear implantation and so its cost effectiveness must be estimated so that comparison can be made with other healthcare provisions competing for the same resources.

Setting aside financial considerations, even if cochlear implants and implant surgery were to cost nothing, most clinicians would wish to be able to predict the outcome of an implant just as they would for any other surgical intervention. Most prospective adult implant recipients are aware of the inherent difficulty in predicting with any accuracy the outcome of their implant, but probably privately harbour hopes of being a 'star' result, so being able to counsel them about likely outcomes is clearly important. When they are actually managing reasonably well with hearing aids (frequently referred to as a marginal hearing aid user), it becomes even more important to be able to predict the probability of an implant giving them something significantly better.

For parents of a deaf child, the decision to put their child through implant surgery is clearly a major one, and no parent would wish to proceed unless they believed that the benefits were likely to be tangible, worthwhile and in the best long-term interests of their child. Most surgeons and implant teams can confidently predict that, assuming the surgery, electrode insertion and device programming are achieved successfully, an implanted child will detect sounds at reasonably predictable levels following switch-on. The extent to which each child can make use of the new auditory input, develop spoken language and flourish in the hearing world clearly varies and is affected by a range of factors – only some of which are within the control of the child's parents and implant team.

Over recent years in which the outcomes of paediatric cochlear implantation have become more widely known, a consensus has emerged that for children implantation at a very young age is likely to lead to the best results in terms of speech and language development and other important outcomes (e.g. O'Neill et al., 2002); Chapter 5 in this book provides greater detail about the challenge that assessment of such young children poses.

Many other studies have attempted to calculate the predictive value of pre-operative variables in adults. The duration of deafness is the factor most frequently cited as having predictive value (e.g. Blamey et al., 1992; van Dijk et al., 1999; Rubinstein et al., 1999; Geier et al., 1999): longer duration of deafness is usually associated with poorer speech recognition outcomes in adults. The explanation generally accepted for this finding is that performance with an implant depends to a degree on the number of surviving spiral ganglion cells in the implanted cochlea, and this number is likely to reduce with increased duration of profound deafness. Nadol et al. (1989) report a temporal bone study which showed that total spiral ganglion cell counts tended to be lower in older people and those with a longer duration of deafness. Interestingly, they also found a significant effect of aetiology on spiral ganglion cell counts, which might lead one to expect aetiology to be a significant factor in performance with an implant. However, this has not been borne out in subsequent studies.

Geier et al. (1999) express the duration of deafness in terms of the percentage of a person's life with deafness instead of an absolute number of years of profound deafness, and found a significant negative correlation with 6-month post-implant speech recognition scores. They also suggest that adults who had been deaf for more than 60% of their lives require longer to achieve their optimum performance with an implant than those with a smaller percentage. The numbers in their study were relatively small, but certainly their finding coincides with our own clinical experience in Birmingham.

Rubinstein et al. (1999) also suggest that if 'substantial' pre-operative speech reception is present this implies a greater population of surviving hair cells which should protect the spiral ganglion from the degenerative effects of long-term deafness and also maintain the viability of central auditory pathways. If this is true, better post-operative results should generally be expected in ears which provided some speech recognition ability pre-operatively; this supports a policy of implanting the 'better ear' as it would therefore be expected to give the better outcome with an implant. Some support for the theory that pre-operative speech recognition acts as a 'trophic factor' which protects the spiral ganglion and/or central auditory pathways from degeneration came from the study reported by Gomaa et al. (2003). They found a direct correlation between pre-operative sentence recognition performance and post-operative word recognition scores. However, Francis et al. (2004) report results from groups of adults classified according to their degree of hearing loss and the degree of symmetry or asymmetry in their hearing levels. They found no significant difference in the speech perception scores obtained by patients implanted in their worse, profoundly deaf ear (with only a severe loss in the contralateral ear) and those patients with a symmetrical severe hearing loss; the conclusion was that the presence of residual hearing in the non-implanted ear confers a functional advantage, implying a central benefit of auditory stimulation.

Although the duration of deafness is likely to be a significant factor for the reasons outlined above, most clinicians would agree that a long period of auditory deprivation does not necessarily result in poor outcome with an implant. A recent study by Hamzavi et al. (2003) found little effect of deafness duration on outcomes in a group of 66 adult implant users; they point out that similar scores can be obtained by a patient who has been deaf for 30 years to one deaf less than 3 years. The duration factor should perhaps be considered as a strong influence but there is no hard and fast rule which can relate it to implant outcome with great reliability.

Other studies have tried to examine a number of variables at once to determine their relative contribution to the variance in performance found. Gantz et al. (1993) applied a pre-operative battery of measures in a randomized clinical trial and then used a multivariate analysis to create a 'predictive index' to estimate the 9-month post-implant point performance (this point in time is chosen because prior experience has indicated that for most implant users performance and benefit have reached an asymptote after this period of implant use). The index included duration of deafness, speech-reading ability, residual hearing, cognitive ability, measures of compliance with treatment and use of non-verbal communication strategies. The reported result was a correlation of 0.81 with performance on a sound-alone sentence recognition test. Clearly, the contribution of each of these variables to outcomes varies considerably and the duration of deafness probably still has the greatest effect; the relative importance of other variables is less.

The 'Iowa formula' described above has been validated more recently. Friedland et al. (2003) used it to predict outcomes in a group of patients implanted in the poorer ear and reported a significant ($r = 0.5$) correlation between the predicted and actual performance achieved. Their conclusion was that the outcome of implantation is closely related to duration of deafness but that this effect may not be ear-specific, i.e. the deafness duration relates not only to the neural survival in the implanted ear but also to the total 'auditory receptivity' of the implant user and so can help to predict outcomes regardless of whether the better or poorer ear is implanted.

The 'POCIA' (Predicting Outcomes of Cochlear Implantation in Adults) study, referred to in the three papers by the UK Cochlear Implant Study Group (2004), gave an opportunity for an analysis of the potential predictive value of a number of pre-operative variables for the results of implantation in a large group of adult patients. This was a prospective cohort study in 13 UK cochlear implant clinics using a battery of computer-based performance tests and questionnaires. The pre-operative factors assessed were taken from the study reported by Gantz et al. (1993) and discussed above, namely:

- *physiological*, e.g. duration of deafness, residual hearing thresholds in the implanted ear;
- *cognitive*, e.g. pre-operative lipreading ability, performance on a visual monitoring task;
- *motivation*, e.g. reported level of involvement in own health care (derived from scores on the Krantz Health Opinion Survey).

Also, a number of outcome variables were recorded at the 9-month post-implant point, including:

- *open-set speech discrimination*: BKB sentences scores;
- *self-reported benefit*: Glasgow Benefit Inventory (this measures the perceived benefit provided by an intervention, i.e. the change in status between pre- and post-implantation);
- *self-reported changes in overall health status*: Glasgow Health Status Inventory (this measures the 'current' health status of the individual).

Regression analyses of individual variables with each of the outcome measures produced a number of statistically significant although generally small correlation coefficients (see Tables 6.1, 6.2, 6.3). Table 6.1 shows the correlations with speech discrimination performance (BKB sentences) at 9 months post-implantation, ranked in decreasing order of the adjusted R-squared (amount of variance explained). The largest individual correlation was with the duration of deafness in the implanted ear ($r = -0.429$, $p < 0.001$), followed closely by the duration of deafness in the other ear. Figure 6.1 shows a scatter plot between BKB scores and the duration of deafness in the implanted ear. This illustrates the fact that the great majority of patients obtaining the highest scores on speech recognition testing are clustered around low durations of deafness, although there remains considerable scatter in the data. Interestingly, small but significant correlations were also found with scores obtained on both the 'digits' and 'letters' version of the Visual Monitoring Task. This was a computer-based test of attention and short-term memory requiring monitoring and responding to visually presented sequences of either digits or letters. One might postulate that performance on a task of this nature could measure similar cognitive skills to those required for speech recognition via an implant. The number of recordable hearing thresholds in the implanted ear, the 'involvement' score from the Krantz Health Opinion Survey and age at the time of implantation also showed very small but significant correlations.

A stepwise multiple regression analysis provided a more detailed picture of the relative contribution of each of the variables to each of the outcomes.

**Table 6.1** Pearson's correlations between selected variables and speech recognition performance at 9 months post-implantation (BKB sentences)

|  | R | Adjusted R squared | Sig | N |
|---|---|---|---|---|
| Duration of deafness in implanted ear | −0.429 | 0.181 | 0.000 | 317 |
| Duration of deafness in other ear | −0.289 | 0.081 | 0.000 | 317 |
| Score achieved on the 'digit' version of the visual monitoring task | 0.162 | 0.022 | 0.009 | 215 |
| Score achieved on the 'letters' version of the visual monitoring task | 0.138 | 0.014 | 0.023 | 208 |
| Number of thresholds recordable in implanted ear | 0.117 | 0.011 | 0.019 | 313 |
| Involvement score from Krantz Health Opinion Survey | 0.124 | 0.011 | 0.026 | 247 |
| Age at time of implant | −0.112 | 0.010 | 0.022 | 323 |
| 4-frequency average hearing level in implanted ear | −0.090 | 0.005 | 0.056 | 313 |
| Annoyance due to tinnitus at 9 months post-implantation | −0.074 | 0.002 | 0.105 | 288 |
| Positive expectations | 0.047 | 0.002 | 0.208 | 309 |
| Annoyance due to tinnitus pre-operatively | 0.020 | 0.000 | 0.363 | 311 |
| Pre-operative depression score (Beck inventory) | −0.055 | 0.000 | 0.175 | 294 |
| Pre-operative lipreading score (CUNY sentences) | −0.054 | 0.000 | 0.177 | 301 |

**Table 6.2** Pearson's correlations between selected variables and overall scores obtained on the Glasgow Benefit Inventory 9 months post-implantation

|  | R | Adjusted R squared | Sig | N |
|---|---|---|---|---|
| Annoyance due to tinnitus at 9 months post-implantation | −0.284 | 0.077 | 0.000 | 268 |
| Duration of deafness in implanted ear | −0.229 | 0.049 | 0.000 | 281 |
| Positive expectations | 0.161 | 0.022 | 0.004 | 273 |
| Pre-operative depression score (Beck inventory) | −0.152 | 0.020 | 0.007 | 265 |
| Number of thresholds recordable in implanted ear | 0.129 | 0.013 | 0.016 | 274 |
| 4-frequency average hearing level in implanted ear | −0.130 | 0.013 | 0.016 | 274 |
| Annoyance due to tinnitus pre-operatively | −0.111 | 0.009 | 0.033 | 276 |
| Duration of deafness in other ear | −0.058 | 0.003 | 0.166 | 281 |
| Pre-operative lipreading score (CUNY sentences) | 0.066 | 0.001 | 0.142 | 269 |
| Age at time of implant | 0.004 | 0.000 | 0.474 | 282 |
| Involvement score from Krantz Health Opinion Survey | 0.022 | −0.004 | 0.372 | 26 |
| Score achieved on the 'digit' version of the visual monitoring task | 0.002 | −0.005 | 0.492 | 198 |
| Score achieved on the 'letters' version of the visual monitoring task | 0.027 | −0.005 | 0.354 | 192 |

**Table 6.3** Pearson's correlations between selected variables and overall scores obtained on the Glasgow Health Status Inventory 9 months post-implantation

| | R | Adjusted R squared | Sig | N |
|---|---|---|---|---|
| Annoyance due to tinnitus at 9 months | −0.393 | 0.151 | 0.000 | 258 |
| Pre-operative depression score (Beck inventory) | −0.278 | 0.074 | 0.000 | 253 |
| Age at time of implant | −0.215 | 0.043 | 0.000 | 269 |
| Pre-operative lipreading score (CUNY sentences) | 0.191 | 0.033 | 0.001 | 259 |
| Annoyance due to tinnitus pre-operatively | −0.184 | 0.030 | 0.001 | 263 |
| Duration of deafness in implanted ear | −0.129 | 0.017 | 0.017 | 268 |
| Positive expectations | 0.127 | 0.012 | 0.021 | 261 |
| Number of hearing thresholds recordable in the implanted ear | 0.102 | 0.007 | 0.050 | 262 |
| Involvement score from Krantz Health Opinion Survey | −0.049 | 0.002 | 0.235 | 218 |
| Duration of deafness in other ear | −0.017 | 0.000 | 0.391 | 268 |
| Score achieved on the 'letters' version of the visual monitoring task | 0.073 | 0.000 | 0.160 | 188 |
| 4-frequency average hearing level in implanted ear | −0.062 | 0.000 | 0.160 | 262 |
| Score achieved on the 'digits' version of the visual monitoring task | 0.016 | −0.005 | 0.412 | 192 |

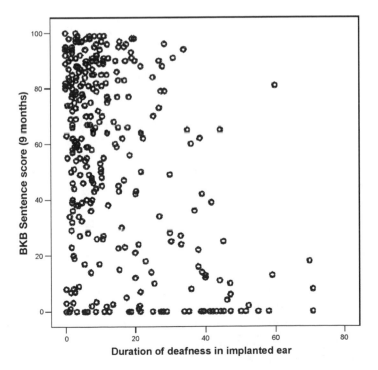

**Figure 6.1** Open-set speech discrimination (% correct with BKB sentences) vs. duration of profound deafness in the implanted ear, n = 317.

The model giving the largest value of R (0.551) for prediction of BKB sentence test scores at 9 months includes three predictors, namely the duration of deafness in the implanted ear, the score on the letters version of the visual monitoring task and the 'involvement' score from the Krantz Health Opinion Survey; this formula explains 29% of the variance. A larger number of variables are excluded from the formula as they do not contribute any further to its predictive value, including for example age and the average pre-operative hearing level in the implanted ear. Figure 6.2 shows a scatter plot of observed vs. predicted values using this formula.

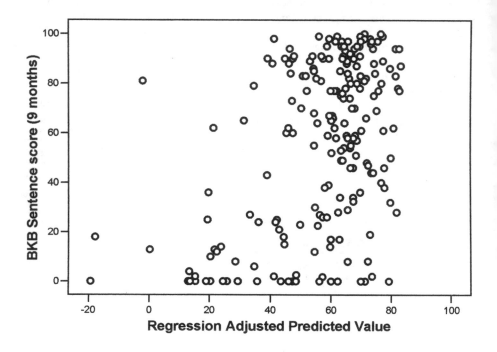

**Figure 6.2** Observed vs. predicted values for open-set speech discrimination scores at 9 months (n = 203).

Correlations with the Glasgow Benefit Inventory (GBI) showed a slightly different pattern. The GBI is a self-reported measure of the perceived benefit from the cochlear implant, and so should take into account other benefits aside from speech discrimination. Table 6.2 shows the correlations with each of the pre-operative variables, again ranked in decreasing order of the size of the adjusted R-squared.

Again, there is a significant negative correlation with the duration of deafness; however, the largest correlation (R = −0.284) is with the reported annoyance due to tinnitus at 9 months, and there was also a smaller but significant negative correlation with the pre-operative tinnitus annoyance measure, illustrating the negative influence that tinnitus can have on the perceived benefit derived from an implant. Also interesting to note is the small but significant correlation between reported positive expectations and the GBI score (R = 0.161), and the small negative correlation with the pre-operative depression inventory score (R = −0.152).

A stepwise multiple regression analysis including only pre-operative variables and the 9 months post-implant GBI score produces a model (R = 0.362, 12% of variance explained) including only two predictors: duration of deafness in the implanted ear and the pre-operative Beck depression inventory score. If the tinnitus annoyance score at 9 months is also included, this increases to R = 0.488, explaining 22.3% of variance, thus showing again the significant negative effect that tinnitus may have on self-reported benefit.

The negative influence of tinnitus on quality of life is also demonstrated by the negative correlations between tinnitus annoyance recorded pre-operatively or at 9 months post-implant (R = −0.111 and −0.284 respectively) and the overall score from the Glasgow Health Status Inventory (GHSI) at 9 months post-implant. As one might expect, both age and the pre-operative depression inventory score both also show a negative correlation with this measure of quality of life, which is not very surprising. Interesting to note also is that the pre-operative lipreading score also showed a small positive correlation with the GHSI, suggesting that the ability to lipread may contribute to overall quality of life. The stepwise multiple regression with 9 months post-implant GHSI as the dependent variable provided a model including two pre-operative predictors, namely the pre-operative depression Beck depression score and age at the time of implantation (R = 0.461, variance explained = 20.3%); if annoyance due to tinnitus at 9 months is also included in the regression, this increases to R = 0.605 (variance explained = 34.4%).

It is somewhat disappointing that the individual correlations obtained from an analysis of a large amount of outcome data such as this are small, and this clearly limits the usefulness of the individual variables examined in the selection of candidates for implantation. However, these data do help our understanding of the physiological and psychological determinants of outcomes. The differences in the correlations with the performance measure and subjective benefit also illustrate how different pre-operative factors relate to different measures of outcome; self-reported post-implant outcomes are apparently much more influenced by variables such as tinnitus and depression, while speech recognition with the implant is most heavily influenced by the duration of deafness, as previously often found. Table 6.4 shows the correlations (all significant at p < 0.001) between the three outcome measures, all at 9 months post-implant; the largest is between the GBI and GHSI score, while the weakest (R = 0.224) is between BKB sentences scores and the GHSI score, reflecting a weak link only between speech recognition ability with an implant and self-reported quality of life.

**Table 6.4** Pearson's correlations between the three 9 months post-operative outcome measures

|        | BKB   | GBI   | GHSI  |
|--------|-------|-------|-------|
| BKB    | 1     | 0.371 | 0.224 |
| GBI    | 0.371 | 1     | 0.512 |
| GHSI   | 0.224 | 0.512 | 1     |

A similar analysis of the outcomes of paediatric implantation was reported in the study by O'Neill et al. (2002), in which they statistically analysed the relationship between a number of variables and gains in auditory performance as measured with the Categories of Auditory Performance (CAP) method. They found a negative correlation between the age at implantation and the gains in CAP scores: none of the other variables studied, e.g. aetiology, were significantly related to CAP gains, apart from the number of medical consultations the child received.

In summary: is it possible to predict outcomes? We are still not able to predict with great certainty the precise outcome of an implant for each individual, but our understanding of the important variables that influence outcomes is much greater than when implants first came on the scene around 20 years ago. There is no 'magic formula' that can precisely predict a result, but it is possible to gain a general idea of the likely outcome: pre-implant duration of deafness remains the dominant factor with other variables clearly making smaller but interesting contributions. The role of pre-operative hearing levels and speech recognition ability as an indication of spiral ganglion cell survival will no doubt become more apparent as selection criteria relax and larger numbers of patients with better pre-operative hearing receive implants.

# Development of selection criteria

Factors that must be considered in the process of assessment of adults and children are described in detail in Chapter 4 and Chapter 5. The possible approaches to defining criteria for candidacy for cochlear implantation are described in detail in the papers by the UK Cochlear Implant Study Group (2004a, b and c); these include an equivalent-effectiveness approach, a health-economic approach and an actuarial approach. The basic premise suggested for defining a criterion is to avoid crossing a boundary, beyond which the disadvantages of the procedure outweigh the advantages. The domain of speech recognition is chosen for the definition of the criterion (as opposed, for example, to a minimum hearing level) because (a) speech recognition scores are now almost universally used to define selection criteria and (b) the 'main force that has driven the relaxation of the criterion has been the desire of clinicians and patients to maximize speech intelligibility' (UK Cochlear Implant Study Group, 2004a).

The definition of acceptable odds that an implant will improve on a pre-operative speech recognition score is explored by the UK Cochlear Implant Study Group (2004c), and the conclusion stated was that cochlear implantation is an effective and cost-effective intervention, provided that implantation occurred in ears with a priori odds at least as favourable as 4 chances out of 5 of improving speech recognition post-implant as compared to pre-implant. In the study reported by Dowell et al. (2004) a 75% likelihood that post-operative performance will be better than pre-operative performance is used as the basis to define new selection criteria. This is equivalent to accepting odds of 3 chances out of 4, which is slightly less than the 4:1 odds recommended by the UKCISG. In the Dowell study, a retrospective analysis of post-operative speech perception scores from implant users implanted in their clinic in Melbourne was used to create a comparative set of data. To be included, patients needed to have a pre-operative open-set sentence score of 10% or more. The 6-month post-implant scores from 92 such patients were then analysed and the 25th percentile (first quartile) point in the distribution of scores was calculated as 68% correct (i.e. 75% of this group of implant users scored above 68% correct on an open-set sentence test after 6 months' implant use). This led to a redefinition of the selection criteria for adults in Melbourne; adults are considered as candidates for an implant if they obtain open-set sentence scores of up to 70% in the best aided condition and up to 40% in the ear to be implanted. The results obtained in a group of 45 adults applying this criterion were reported and 95% of the patients had higher scores post-operatively when comparing pre- and post-operative scores in the implanted ear; this was taken as evidence that the new selection criteria were appropriate.

A similar approach is described by Blamey and Sarant (2002). They used a combination of speech perception scores with spoken language measures to develop a criterion for estimating the probability that a child would perform better with an implant than with a hearing aid; the data used came from a group of 50 children with implants and 43 children using hearing aids. They point out, quite rightly, how difficult it is to predict the eventual outcomes of cochlear implants in children and how much the distribution of scores for paediatric implant and hearing aid users overlap; any such analysis will inevitably include much unpredictable variability.

This method of developing selection criteria for cochlear implantation has the great advantage of being evidence-based, but is of course by no means foolproof; Dowell et al. (2004) do emphasize that, in order for a statistical method such as they describe to be reliable, the data set used to calculate a criterion must be of adequate size and obtained from an unselected sample of implant users. Also, if the data set is large enough, it may be possible to group the implant users according to factors that are known to influence performance and so refine the selection criteria further, for example the influence of duration of pre-implant profound deafness on outcomes for adults is well documented, as already discussed. This is well illustrated in the paper by the UKCISG (2004c); they show that the odds of exceeding any particular sentence score post-implant decline rapidly with an increased duration of deafness. For example, for a duration of deafness of around 4 years the odds of exceeding a sentence score of 40% correct are 4:1; for a duration of deafness of 30 years, the odds ratio falls to 1:1, which would be considered unacceptably low for the vast majority of patients or clinicians. Thus, any method for defining a criterion for cochlear implant candidature in adults should take into account duration of deafness. To exclude this factor risks greatly weakening the usefulness of a criterion. The results reported by Dowell et al. (2004) do not take this into account. However, Summerfield and Barton (2004, personal communication) make recommendations for the criteria of candidature for cochlear implantation in adults, based on the results of the UKCISG study discussed above. In particular, they suggest that the MRC-IHR actuarial equation described in UKCISG (2004c) is used to calculate the odds of improving on a pre-operative score. This calculation takes into account both pre-operative speech recognition scores and the duration of profound deafness.

# Changing criteria and the future

As mentioned at the beginning of this chapter, outcomes of cochlear implantation have improved enormously over recent years, and the expectation of achieving open-set speech recognition post-implantation is now commonplace in adults. The expectations of great gains in speech and language development and educational achievement in implanted children are far greater now than when paediatric implants were first available. Inevitably, this has led to an almost continuous shift in selection criteria which one might expect to eventually reach an asymptote. There is, after all, no likelihood that cochlear implants will ever be considered for adults or children with only mild hearing loss. However, further gains in performance with implants, particularly in background noise, are to be expected as further improvements to various aspects of implant design are achieved, and so the evidence-based approach to defining selection criteria as exemplified by Dowell et al. (2004) could well lead to further upward shifts in criteria. Continuous collation or large amounts of outcomes data are therefore required. This will require significant collaboration between implant clinics to facilitate this process. As the pool of results from cochlear implantation continues to grow, so, it is hoped, will our understanding of the complexities of why the variability in performance is so great, and our skill in predicting results will improve.

# References

Archbold S, Lutman ME, Marshall DH (1995) Categories of auditory performance. Annals of Otology, Rhinology and Laryngology (suppl. 166): 312–14.

Blamey P, Sarant J (2002) Speech perception and language criteria for paediatric cochlear implant criteria. Audiology and Neuro-otology 7(2): 114–21.

Blamey PJ, Pyman BC, Gordon M et al. (1992) Factors predicting postoperative sentence scores in postlinguistically deaf adult cochlear implant patients. Annals of Otology, Rhinology and Laryngology 101(4): 342–8.

David EE, Ostroff JM, Shipp D et al. (2003) Speech coding strategies and revised cochlear implant candidacy: an analysis of post-implant performance. Otology and Neurotology 24(2): 228–33.

Dowell RC, Hollow R, Winton E (2004) Outcomes for cochlear implant users with significant residual hearing: implications for selection criteria in children. Archives of Otolaryngology: Head and Neck Surgery 130(5): 575–81.

Francis HW, Yeagle JD, Brightwell T et al. (2004) Central effects of residual hearing: implications for choice of ear for cochlear implantation. Laryngoscope 114(10): 1747–52.

Friedland DR, Venick HS, Niparko JK (2003) Choice of ear for cochlear implantation: the effect of history and residual hearing on predicted postoperative performance. Otology and Neurotology 24(4): 582–9.

Gantz BJ, Woodworth GG, Knutson JF et al. (1993) Mulitvariate predictors of audiological success with multi-channel cochlear implants. Annals of Otology, Rhinology and Laryngology 102: 909–16.

Geier L, Barker M, Fisher L et al. (1999) The effect of long-term deafness on speech recognition in post-lingually deafened adult Clarion cochlear implant users. Annals of Otology, Rhinology and Laryngology 108: 80–4.

Gomaa NA, Rubinstein JT, Lowder MW et al. (2003) Residual speech perception and cochlear implant performance in postlingually deafened adults. Ear and Hearing 24(6): 539–44.

Hamzavi J, Baumgartner W-D, Pok SM et al. (2003) Variables affecting speech perception in postlingually deaf adults following cochlear implantation. Acta Otolaryngologica 123: 493–8.

Kileny P, Zimmerman-Phillips S, Kemink J et al. (1991) Effects of preoperative electrical stimulability and historical factors on performance with multichannel cochlear implant. Annals of Otology, Rhinology and Laryngology 100(7): 563–8.

Knutson JF, Hinrichs JV, Tyler RS et al. (1991) Psychological predictors of audiological outcomes of multichannel cochlear implants: preliminary findings. Annals of Otology, Rhinology and Laryngology 100: 817–22.

Nadol JBJ, Young YS, Glynn RJ (1989) Survival of spiral ganglion cells in profound sensorineural hearing loss: implications for cochlear implantation. Annals of Otology, Rhinology and Laryngology 98(6): 411–16.

O'Neill C, O'Donoghue GM, Archbold SM et al. (2002) Variations in gains in auditory performance from pediatric cochlear implantation. Otology and Neuro-otology 23(1): 44–8.

Pisoni DB (2000) Cognitive factors and cochlear implants: some thoughts on perception, learning and memory in speech perception. Ear and Hearing 21(1): 70–8.

Rubinstein JT, Parkinson WS, Tyler RS et al. (1999) Residual speech recognition and cochlear implant performance: effects of implantation criteria. American Journal of Otology 20: 445–52.

Shipp DB, Nedzelski JM (1994) Prognostic value of round-window psychophysical testing with cochlear-implant candidates. Journal of Otolaryngology 23(3): 172–6.

Tait M, Lutman ME, Robinson K (2000) Preimplant measures of preverbal communicative behaviour as predictors of cochlear implant outcomes in children. Ear and Hearing 21(1): 18–24.

Tyler RS (1994) Advantages and disadvantages expected and reported by cochlear implant patients. American Journal of Otology 15(4): 523–31.

UK Cochlear Implant Study Group (2004a) Criteria of Candidacy for Unilateral Cochlear Implantation in Postlingually Deafened Adults I: Theory and Measures of Effectiveness. Ear and Hearing 25(4): 310–35.

UK Cochlear Implant Study Group (2004b) Criteria of Candidacy for Unilateral Cochlear Implantation in Postlingually Deafened Adults II: Cost-effectiveness Analysis. Ear and Hearing 25(4): 336–60.

UK Cochlear Implant Study Group (2004c) Criteria of Candidacy for Unilateral Cochlear Implantation in Postlingually Deafened Adults III: Prospective Evaluation of an Actuarial Approach to Defining a Criterion. Ear and Hearing 25(4): 361–74.

van Dijk JE, van Olphen AF, Langereis MC et al. (1999) Predictors of cochlear implant performance. Audiology 38(2): 109–16.

# CHAPTER 7

# Psychological aspects of cochlear implantation

JOHN F. KNUTSON

## Introduction

Over the two decades since cochlear implants became available as an approved clinical prosthesis, considerable evidence has demonstrated that multichannel cochlear implants can result in significant audiological and speech perception benefit in postlingually deafened adults and children with congenital or acquired deafness (Fryauf-Bertschy et al., 1992; Miyamoto et al., 1993; Gantz et al., 1994a, 1994b; Waltzman et al., 1995a, 1997). Additionally, there is evidence that cochlear implants can result in other improvements in communicative capacity, such as improved speech intelligibility (Miyamoto et al., 1997b), expressive language skills (Miyamoto et al., 1997a; Svirsky et al., 2002), and turn-taking and attentional gazing (Lutman and Tait, 1995). Going beyond speech perception and audiological measures, there is evidence that implant use can result in the ability to perceive some elements of music (e.g. Gfeller et al., 1997, 2000) and participate in musical activities (Gfeller et al., 1998b). Importantly, however, regardless of the index of benefit, adult and pediatric recipients of contemporary cochlear implants continue to evidence great variability in outcome.

The variability in outcome not only raises important theoretical and practical questions about implant design, it can occasion challenging decisions for adults who consider an implant for themselves or for parents who elect to seek an implant for a child (Kluwin and Stewart, 2000; Wever, 2002). Although the newer generations of implant designs offer considerable optimism, the identification of a need for research on variables that can predict implant outcome by the NIH Consensus Development Conference (NIH, 1995) continues to hold. The variance in outcome not only points to the need to develop strategies to predict and understand variability in outcome but also points to the need to consider indices of outcome that go beyond audiological measures. For predicting benefit and expanding outcome measures, psychological variables have been among the promising candidates.

Although the possibility of using psychological variables to predict implant benefit or to assess implant outcomes was proposed at the time clinical research with cochlear implants was in its infancy (e.g. Vega, 1977; Miller et al., 1978; Crary et al., 1982), investigations of psychological variables in implantation have played a much less salient role than the investigations of other variables. In a technologically sophisticated bio-medical field, it should not be surprising that psychological factors would be investigated less than design and technology factors. However, in some respects the limited research can be attributed, in part, to the controversy as to how psychological variables should be assessed in deaf populations (cf. McKenna, 1986, 1991; Evans, 1989; Pollard, 1996), and in part, to the difficulties in applying standardized instruments to special populations. Although some standardized psychological instruments are clearly not suit-able for use with deaf populations, it is also the case that the use of non-standardized measures can compromise replicability across sites and minimizes the likelihood of publication in archival journals. Consequently, whenever possible, there are clear advantages in the use of standardized measures for assessing psychological variables in adult and child implant recipients. There are, however, circumstances where frankly experimental procedures have provided useful information. Thus, although there is a general advantage to the use of standardized measures, less common and innovative measures may be required.

In considering either the prediction of implant benefit from psycho-logical variables or the measurement of the psychological benefit of implantation, the research literatures can be distinguished as a function of whether the samples are postlingually deafened adults or pre- and peri-lingually deafened children. Although conceptual similarities characterize the literature based on adults and children, significant methodological and population differences largely require separate considerations of adult and child samples. Consequently, this chapter is organized first to consider the role of psychological variables in the prediction of implant outcome in adults and children. Then, the chapter considers the evidence that psychological change can accompany implant use by adult and pedi-atric recipients.

# Predicting implant benefit in postlingually deafened adults

One possible psychological predictor of implant success is intelligence. The general utility of standardized intelligence tests to predict perform-ance in academic contexts and circumstances when a subject needs to learn new material provides general support for the notion that IQ tests might predict how implant recipients would learn to use the new signal and perform on speech recognition tests. Specific support for the notion that intelligence could underlie implant benefit comes from evidence that there is a trajectory of improvement that recipients display. There is also evidence that learning and formal training programs can influence performance (e.g. Gfeller et al., 2002b, 2002c), and that lexical competence is a factor in word recognition tests (e.g. Kaiser et al., 2003). Although Knutson et al. (1991a) failed to establish any link between the Wechsler Adult Intelligence Scale-Revised (WAIS-R) and implant benefit, a paper based on a sample of US veteran hospital patients reported a significant correlation between WAIS-R scores and speech perception (Waltzman et al., 1995b). Differences in findings between studies cannot be reconciled on the basis of methodological differences or implant differences. Thus, the incompatibility of these findings underscores the need for further research. It is important to note that the Knutson et al. (1991a) study included subjects with a range of close to 4 standard deviations, so the lack of correlation between IQ tests and speech recognition is not attributable to a truncated range. At the least, the inconsistencies between studies suggest caution in making assertions that intelligence tests could be useful for establishing implant candidacy.

Although the Knutson et al. (1991a) study did not establish the utility of standardized intelligence tests as a predictor of implant outcome, it did provide evidence that some more specialized cognitive abilities were predictive of the audiological outcome of implants. Based on a prospective sample of consecutively implanted recipients of multichannel devices, findings indicated that three different experimental cognitive tasks accounted for 16–30% of the variance in standardized speech recognition tests. These tasks assessed attentional processes by requiring subjects to identify features in sequentially arrayed information, and to do so rapidly. Additionally, the tasks that predicted implant outcome included a working memory component. In addition to identifying the important role of cognitive factors in implant outcome, Knutson et al. (1991a) established that a pre-implant measure of participatory compliance with healthcare regimens was predictive of audiological benefit. Perhaps the most important aspect of this research was the fact that the cognitive and compliance variables could be combined with historical, electrophysiological and demographic variables in a multivariate predictive model accounting for up to 75% of the variance in audiological implant benefit (Gantz et al., 1993a, 1993b). Such early findings suggested the importance of psychological variables in predicting implant outcomes using variables that were not statistically redundant with other readily assessed subject attributes, such as age or duration of profound deafness.

One of the better predictors of audiological benefit in the Knutson et al. (1991a) study was the Visual Monitoring Task. The task required subjects to view single numbers presented at either a 1-per-second rate or a 1-per-2-second rate. When the currently presented number, combined with the preceding two numbers, produced an even–odd–even pattern, the subject was required to strike the space bar on a PC keyboard. The obtained $d'$ VMT score reflected correct responses and correct rejections, taking into account both false positive responses and false rejections. The generality of the VMT as a predictor of implant benefit was also established in a study of music perception. Specifically, Gfeller et al. (1998a, 2002d) demonstrated that both the timbral appraisal and accurate recognition of the sounds of musical instruments by implant recipients was significantly correlated with the VMT. Importantly, speech perception scores did not correlate with the ability to correctly identify timbral differences among instruments. Thus, these findings suggest that the subject attributes measured with the VMT account for unique variance in audiological implant benefit. Extending the generality of cognitive processing as a predictor of implant benefit, the Sequence Completion Task (Simon and Kotovsky, 1963) significantly predicted timbral recognition and appraisal of musical instruments in the Gfeller et al. (2002d) study. Importantly, those cognitive measures also predicted musical listening and the enjoyment of music by implant users (Gfeller et al., 2000), and the appraisal of complex songs (Gfeller et al., 2003). Although these studies suggest the importance of cognitive abilities in determining implant benefit, they do not predict all aspects of implant outcome. For example, in a study of the recognition of familiar melodies, the cognitive measures were not effective predictors (Gfeller et al., 2002a).

The Knutson et al. (1991a) study and the studies predicting music perception established that cognitive measures effectively predict *some* audiological outcomes following implant use. In that work, the investigators had hypothesized that working memory would be among the cognitive abilities related to implant benefit. Although the VMT does include a memory component, a test of memory that was included in the protocol (Wechsler Memory Scale – WMS) did not correlate with the audiological outcome measures in the Knutson et al. (1991a) study. Thus, the Knutson et al. data raised questions about the role of memory in implant success. Owing to the verbal loading and the modifications that are necessary to use the WMS with deafened subjects, it is possible that the WMS might have been a poor measure for implant candidates. For a new experimental test of associative memory that would not be compromised by the limitations of the WMS, a nonverbal Paired Associate Test (PAT) was developed in our laboratory. The PAT presents 12 two-dimensional monochromatic geometric figures on a computer screen; each geometric figure is paired with a single number (8 numbers are associated with one figure each and 2 numbers are associated with two figures each). The subject is required to learn the number that goes with each figure. The subject determines the duration of figure presentation. Immediately following the subject's response, feedback (correct/incorrect) is given and the subject is given 8 seconds to view the figure and the correct number before the next figure is presented. The entire series of figure-number pairings is repeated 10 times.

To determine whether the PAT would be predictive of audiological benefit of implantation, it was administered presurgically to a pool of consecutively implanted recipients of a newer Continuous Interleaved Sampling (CIS) device (Clarion) and to all available subjects (n = 45) from the Knutson et al. (1991a) study who had more than 30 months' experience with their implants. Some data suggest the CIS processing might result in more rapid benefit (e.g. Battmer et al., 1995a, 1995b; Gantz et al., 1995; Tyler et al., 1996). In addition to testing the possible utility of the PAT in predicting audiological outcomes of implants, all of the psychological variables that were predictive of implant outcome in the Knutson et al. (1991a) study were administered to the CIS implant recipients. Although the PAT was administered to the Nucleus and Ineraid recipients after long-term implant use, it is unlikely that implant use would influence performance on the PAT, because it is presented visually and has no verbal content. Since the outcome of the Nucleus and Ineraid devices did not differ significantly and because no other published studies have established differences in performance between those two devices, the data from the Nucleus and Ineraid devices were combined. Scores from 24-month follow-up sessions of the Clarion subjects and the mean of all scores obtained 30 months and beyond for the Nucleus 22 and Ineraid subjects were used in the analyses.

**Table 7.1** Correlations between psychological predictors and audiological measures

| 24-month Follow-up Tests, CIS Users (n=36) | | | | | | Mean scores after 30 months of use by Nucleus 22 and Ineraid Users (n=45) | | | | |
|---|---|---|---|---|---|---|---|---|---|---|
| Psychological Predictors | NU-6 Cons. | NU-6 Sen. | NU-6 Vow. | NU-6 Words | Phon. | Cons. | Sen. | Vow. | Words | Phon. |
| Visual Monit. | .53 | .51 | .45 | .43 | .49 | .43 | .34 | .44 | .40 | .39 |
| Seq. Learn. | .40 | .43 | .44 | .38 | .35 | .53 | .41 | .56 | .39 | .40 |
| Raven's | .51 | .57 | .52 | .56 | .53 | .36 | .36 | .35 | .35 | .37 |
| PAT | .36 | .35 | .28 | .44 | .44 | .24 | 17 | .28 | .25 | .18 |
| DAS | −.13 | −.18 | −.14 | −.02 | .05 | .37 | .44 | .36 | .35 | .35 |
| HOS | .01 | .13 | .18 | .03 | .00 | .35 | .47 | .31 | .25 | .51 |

Visual Monitoring is an experimental laboratory test of attention and working memory. Seq. Learning is the Sequence Learning Test of Simon and Kotovsky (1963). Raven's is the Raven Progressive Matrices (Raven et al., 1977). The PAT is a nonverbal laboratory test of short-term associative memory. The DAS is the Dyadic Adjustment Scale (Spanier, 1976). The HOS is the Health Opinion Survey (Krantz et al., 1980).

The correlations between each of the psychological variables and the scores on five speech perception tests (administered by means of a computer-controlled laser videodisc system sound-only in a sound field at 65 dB SPL within a sound-attenuated chamber) from the Iowa Phoneme and Sentence Test (Tyler et al., 1986) are shown in Table 7.1 for the two samples. Three of the scores are derived from two open-set tests (Word and Phoneme reproduction scores NU-6 Monosyllabic Word List; word reproduction score from the Sentences Without Context Test). The consonant reproduction (Cons.) and vowel reproduction (Vow.) scores were closed-set tests. Importantly, the cognitive measures that predicted early audiological benefit (i.e. 18-month) with the Nucleus and Ineraid devices in the Knutson et al. (1991a) study also predicted long-term outcomes with those devices and 24-month outcomes with the Clarion device. Three cognitive measures all require the subject to identify targeted information in sequentially arrayed stimuli. Although the VMT and the SLT put a premium on rapid responding, the Raven's (Raven et al., 1977) does not require speed. The fact that these cognitive variables are effective predictors of audiological benefit achieved from very different implant designs is consistent with the hypothesis that some cognitive processes play a central role in determining implant benefit in adult recipients.

Although the PAT predicted some long-term speech perception scores for the Nucleus 22 and Ineraid recipients, the memory measure was considerably better predicting performance with the Clarion recipients. Thus, although the CIS processing might be superior to the early multichannel devices, its superiority did not invalidate the predictive utility of the cognitive measures. Given the probable importance of working memory in the VMT and the PAT, the findings are consistent with the theoretical model of Roennberg et al. (1998) in which working memory plays a critical role in determining how implant recipients are able to recognize the degraded language signal that is provided by the cochlear implant.

In contrast to the utility of the cognitive measures to predict speech recognition scores with all devices, the participation and compliance score (Health Opinion Survey – HOS) that had predicted early (Knutson et al., 1991a) and long-term outcomes with the Nucleus 22 and Ineraid devices did not predict outcomes for Clarion users. Moreover, for married subjects, the Dyadic Adjustment Scale (DAS) predicted mean long-term implant performance with the Ineraid and Nucleus devices but did not predict 24-month audiological performance of Clarion users. Thus, while the cognitive variables predicted outcomes for all multichannel implant designs tested in our laboratory to date, the measures related to participatory engagement and supportive relationships did not.

The parallels and differences between the two samples have important implications for using psychological variables to predict speech perception in implant users. The CIS strategy seems to result in more rapid benefit than the earlier multichannel devices (Battmer et al., 1995a; Gantz et al., 1995) and so it is not surprising that participatory engagement (HOS) may play less of a role in implant outcome. That is, with more rapid realization of success, less effort may be required in learning to use the device. Perhaps more importantly, even if more rapid benefit is realized from CIS processing, the importance of cognitive factors in predicting audiological benefit is at least equal to that with earlier multichannel device designs. In short, for postlingually deafened adults, cognitive variables involving attention and working memory would seem to be important in maximizing benefit from contemporary implant designs, but personality and social factors may not be important. Research from other laboratories also suggests that standardized personality measures, attitude scales and aptitude tests do not predict implant benefit (van Dijk et al., 1999).

Like the findings previously reported (i.e. Knutson et al., 1991a), the longer-term audiological outcomes were not predicted by WAIS-R IQ regardless of device type. It should be noted, however, that the significant correlation between the Raven's Progressive Matrices and the audiological outcome measures could be taken as evidence of intelligence predicting implant benefit. Although the Raven's was developed to be a nonverbal measure of intelligence, it was not adopted in the protocol as a measure of intelligence. Its selection was based on the Carpenter et al. (1990) studies of eye-tracking that documented that Raven's performance reflects the identification of sequential patterns. Thus, the Raven's was included as a test of the ability to identify meaningful sequential patterns and not as an index of intelligence. Thus, it would seem that the evidence in support of using IQ to predict implant benefit is limited.

# Predicting implant use and benefit in child implant recipients

The available evidence indicates that implant benefit is achieved slowly over a long period of time and it is clear that functional experience with the implant contributes to the ultimate outcome. Whether reflected in speech perception, expressive language or speech production, the trajectory of change follows a time course that may not reach an asymptote until three or more years post-implantation (Tye-Murray et al., 1995; Kiefer et al., 1996; Miyamoto et al., 1996, 1997b: Mondain et al., 1997; Kirk et al., 2000; Tyler et al., 2000a, 2000b). The actual hours of implant use per day correlates with long-term implant benefit (Fryauf-Bertschy et al., 1997), so it is reasonable to hypothesize a causal link between experience and benefit. Thus, there is good reason to consider variables that are likely to influence hours of daily use of the implant.

Although it would also seem possible that audiological benefit could facilitate early use of the device, the time course for achieving benefit suggests that benefit-facilitated early use is improbable. That is, the time course of audiological benefit suggests that benefit-facilitated use would occur *after* a relatively long period of implant use. Thus, for prelingually deafened children, it is probable that reliable use must precede benefit. Hence, seeking psychological factors that could predict use may be important in developing models to predict benefit. The probable role of family factors in determining the use of implants and, ultimately, the audiological outcomes in children is supported by a number of different lines of evidence. For example, in a recent study based on a large sample of children implanted by age five with three or more years of active implant use, Geers et al. (2003a) note that children from smaller families, better educated families and higher socioeconomic status families evidenced greater speech perception on standardized measures. As the study was not based on a prospective sample, strong conclusions about factors that predict outcome cannot be made, but it does point to the probable role of parenting in determining implant outcome. For example, since family size per se is not likely to be an active variable determining implant outcome, it can be considered a proxy variable for family-based factors that could influence implant use. Since a simple probabilistic model would indicate that parents can provide more attention, supervision and resources to each child within smaller families relative to larger families, the Geers et al. (2003a) findings point to some parent-specific factors playing a process role in determining implant use.

### Parenting and child behavior as a predictor of implant use

For young children, the reliable use of the implant is likely to be a function of the actions of parents. The use of the implant during the initial period following connection can play a critical role in implant outcomes (Te et al., 1996). The parent plays a critical role in assuring initial use of the implant because the child does not necessarily appreciate it at first. There is evidence that some recipients cease implant use, with the rate of termination apparently greater among implanted children than among implanted adults (Rose et al., 1996; West and Stucky, 1995). Although termination of use in the context of no audiological benefit should not be surprising, some termination of use by children occurs long before maximum benefit is likely to be achieved. Additionally, some children who use implants can be characterized as unreliable users, with parents of unreliable users failing to adequately maintain the speech processor. Termination of implant use prior to asymptotic benefit or unreliable implant use occasions considerable concern because unreliable use is likely to result in limited audiological benefit.

To determine whether psychological variables could predict unreliable use or premature termination of use, Knutson et al. (2000a) analyzed a constellation of pre-implant psychological variables and implant use by 69 consecutively implanted children. The audiologists working with the children identified reliable and unreliable users. The unreliable users were those children who had either completely ceased using the implant within 12 months of implant surgery or who used the implant only at school. For unreliable subjects, implant use at school was often inconsistent, with teachers reporting poor speech processor maintenance. The unreliable users were significantly older than the reliable users (t = 2.61, p < .05).

Although age of implantation is important in determining open-set and closed-set speech perception (e.g. Harrison et al., 2001), among unreliable users in the Knutson et al. (2000a) study, intermittent use occurred shortly after connection and well before substantial benefit would be likely to be achieved. Thus, it is probable that the lack of use would affect audiological benefit rather than limited audiological benefit resulting in unreliable use.

To determine whether the reliable and unreliable users differed on psychological variables, contrasts were conducted on a set of variables selected *a priori*. Reliable users and non-reliable users did not differ on measured intelligence (mean IQ scores from the Leiter International Performance Scale (Arthur, 1949) and Hiskey-Nebraska Test of Learning Aptitude (Hiskey, 1955)). Based on the mothers' pre-implant completion of the Achenbach Child Behavior Checklist (CBC; Achenbach and Edelbrock, 1991), the group of reliable users evidenced significantly fewer externalizing behavioral problems prior to implantation. Thus, the data suggested that mothers of unreliable users reported a general pattern of difficulty with their children prior to implantation and that the difficulties primarily reflected the child externalizing problems.

Often clinicians and researchers need to gather information from parents about a range of child behaviors, including hours of daily implant use. The Parental Daily Report (PDR), a procedure pioneered by Chamberlain and Reid (1987), provides a means of gathering information that is not compromised by long-term recall. The PDR involves contacting a parent by phone on five consecutive evenings to inquire as to whether the child displayed various behaviors. To determine reliability of implant use, the PDR can be used to secure information from the parents as to the number of hours the child had worn the implant that day. Administered quarterly, a PDR assessment of hours of daily implant use can be used in tests of implant use and outcome. Using quarterly PDRs, Knutson et al. (2000a) correlated pre-implant psychological measures with hours of implant use during the first three years following implantation. Results indicated no significant correlations between hours of use and age at implantation or intelligence. From the CBC, only the correlation between hours of use and the Anxious/Depressed Scale was significant. Based on the mother's presurgical response to the Home Environment Questionnaire (HEQ, Laing and Sines, 1982), the hours of implant use were significantly and positively correlated with the Affiliation, Sociability and Social Status Scales, accounting for 16–25% of the variance. Paralleling the HEQ scales, the mothers' rating of the child's sociability on the Missouri Children's Behavior Checklist (MCBC, Sines, 1986), correlated significantly with hours of use. In short, mothers who described their children and their homes as more sociable and with more affiliation at pre-implant had children who were more reliable users during the three years following implantation. Children who used the implant less were reported by their mothers to have more symptoms of anxiety and depression than those children who used the implant routinely. In general, these findings suggest that some pre-implant child variables and characteristics of the home environment might be predictive of implant use.

The Knutson et al. (2000a) study correlated presurgical psychological measures with standardized speech perception measures at 12-, 24- and 36-month follow-ups. Standardized nonverbal tests of intelligence administered presurgically did not predict implant benefit. Similarly, there was no consistent pattern of correlations between the speech perception measures and the CBC Internalizing Scale. Although correlations between the CBC Externalizing Score and the 12-month audiological scores only approached statistical significance, all but two correlations were statistically significant at the 24- and 36-month follow-up sessions (all $r \geq 0.33$). When considered in the context of the finding that the CBC Externalizing Score was related to unreliable use, these correlations suggest children who present with externalizing behavioral problems realize less benefit from implants, even when used for up to 36 months post-implant. As non-users and unreliable users were not represented in the sample upon which the correlations were based, the findings cannot be attributed to non-users who would, of course, perform poorly. Thus, the Knutson et al. (2000a) study demonstrated that some maternal ratings of child behavior prior to implantation were predictive of hours of implant use and speech perception scores after 36 months of implant use.

Although the Knutson et al. (2000a) study failed to show a relation between presurgical nonverbal IQ and speech perception measures, more recently Geers et al. (2003a) reported that the WISC Performance IQ score predicted speech perception in children implanted by age five with several years of implant experience. Similarly, based on the same sample of subjects, Toby et al. (2003) reported that the WISC Performance IQ score predicted the speech production of the children. There are, however, methodological limitations in that research that cast doubt on whether the WISC Performance IQ score can be used presurgically to predict implant benefit. First, the sample used in the Geers et al. (2003a) and Toby et al. (2003) studies was not a prospective sample. Although the sample was very large, it is impossible to develop a predictive model without establishing a prospective random sample. Secondly, the WISC Performance score was obtained after years of implant use. In a recent study by Knutson et al. (2000b), 46% of pediatric implant recipients showed a 0.5 standard deviation increase in Performance IQ after long-term implant use. While Knutson et al. (2000b) did not report the correlations between the post-implant Performance IQ and the post-implant speech perception measures because they were not statistically significant, the absolute magnitude of the correlation approximated that of the Geers et al. (2003a) study. In short, recognizing the power difference between the two studies, it seems probable that the Geers et al. (2003a) and Toby et al. (2003) correlations are more likely to be due to improvements in Performance IQ associated with the speech and language benefits of the implant than due to the effective prediction of implant outcome with an IQ measure.

Several studies identified additional family-based factors that could play an active role in the child's adaptation to the implant, its use and the ultimate benefit that is obtained. For example, Preisler et al. (2003), using analyses of video records of interactions in the home and in the school, detail the complexity of predicting implant benefit from those observations. That study did, however, underscore the importance of the communicative interaction between the child and the parent(s) *prior* to implantation as a possible factor in implant outcome. Preisler et al. (2003) also identified patterns of conflict that could arise between parents and children in the context of implant use. Bat-Chava and Martin (2002) use qualitative methods to detail how parenting and child characteristics play a role in the sibling interactions in homes of children using implants or hearing aids. It should be noted that familial influences on implant outcome are not necessarily fixed at the time a child is implanted. For example, Paganga et al. (2001) describe an intervention that facilitated the parent–child communication among pediatric implant users. Those findings suggest the possibility of improving the home environment for implant recipients and also the prospect of experimentally testing hypotheses regarding parenting factors that could determine implant use and outcome.

Communicative effectiveness and behavior management of the child has been implicated as a factor in determining implant benefit. It is also the case that the language environment of the child could play a role in determining implant outcome. For example, Stallings et al. (2000) document that parental word familiarity was associated with the child's receptive vocabulary and their receptive and expressive language. Although such findings can be placed in the context of educational level and socioeconomic strata of the family, the aforementioned studies strongly suggest that these findings are another example of how active parental involvement and their communicative effectiveness plays a central role in determining implant outcome in children.

In view of the utility of cognitive measures in predicting implant benefit in adult users, it is not surprising that there have been efforts to determine whether some cognitive measures might play a role in the outcome of pediatric implantation. Testing young children who cannot use acoustic stimuli and who do not read or recognize standard characters occasions a great challenge for investigators attempting a downward extension of the measures used successfully with adults. For example, in an attempt to develop a measure of working memory that would be suitable for very young children, Cleary et al. (2000) attempted to use a task that required children to reproduce sequential patterns of lighted signals. Although this paradigm seemed to be an ideal test of working memory for the cochlear implant population, available data indicate it did not predict implant outcome when administered in a vision-only version. Thus, to date, investigators have not been successful in devising measures of cognitive function that are suitable for use presurgically with young pediatric implant candidates. There are, however, other data based on child implant users that strongly support the notion that working memory is an important factor in implant outcome.

In several studies David Pisoni and his colleagues (Cleary et al., 2000; Pisoni and Geers, 2000; Pisoni and Cleary, 2003), testing samples of children from different sites who were using several different implant designs, have successfully used the Digit Span test to assess working memory in children and then relate performance on that measure to speech recognition scores. Digit Span involves the presentation of a series of numbers at the rate of 1 per second. The score is the length of the string that the subject can reproduce in correct order forward (as presented) or backward (reverse sequence of presentation). Presented aurally and included as part of such standardized tests as the Wechsler Adult Intelligence Scale (WAIS) and the Wechsler Intelligence Scale for Children (WISC) as well as in laboratory tests of memory, the Digit Span is relatively easy to administer and it is generally acknowledged to be a reliable and valid test of auditory working memory. Although researchers have obtained the Digit Span scores post-implantation, there is no reason to believe that a cochlear implant would affect the short-term working memory that is assessed with that test. Thus, on the basis of the correlation between Digit Span performance and speech recognition tests, Pisoni and colleagues have concluded that working memory used to encode and manipulate the phonological representation of words is critical for implant success. In findings consistent with the Digit Span studies, Dawson et al. (2002), using subtests derived from the Kaufman Assessment Battery for Children (Kaufman and Kaufman, 1983), established short-term memory as a significant predictor of receptive language in child implant users. In short, as with data from adult users, there is considerable evidence that working memory is important in achieving implant benefit. Unfortunately, there are no available measures of short-term working memory that can be administered to young pediatric implant candidates to prospectively predict outcomes.

The adult prediction work described above also implicates the role of attention in implant benefit. Such data have not been described with pediatric implant users. It should be noted, however, that studies of attentional processes in deaf children and implant recipients have established the feasibility of assessing attention in young deaf children (e.g. Quittner et al. 1994; Mitchell and Quittner, 1996; Tharpe et al., 2002). Thus, research on a combination of attentional processes and working memory as predictors in pediatric implant outcome might be a fertile area to explore.

# Psychological consequences of implantation in adults

Although the call for research on the psychological sequelae of cochlear implants was articulated over 20 years ago (Crary et al., 1982) and reiterated more recently (Aplin, 1993), there has been relatively little published work on the psychological consequences of implant use by adults or children. One justification for implantation has been the prospect of improving the 'quality of life' of the implant recipient and so early researchers argued for the inclusion of psychological variables when evaluating the utility of implants. Such a notion is not unlike other areas of medical intervention, in which an interest in assessing the impact of the intervention on the quality of life has been manifested (cf. De Bruin et al., 1992; Frisch et al., 1992) and where quality of life is central to cost-benefit assessments (Summerfield and Marshall, 1995; Summerfield et al., 1995; Wyatt et al., 1995).

Research on the psychological status of deafened adults (e.g. Thomas, 1984; Knutson and Lansing, 1990) can provide a framework for selecting target domains when attempting to determine the psychological consequences of implantation. These domains include depression, loneliness, social anxiety, social isolation and suspiciousness (see Mykelbust, 1966; Rosen, 1979; Thomas, 1984; Cowie and Douglas-Cowie, 1992). Importantly, even when those domains are selected, the empirical evidence regarding the psychological outcome of implantation in adults can be viewed as somewhat mixed. Some studies (e.g. Crary et al., 1982; Miller et al., 1978), which included subjects receiving the less effective single-channel devices, do not report positive findings. Other studies report somewhat mixed psychological outcomes (e.g. Haas, 1990). More positive reports, however, have emerged, based on standardized and nonstandardized measures of psychological function. Knutson et al. (1991b) and Spitzer et al. (1992) report positive outcomes in the areas of affective state (e.g. depression, anxiety). Faber and Grontred (2000) report improved indices of quality of life that included improved communication and familial function. Using the *Communication Profile for the Hearing Impaired*, Binzer (2000) reports significant improvements in the Personal Adjustment Scale after only three months of implant use. Since the combined Personal Adjustment scales are highly correlated with indices of social introversion, loneliness, depression and social anxiety (see Knutson and Lansing, 1990), the Binzer study can be seen as largely consistent with the Knutson et al. (1991b) and Spitzer et al. (1992) studies.

Based on users with at least 54 months of implant use, a study by Knutson et al. (1998) established the sustained psychosocial benefits that accompany multichannel implant use in postlingually deafened adults. In that study, reductions in social anxiety, social isolation and loneliness were reported for long-term implant users who completed annual assessments with standardized measures of known reliability and validity. Although statistically significant and clinically meaningful reductions in loneliness and social anxiety were achieved, mean scores indicated that cochlear implant recipients continued to evidence significant loneliness and social anxiety after extended implant use. Those findings were essentially replicated using the Nottingham Health Profile in a sample of Finnish implant recipients, where elevated loneliness persisted after long-term implant use (Karinen et al., 2001).

One important point that emerged from the Knutson et al. (1998) study is the relatively long period of time required before statistically significant changes were detected in social behaviors. Although reductions in negative mood and emotion were evidenced within a year to 18 months of implant use, reports of improvements in marital and familial relationships and assertiveness were only realized after more than four years of implant use. Such findings suggest that psychological benefit in the areas of social competence and familial interaction will require long-term follow-up protocols and that neither researchers nor clinicians can be limited to 12- or 24-month follow-ups.

Importantly, the Knutson et al. (1998) study documented that the improvements in emotional and psychosocial function that are associated with extended implant use are significantly, albeit imperfectly, correlated with indices of audiological benefit. Thus, while psychological benefits are related to audiological benefits, it is also clear that the psychological benefits are not redundant with audiological benefits. Indeed, the data reported by Knutson et al. (1998) indicate that the utility of implants can be assessed in domains outside of audiological function. Thus, a case can be made to include psychosocial outcomes of implants in efforts to establish cost-benefit analyses of cochlear implantation such as that described by Cheng et al. (2000).

## Psychological status and outcomes of child implant recipients

Like the adult literature, research on the psychological status of deaf children can guide the selection of psychological measures for use in evaluating the outcome of cochlear implants. The literature on the psychological characteristics of deaf children tends to be focused in two broad domains: (1) psychosocial competence and (2) cognitive development, including language development and academic progress. Increasingly, these domains are placed in a developmental-interactive context, which takes into account the impact of the child's sensory status at various developmental stages while the child participates in a communicative environment that has both social and educational functions (see Marschark, 1993a). Such a framework is congruent with contemporary models of development that place child behavior in a broader systems context (e.g. Cox and Paley, 1997) and supports the notion of including age-appropriate, setting-specific and interactive variables in the assessment of implant outcomes.

With respect to psychosocial competence, difficulties in communication have been shown to compromise interactions with peers and the development of interpersonal relationships (Rasing and Duker, 1992; Rasing, 1993). Thus, it is not surprising that hearing impairment has been associated with compromised social competence. Indices of compromised psychological and social competence among hearing-impaired children have included impulsivity, distractibility, social immaturity and tantrums (Meadow, 1980; Greenberg and Kusche, 1989, 1993; Watson et al., 1990; Marschark, 1993b; Quittner et al., 1994; Mitchell and Quittner, 1996). In general, the contemporary literature underscores the importance of focusing on social competence and behavioral problems as psychological outcome variables of cochlear implants. Moreover, because Levy-Schiff and Hoffman (1985) found that the degree of social competence was related to the degree of hearing loss, it is reasonable to hypothesize that the degree of improvement in social competence following implantation should co-vary, albeit not perfectly, with the degree of audiological benefit.

Evidence also exists that familial interaction can be influenced by the presence of a deaf child. Over 90% of congenitally deaf children have hearing parents. Research has indicated that hearing parents of deaf children are more likely to use directing and controlling behaviors (Brinich, 1980; Greenberg, 1980) and to rely more on physical discipline (Schlesinger and Meadow, 1972) than parents of hearing children. This pattern of greater reliance on physical discipline is also thought to be reflected in the association between physical child abuse and communication impairments (Fox et al., 1988; Knutson and Sullivan, 1993). Recently completed analog tests of disciplinary preferences indicate that mothers of child implant candidates and mothers of deaf children are more likely to endorse the use of physical discipline than mothers of normal hearing children (Knutson et al., 2004). Moreover, because familial stressors have been shown to magnify risk factors for poor adjustment (O'Grady and Metz., 1987; Abidin et al., 1992) and because the presence of a deaf child can be identified as a chronic stressor (Quittner, 1990), there is reason to hypothesize that familial adjustment and interaction could be affected by the presence of a deaf child and that implantation could influence how the family functions (See Quittner et al., 1991). Conversely, if cochlear implants affect communicative skills displayed with familiar adults (Lutman and Tait, 1995), it is reasonable to hypothesize that cochlear implants could positively influence familial interactions.

Questions have been raised regarding the degree to which child implant candidates and their parents are psychologically different than deaf children and parents who are not seeking an implant. While critics of implantation often pose such questions, the question pertains directly to the identification of domains in which psychological outcomes of pediatric implantation could be established. In one study relevant to that question, Knutson et al. (1996) determined whether implant candidates presented with significant behavioral problems by comparing them to a behaviorally deviant sample and a control sample. Parents of cochlear implant candidates were administered a number of standardized psychological tests, personality inventories and child behavior rating scales. The instruments were selected because of their widespread use in research on child behavior and their established reliability and validity. Parents completed the Minnesota Multiphasic Personality Inventory (MMPI, Hathaway and McKinley, 1943), the Home Environment Questionnaire (HEQ, Laing and Sines, 1982), the Child Behavior Checklist (CBC, Achenbach and Edelbrock, 1991) and the Missouri Child Behavior Checklist (Sines, 1986). In addition, these same instruments were administered to two comparison groups. One comparison group consisted of parents of children, matched to the cochlear implant candidates with respect to gender, age and measured IQ, who had been referred to a psychological clinic because of behavioral problems. The second group consisted of mothers of children who had been referred to the Department of Otolaryngology for services generally unrelated to hearing loss. Most importantly, on most measures, the implant candidates and their parents were more like the otolaryngological comparison group than the psychology clinic comparison group. In brief, the analyses generally supported the notion that child implant candidates and their families were *not* characterized by significant behavioral deviance and the study established the general absence of psychopathology among child implant candidates.

There were, however, several findings that suggested child implant candidates had significant *social* difficulties. On the HEQ, the mothers of the implant candidates indicated that their children experienced more rejection and inhospitable interactions outside the home than did children referred to the psychology clinic. While it might be expected that children referred for behavioral problems would be rejected in their communities, it is not obvious that deaf children would experience even greater rejection. On the CBC, social participation and social competence ratings of the implant candidates were extremely low. Thus, although the implant candidates were not evidencing psychopathology, they were experiencing difficulties in social interactions with their peers. Such findings point to improved social function as a possible psychological outcome measure of implant success.

Interparent consistency is important in discipline and supervision, and another potentially important finding reported by Knutson et al. (1996) related to the degree of agreement between mothers and fathers. When the responses of mothers and fathers were compared on the various scales, there were greater discrepancies between the reports of mothers and fathers from the implant group than between mothers and fathers in the other groups. Indeed, Knutson et al. (1996) report that there was less concordance in parental reports within the implant group than would be expected on the basis of the available literature on mother–father agreement (Christensen et al., 1992; Hinshaw et al., 1992; Greenbaum et al., 1994).

The Knutson et al. (1996) study established the lack of psychopathology among families of child implant candidates, but it did not contrast children and families who had sought an implant from those who had not sought an implant. Knutson et al. (1997a) contrasted implant candidates and their parents with a sample of deaf children and their parents who had elected not to seek a cochlear implant prior to the study or during the three years following data collection. The comparison children and their parents completed the same protocol that was completed by candidates for a cochlear implant. The results of this study were straightforward. There were no important differences between the children whose parents sought a cochlear implant and the children whose parents elected not to seek an implant on measures of intelligence, behavior and the home environment. While some statistically significant differences were detected, the absolute differences were clinically unimportant.

Although embracing a null hypothesis is not often appropriate in contemporary science, Knutson et al. (1997a) concluded that it was quite appropriate in the comparison between implant-seeking families and those who did not seek an implant. With ample power, virtually identical means on most scales, and equal variance on each of the measures, the findings strongly supported the notion that children seeking an implant and their families are not behaviorally distinguishable from families who choose not to seek an implant for a congenitally deaf child. More importantly, the Knutson et al. (1996) and Knutson et al. (1997a) studies form a basis for arguing that assessment of the psychological outcomes of implants should focus on social competence and social interactions rather than indices of psychopathology.

## Direct observational analyses of family and peer interaction

The lack of concordance between mother and father reports in the study above, as well as in other areas of psychological research, can be used to cast doubt on the veracity of parental reporting. As a result, direct observational methodologies have evolved as an important strategy for psychological assessment. Using micro- and macro-level direct observational assessments of families of child implant candidates and those of deaf children who were not implant candidates, Knutson et al. (1997b) documented the methodological feasibility of laboratory tests of family interaction with implant candidates and recipients and provided substantive information about those families.

Knutson et al. (1997b) provided data that could have direct relevance to predicting implant outcome and assessing change following implantation. One important finding was that, like the Knutson et al. (1997b) study, there were no reliable differences between the sample of consecutively referred implant candidates and the comparison sample of families of deaf children who were not implant candidates. Thus, like the studies that used psychological tests and questionnaires, the implant-seeking families were observationally similar to families who chose not to seek an implant for their child.

The Knutson et al. (1997b) study also reports findings which suggest areas of parent–child interaction that can provide a specific focus for studies of the impact of cochlear implants on familial function. When the observational data from the two samples were contrasted with a large normative sample of families, important differences were identified between families of deaf children and families without a deaf child. While differences between the samples in the overall mean rate of some behaviors were interesting (e.g. more frequent verbalizations by parents of deaf children), it was the lack of synchrony between the behavior of the parents and the behavior of the children that was most striking. Lack of synchrony refers to a circumstance where a child behavior (e.g. compliance) does not co-vary with the same parent behavior or a related behavior (physical positive). On the basis of theory and prior observational research with normative samples, it is possible to identify child and parent behaviors that evidence such synchrony. Importantly, in the Knutson et al. (1997b) study, such synchrony was quite apparent in the normative families but was not apparent in the families of deaf children. As a result, Knutson et al. (1997b) suggest that patterns of increased synchrony in familial interaction might be an outcome of implant use. Data related to that hypothesis are not available, however.

In addition to detailing patterns of familial interactions, Knutson et al. (1997b) also describe observations of implant candidates and recipients interacting with hearing peers in the standardized laboratory paradigm, pioneered by Gottman (1983) and Dodge et al. (1986). This observational methodology is a well-established strategy for assessing the social competence and friendships of children of at least six years of age. In the paradigm used in Knutson et al. (1997b), two normal-hearing children engage in social play in a small room supplied with age-appropriate toys. After the two 'host' children have played for 10 minutes, the implant candidate or recipient enters the room and is introduced to the host children. The experimenter departs and the three children are given an opportunity to play. Coded video records of the play provide an assessment of the overtures the entering child makes to gain entry to the group and how they interact with age- and gender-matched peers. Moreover, it is a direct test of the challenges that deaf children and implant recipients confront when they are required to engage hearing children in a variety of contexts (e.g. Archbold et al., 2002; Spencer et al., 1994).

In the Knutson et al. (1997b) study, approximately 40% of the children at pre-implant, or after 12 months of implant use, failed to engage effectively in interaction with their peers. The social behaviors of the children who failed to enter and the children who entered less successfully were characterized by a pattern of social immaturity. Although efforts to identify variables that distinguished between the successful and unsuccessful entry was compromised by the lack of statistical power, age emerged as an important variable. That is, older children were more likely to enter than younger children. In a follow-up study, Boyd et al. (2000) report that short-term (less than 24 months) or long-term (more than 24 months) implant use was not associated with improved social competence in the peer entry task. Such findings are discouraging if enhanced social competence with hearing peers is a goal of implantation. However, Bat-Chava and Deignon (2001) provide some evidence based on qualitative and quantitative assessments that peer relationships can evidence some improvement following implantation. While these authors caution that peer communication difficulties persist post-implantation, they also note the potential benefit in peer relationships that comes with implantation.

There are additional data to indicate that psychological benefit can be associated with pediatric implantation. For example, Knutson et al. (2000b) examined changes in verbal and performance IQ (Wechsler Intelligence Scale for Children – Third Edition) and changes in internalizing and externalizing behavioral problems, as measured with the CBC administered to the mothers. Standardized speech perception scores at 12-, 24- and 36-month follow-up sessions were significantly correlated with mean verbal IQ scores. Importantly, 56% of the sample evidenced a one-half standard deviation increase in verbal IQ across the follow-up period. As previously noted, 46% evidenced a one-half standard deviation increase in performance IQ across the follow-up period. Thus, although pre-implant IQ scores were not correlated with audiological benefit, improved audiological performance was associated with improved measured intelligence. Paralleling the findings with respect to measured intelligence, audiological benefit was highly, but negatively, correlated with Externalizing and Total Problem scores at follow-up. The authors concluded that this pattern probably was an extension of the finding that parents who report externalizing problems with their children are likely to realize only modest benefit from implantation. Such findings are consistent with Robbins' (2003) recent identification of compliance and behavioral management as an important consideration for clinicians working with young implant recipients.

Although not based on a longitudinal assessment or a prospective sample, research by Geers et al. (2003b) and Nicholas and Geers (2003) provides data that are consistent with the conclusions of the Knutson et al. (2000a) study. Geers et al. (2003b), using the WISC-III Similarities subtest as an index of verbal reasoning, provide evidence that speech perception benefit was associated with improved language skills. Additionally, based on a modified index of perceived competence and social acceptance and parental ratings of emotional status, Nicholas and Geers (2003) were able to characterize their large sample of pediatric implant users as doing well psychologically.

Another factor that must be considered in psychological studies of implant outcome is the possibility that implants could have adverse psychological consequences (Vernon and Alles, 1995). There are no sys-tematic data to support the assertion that implants have pernicious effects on the lives of deaf children, but this has not prevented some critics of cochlear implants from asserting that adverse psychological sequelae will result when prelingually deafened children are implanted (Lane, 1996) or that failures and adverse consequences could be present among unstud-ied samples (Kluwin and Stewart, 2000). It is clearly true that some children and adolescents cease using the implant and can report dissatis-faction with the implant. However, such an outcome is not commensurate with evidence that implants have adverse psychological effects. Some crit-ics of implantation of prelingually deafened children have raised questions about the impact of implantation on the cultural identity of children and adolescents, but a study by Wald and Knutson (2000) indi-cated that deaf adolescents with and without implants were comparable with respect to deaf and bicultural identities. The implanted adolescents had great hearing identity, but it was not associated with problems in social adjustment or behavior. While it may be appropriate for clinicians and researchers to continue to include measures that can detect adverse effects of implantation, it is worth underscoring the fact that this author has not been able to locate any reports of adverse effects published in peer-reviewed archival journals.

## Conclusions

There are enduring gaps in our knowledge, but the existing evidence sug-gests that psychological variables, especially working memory, may be important in determining the outcome of the current generation of cochlear implants used by both postlingually deafened adults and young children. Moreover, there is also some evidence that implants can have a salutary influence on the psychological status of deafened adults and chil-dren. Still, it is important to note that the common psychosocial problems that have been associated with profound deafness are not necessarily totally resolved by successful implant use. Such an outcome would, how-ever, be an unreasonable standard to apply to any prosthesis. Regardless, it is important for clinicians working with implant recipients to recognize the limitations that exist.

### Acknowledgements

The development of this chapter was supported, in part, by a research grant awarded to Department of Otolaryngology – Head and Neck Surgery, University of Iowa (Grant Number 5 P50 DC000242) from the National Institute of Deafness and Other Communication Disorders, National Institutes of Health, in part by grant RR00059 from the General

Clinical Research Centers Program, Division of Research Resources, NCRR, NIH and, in part, by the Lions Clubs International Foundation and the Iowa Lions Foundation.

# References

Abidin RR, Jenkins CL, McGaughey MC (1992) The relationship of early family variables to children's subsequent behavioral adjustment. Journal of Clinical Child Psychology 21: 60–9.

Achenbach TM, Edelbrock C (1991) Manual for Child Behavior Checklist. Burlington, VT: University of Vermont.

Aplin YD (1993) Psychological evaluations of adults in a cochlear implant program. American Annals of the Deaf 138: 415–19.

Archbold SM, Nikolopoulos TP, Lutman ME et al. (2002) The educational settings of profoundly deaf children with cochlear implants compared with age-matched peers with hearing aids: implications for management. International Journal of Audiology 41(3): 157–61.

Arthur, G (1949) The Arthur Adaptation of the Leiter International Performance Scale. Journal of Clinical Psychology 5: 345–349.

Bat-Chava Y, Deignan E (2001) Peer relationships of children with cochlear implants. Journal of Deaf Studies and Deaf Education 6: 186–99.

Bat-Chava Y, Martin D (2002) Sibling relationships for deaf children: the impact of child and family characteristics. Rehabilitation Psychology 47: 73–91.

Battmer RD, Gnadeberg D, Allum-Mecklenburg DJ et al. (1995a) Matched-pair comparisons for adults using the Clarion or Nucleus devices. Annals of Otology, Rhinology and Laryngology 166: 251–4.

Battmer RD, Lenarz T, Allum-Mecklenburg DJ et al. (1995b) Postoperative results for adults and children implanted with the Clarion device. Annals of Otology, Rhinology and Laryngology 166: 254–5.

Binzer SJ (2000) Self-assessment with the communication profile for the hearing impaired: pre- and post-cochlear implantation. Journal of the Academy of Rehabilitative Audiology 33: 91–114.

Brinich P (1980) Childhood deafness and maternal control. Journal of Communication Disorders 13: 75–81.

Boyd RC, Knutson JF, Dahlstrom AJ (2000) Social interaction of pediatric cochlear implant recipients with age-matched peers. Annals of Otology, Rhinology and Laryngology 109: 105–9.

Carpenter PA, Just MA, Shell P (1990) What one intelligence test measures: a theoretical account of the processing in the Raven Progressive Matrices Test. Psychological Review 97: 404–31.

Chamberlain P, Reid JB (1987) Parent observation and report of child symptoms. Behavioral Assessment 9: 97–109.

Cheng AK, Rubin HR, Powe NR et al. (2000) Cost-utility analysis of the cochlear implant in children. Journal of the American Medical Association 284(7): 850–6.

Christensen A, Margolin G, Sullaway M (1992) Interparental agreement on child behavior problems. Psychological Assessment 4: 419–25.

Cleary M, Pisoni DB, Kirk KI (2000) Working memory spans as predictors of spoken word recognition and receptive vocabulary in children with cochlear implants. Volta Review 102: 259–80.

Cowie R, Douglas-Cowie E (1992) Post-lingually Acquired Deafness: Speech Deterioration and Wider Consequences. Berlin: Mouton de Gruyter.

Cox MJ, Paley B (1997) Families as systems. Annual Review of Psychology 48: 243–67.

Crary WG, Berliner KI, Wexler M et al. (1982) Psychometric studies and clinical interviews with cochlear implant patients. Annals of Otology, Rhinology and Laryngology 91: 55–81.

Dawson PW, Busby PA, McKay CM et al. (2002) Short-term auditory memory in children using cochlear implants and its relevance to receptive language. Journal of Speech, Language and Hearing Research 45: 789–801.

De Bruin AF, De Witte LP, Stevens F et al. (1992) Sickness impact profile: the state of the art of a generic functional status measure. Social Science and Medicine 35: 1003–14.

Dodge KA, Pettit GS, McClaskey CL et al. (1986) Social competence in children. Monographs of the Society for Research in Child Development 51(2, Serial No. 213).

Evans JW (1989) Thoughts on the psychosocial implications of cochlear implantation in children. In E Owens, DK Kessler (eds), Cochlear Implants in Young Deaf Children. Boston: College-Hill Press, pp. 307–14.

Faber CE, Grontved AM (2000) Cochlear implantation and change in quality of life. Acta Oto-Larynologica 120(543): 151–3.

Fox L, Long SH, Langlois A (1988) Patterns of language comprehension deficit in abused and neglected children. Journal of Speech and Hearing Disorders 53: 239–44.

Frisch MB, Cornell J, Villanueva M et al. (1992) Clinical validation of the Quality of Life Inventory: a measure of life satisfaction for use in treatment planning and outcome assessment. Psychological Assessment 4: 92–101.

Fryauf-Bertschy H, Tyler RS, Kelsay DM et al. (1992) Performance over time of congenitally deaf and postlingually deafened children using a mulitchannel cochlear implant. Journal of Speech and Hearing Research 35: 913–20.

Fryauf-Bertschy H, Tyler RS, Kelsay DM et al. (1997) Cochlear implant use by prelingually deafened children: the influences of age at implant and length of device use. Journal of Speech and Language Research 40(1): 183–99.

Gantz BJ, Woodworth G, Abbas P et al. (1993a) Multivariate predictors of audiological success with cochlear implants. Annals of Otology, Rhinology and Laryngology 102: 909–16.

Gantz GJ, Woodworth G, Knutson JF et al. (1993b) Multivariate predictors of success with cochlear implants. Advances in Oto-Rhino-Laryngology 48: 153–67.

Gantz BJ, Tyler RS, Tye-Murray N et al. (1994a) Long-term results of mulitchannel cochlear implants in congenitally deaf children. In IJ Hochmair-Desoyer, ES Hochmair (eds), Advances in Cochlear Implants. Vienna: Manz, pp. 528–33.

Gantz BJ, Tyler RS, Woodworth GG et al. (1994b) Results of multichannel cochlear implants in congenital and acquired prelingual deafness in children: five-year follow-up. The American Journal of Otology 15(2): 1–7.

Gantz BJ, Tyler RS, Woodworth GG (1995) Preliminary results with the Clarion cochlear implant in postlingually deaf adults. Annals of Otology, Rhinology and Laryngology 104: 268–9.

Geers AE, Brenner C, Davidson L (2003a) Factors associated with development of speech perception skills in children implanted by age five. Ear and Hearing 24: 24S–35S.

Geers AE, Nicholas JG, Sedey AL (2003b) Language skills of children with early cochlear implantation. Ear and Hearing 24: 46S–58S.

Gfeller K, Woodworth G, Robin DA et al. (1997) Perception of rhythmic and sequential pitch patterns by normally hearing adults and adult cochlear implant users. Ear and Hearing 18(3): 252–60.

Gfeller K, Knutson JF, Woodworth G et al. (1998a) Timbral recognition and appraisal by adult cochlear implant users and normally hearing adults. Journal of the American Academy of Audiology 9: 1–19.

Gfeller K, Witt S, Spencer LJ et al. (1998b) Musical involvement and enjoyment of children who use cochlear implants. Volta Review 100: 213–33.

Gfeller K, Christ A, Knutson JF et al. (2000) Musical backgrounds, listening habits, and aesthetic enjoyment of adult cochlear implant recipients. Journal of the American Academy of Audiology 11: 390–406.

Gfeller K, Turner C, Mehr M et al. (2002a) Recognition of familiar melodies by adult cochlear implant recipients and normal-hearing adults. Cochlear Implants International 3(1): 29–53.

Gfeller K, Witt S, Adamek M et al. (2002b) Effects of training on timbre recognition and appraisal by postlingually deafened cochlear implant recipients. Journal of the American Academy of Audiology 13(3): 132–45.

Gfeller K, Witt S, Stordahl J et al. (2002c) The effects of training on melody recognition and appraisal by adult cochlear implant recipients. Journal of the Academy of Rehabilitative Audiology 22: 115–38.

Gfeller K, Witt S, Woodworth G et al. (2002d) Effects of frequency, instrumental family and cochlear implant type of timbre recognition and appraisal. Annals of Otology, Rhinology and Laryngology 111: 349–56.

Gfeller K, Christ A, Knutson JF et al. (2003) The effects of familiarity and complexity of appraisal of complex songs by cochlear implant recipients and normal hearing adults. Journal of Music Therapy 40(2): 78–112.

Gottman JM (1983) How children become friends. Monographs of the Society for Research in Child Development 48(3, Serial No. 201).

Greenbaum PE, Decrick RF, Prange ME et al. (1994) Parent, teacher, and child ratings of problem behaviors of youngsters with serious emotional disturbances. Psychological Assessment 6: 141–8.

Greenberg MT (1980) Social interactions between deaf preschoolers and their mothers: the effects of communication method and communication competence. Developmental Psychology 16: 465–74.

Greenberg MT, Kusche CA (1989) Cognitive, personal, and social development of deaf children and adolescents. In: MC Wang, HJ Walberg, MC Reynolds (eds), The Handbook of Special Education: Research and Practice (Vols. 1–3). Oxford: Pergamon Press.

Greenberg MT, Kusche CA (1993) Promoting Social and Emotional Development in Deaf Children. Seattle: University of Washington Press.

Haas LJ (1990) Psychological safety of a multiple channel cochlear implant device. International Journal of Technology Assessment in Health Care 6: 421–9.

Harrison RV, Panasar J, El-Hakim H et al. (2001) The effects of age of cochlear implantation on research perception outcomes in prelingually deaf children. Scandinavian Audiology 30(53): 73–8.

Hathaway SR, McKinley JC (1943) Minnesota Multiphasic Personality Inventory. Minneapolis: The University of Minnesota.

Hinshaw SP, Han SS, Erhardt D et al. (1992) Internalizing and externalizing behavior problems in preschool children: correspondence among parent and teacher ratings and behavior observations. Journal of Clinical Child Psychology 21(2): 143–50.

Hiskey, HS (1955) Hiskey-Nebraska Test of Learning Aptitude. Lincoln, NE: College View Printers.

Kaiser AR, Kirk KI, Lachs L et al. (2003) Talker and lexical effects on audiovisual word recognition by adults with cochlear implants. Journal of Speech, Language and Hearing Research 46(2): 390–404.

Karinen PJ, Sorri MJ, Vaelimaa TT et al. (2001) Cochlear implant patients and quality of life. Scandinavian Audiology 30(52): 48–50.

Kaufman AS, Kaufman NL (1983) Kaufman Assessment Battery for Children (K-ABC). Circle Pine, MN: American Guidance Service.

Kiefer J, Gall V, Desloovere C et al. (1996) A follow-up study of long-term results after cochlear implantation in children and adolescents. European Archives of Oto-Rhino-Laryngology 253(3): 158–66.

Kirk KI, Miyamoto RT, Ying EA et al. (2000) Cochlear implantation in young children: effects of age at implantation and communication mode. Volta Review 102: 127–44.

Kluwin TN, Stewart DA (2000) Cochlear implants for younger children: a preliminary description of the parental decision process and outcomes. American Annals of the Deaf 145: 26–32.

Knutson JF, Sullivan PM (1993) Communicative disorders as a risk factor in abuse. Topics in Language Disorders 13: 1–14.

Knutson JF, Lansing CR (1990) The relationship between communication problems and psychological difficulties in persons with profound acquired hearing loss. Journal of Speech and Hearing Disorders 55: 656–64.

Knutson JF, Hinrichs JV, Tyler RS et al. (1991a) Psychological predictors of audiological outcomes of multichannel cochlear implants: preliminary findings. Annals of Otology, Rhinology and Laryngology 100: 817–22.

Knutson JF, Schartz HA, Gantz BJ et al. (1991b) Psychological changes following 18 months of cochlear implant use. Annals of Otology, Rhinology and Laryngology 100: 877–82.

Knutson JF, Hinrichs JV, Gantz BJ et al. (1996) Psychological variables and cochlear implant success: implications for adolescent recipients. In PM Sullivan, PE Brookhouser (eds), Deaf Adolescents: Puzzles, Problems and Promises. Proceedings of the Fourth National Conference on the Habilitation and Rehabilitation of hearing impaired adolescents. Omaha, NE: Boys Town Press, pp. 47–67.

Knutson JF, Boyd RC, Goldman M et al. (1997a) Psychological characteristics of child cochlear implant candidates and hearing-impaired children who are not cochlear implant candidates. Ear and Hearing 18(5): 355–63.

Knutson JF, Boyd RC, Reid JB et al. (1997b) Observational assessments of the interaction of implant recipients with family and peers: preliminary findings. Otolaryngology: Head and Neck Surgery 117(3): 196–207.

Knutson JF, Murray K, Husarek S et al. (1998) Psychological change following 54 months of cochlear implant use. Ear and Hearing 19(3): 191–201.

Knutson JF, Ehlers SL, Wald RL et al. (2000a) Psychological predictors of pediatric cochlear implant use and benefit. Annals of Otology, Rhinology and Laryngology 109: 100–3.

Knutson JF, Wald RL, Ehlers SL et al. (2000b) Psychological consequences of pediatric cochlear implant use. Annals of Otology, Rhinology and Laryngology 109: 109–11.

Knutson JF, Johnson C, Sullivan PM (2004) Disciplinary choices of mothers of deaf children and mothers of normally hearing children. Child Abuse and Neglect 28: 925–37.

Krantz DS, Baum A, Wideman MV (1980) Assessment of preferences for self-treatment and information in health care. Journal of Personality and Social Psychology 39: 997–90.

Laing JA, Sines JO (1982) The Home Environment Questionnaire: an instrument for assessing several behaviorally relevant dimensions of children's environments. Journal of Pediatric Psychology 7: 425–49.

Lane H (1996) Ethical consideration of pediatric cochlear implantation. Paper presented at the Sixth Symposium on Cochlear Implants in Children, Miami, FL.

Levy-Schiff R, Hoffman MA (1985) Social behaviour of hearing-impaired and normally hearing preschoolers. British Journal of Educational Psychology 55: 111–18.

Lutman ME, Tait DM (1995) Early communicative behavior in young children receiving cochlear implants: factor analysis of turn taking and gaze orientation. Annals of Otology, Rhinology and Laryngology (suppl.) 166: 397–9.

McKenna L (1986) The psychological assessment of cochlear implant patients. British Journal of Audiology 20: 29–34.

McKenna L (1991) The assessment of psychological variables in cochlear implant patients. In H Cooper (ed.), Cochlear Implants: A practical guide. San Diego: Singular Publishing Group, Inc., pp. 125–45.

Marschark M (1993a) Origins and interactions in the social, cognitive, and language development of deaf children. In M Marschark, MD Clark (eds), Psychological Perspectives on Deafness. Hillsdale, NJ: Lawrence Erlbaum Associates, pp. 7–26.

Marschark M (1993b) Psychological Development of Deaf Children. New York: Oxford University Press.

Meadow KP (1980) Deafness and Child Development. Berkeley, CA: University of California Press.

Miller L, Duvall S, Berliner K et al. (1978) Cochlear implants: a psychological perspective. Journal of Otolaryngology Society of Australia 4: 201–3.

Mitchell TV, Quittner AL (1996) Multimethod study of attention and behavior problems in hearing-impaired children. Journal of Clinical Child Psychology 25: 83–96.

Miyamoto RT, Osberger MJ, Robbins AM et al. (1993) Prelingually deafened children's performance with the nucleus multichannel cochlear implant. American Journal of Otology 14(5): 437–45.

Miyamoto RT, Kirk KI, Robbins AM et al. (1996) Speech perception and speech production skills of children with multichannel cochlear implants. Acta Oto-Laryngologica 116(2): 240–3.

Miyamato RT, Svirsky MA, Robbins AM (1997a) Enhancement of expressive language in prelingually deaf children with cochlear implants. Acta Oto-Laryngologica 117(2): 154–7.

Miyamoto RT, Svirsky M, Kirk KI et al. (1997b) Speech intelligibility of children with multichannel cochlear implants. Annals of Otology, Rhinology and Laryngology (suppl.) 168: 35–6.

Mondain M, Sillon M, Vieu A et al. (1997) Speech perception skills and speech production intelligibility in French children with prelingual deafness and cochlear implants. Archives of Otolarynology: Head and Neck Surgery 123(2): 181–4.

Mykelbust HR (1966) The Psychology of Deafness: Sensory Deprivation, Learning and Adjustment. New York: Grune & Stratton.

National Institute of Health (1995) NIH Consensus Statement (Vol. 13, No. 2). Washington: US Government Printing Office.

Nicholas JG, Geers AE (2003) Personal, social, and family adjustment in school-aged children with a cochlear implant. Ear and Hearing 24: 69S–81S.

O'Grady D, Metz JR (1987) Resilience in children at high risk of psychological disorder. Journal of Pediatric Psychology 12: 3–23.

Paganga S, Tucker E, Harrigan S et al. (2001) Evaluating training courses for parents of children with cochlear implants. International Journal of Language and Communication Disorders 36: 517–22.

Pisoni DP, Geers A (2000) Working memory in deaf children with cochlear implants: correlations between digit span and measures of spoken language processing. Annals of Otology, Rhinology and Laryngology 109: 92–3.

Pisoni DP, Cleary M (2003) Measures of working memory span and verbal rehearsal speed in deaf children after cochlear implantation. Ear and Hearing 24: 106S–120S.

Pollard RQ Jr (1996) Conceptualizing and conducting preoperative psychological assessments of cochlear implant candidates. Journal of Deaf Studies and Deaf Education 1: 16–28.

Preisler G, Tvingstedt AL, Ahlstroem M (2003) A psychosocial follow-up study of deaf preschool children using cochlear implants. Child: Care, Health and Development 28(5): 403–18.

Quittner AL (1990) Chronic parenting stress: moderating versus mediating effects of social support. Journal of Personality and Social Psychology 59: 1266–78.

Quittner AL, Steck JT, Rouiller RL (1991) Cochlear implants of children: a study of parental stress and adjustment. The American Journal of Otology 12: 95–104.

Quittner AL, Smith LB, Osberger MJ et al. (1994) The impact of audition on the development of visual attention. Psychological Science 5(6): 347–53.

Rasing EJ (1993) Effects of a multifaceted training procedure on the social behaviors of hearing-impaired children with severe language disabilities: a replication. Journal of Applied Behavior Analysis 26(3): 405–6.

Rasing EJ, Duker PC (1992) Effects of a multifaceted training procedure on the acquisition and generalization of social behaviors in language-disabled deaf children. Journal of Applied Behavior Analysis 25(3): 723–34.

Raven JC, Court JH, Raven J (1977) Manual for Raven's Progressive Matrices and Vocabulary Scales. London: Lewis.

Robbins AM (2003) Communication intervention for infants and toddlers with cochlear implants. Topics in Language Disorders 23(1): 16–28.

Roennberg J, Andersson J, Andersson J et al. (1998) Cognition as a bridge between signal and dialogue: communication in the hearing impaired and deaf. Scandinavian Audiology 27(49): 101–8.

Rose DE, Vernon M, Pool AF (1996) Cochlear implants in prelingually deaf children. American Annals of the Deaf 141: 258–62.

Rosen JK (1979) Psychological and social aspects of the evaluation of acquired hearing impairment. Audiology 18: 238–52.

Schlesinger H, Meadow K (1972) Sound and sign: child deafness and mental health. Berkeley, CA: University of California Press.

Simon HA, Kotovsky K (1963) Human acquisition of concepts for sequential patterns. Psychological Review 70: 543–6.

Sines JO (1986) Normative Data for the Revised Missouri Children's Behavior Checklist (MCBC). Journal of Abnormal Child Psychology 14: 89–94.

Spanier GB (1976) Measuring dyadic adjustment: new scales for assessing the quality of marriage and dyads. Journal of Marriage and the Family 38: 15–28.

Spencer P, Koester LS, Meadow-Orlans K (1994) Communicative interactions of deaf and hearing children in a day care center. American Annals of the Deaf 139: 512–18.

Spitzer JB, Kessler MA, Bromberg B (1992) Longitudinal findings in quality of life and perception of handicap following cochlear implantation. Seminars in Hearing 13: 260–74.

Stallings LM, Kirk KI, Chin SB et al. (2000) Parent word familiarity and the language development of pediatric cochlear implant users. Volta Review 102: 237–58.

Summerfield AQ, Marshall DH (1995a) Preoperative predictors of outcomes from cochlear implantation in adults: performance and quality of life. Annals of Otology, Rhinology and Laryngology (suppl.) 166: 105–8.

Summerfield AQ, Marshall DH, Davis AC (1995b) Cochlear implantation: demand, costs, and utility. Annals of Otology, Rhinology and Laryngology 104(9): 245–8.

Svirsky MA, Chute PM, Green J et al. (2002) Language development in children who are prelingually deaf who have used the SPEAK or CIS stimulation strategies since initial stimulation. Volta Review 102: 199–213.

Te GO, Hamilton MJ, Rizer FM et al. (1996) Early speech changes in children with multichannel cochlear implants. Otolaryngology: Head and Neck Surgery 115: 508–12.

Tharpe AM, Ashmead DH, Rothpletz AM (2002) Visual attention in children with normal hearing, children with hearing aids, and children with cochlear implants. Journal of Speech, Language and Hearing Research 45: 403–13.

Thomas AJ (1984) Acquired hearing loss: psychological and psychosocial implications. London: Academic Press.

Toby EA, Geers AE, Brenner C et al. (2003) Factors associated with development of speech production skills in children implanted by age five. Ear and Hearing 24: 36S–46S.

Tye-Murray N, Spencer L, Gilbert-Bedia E (1995) Relationships between speech production and speech perception skills in young cochlear-implant users. Journal of the Acoustical Society of America 98: 2454–60.

Tyler RS, Preece JP, Tye-Murray N (1986) The Iowa Phoneme and Sentence Test. Iowa City: The University of Iowa

Tyler RS, Gantz BJ, Woodworth GG et al. (1996) Initial independent results with the Clarion cochlear implant. Ear and Hearing 17(6): 528–36.

Tyler RS, Kelsay DM, Teagle HF et al. (2000a) Seven-year speech perception results and the effects of age, residual hearing and pre-implant speech perception in prelingually deaf children using the Nucleus and Clarion cochlear implants. Advances in Oto-Rhino-Laryngology 57: 305–10.

Tyler RS, Teagle HF, Kelsay DM et al. (2000b) Speech perception by prelingually deaf children after six years of cochlear implant use: effects of age at implantation. Annals of Otology, Rhinology and Laryngology 185: 82–4.

van Dijk JE, van Olphen AF, Langereis MC et al. (1999) Predictors of cochlear implant performance. Audiology 38: 109–16.

Vega A (1977) Present neuropsychological status of subjects implanted with auditory prostheses. Annals of Otology, Rhinology and Laryngology 86(suppl. 38): 57–60.

Vernon M, Alles CD (1995) Issues in the use of cochlear implants with prelingually deaf children. American Annals of the Deaf 139(5): 485–92.

Wald R, Knutson JF (2000) Deaf culture identity of adolescents with and without cochlear implants. Annals of Otology, Rhinology and Laryngology 109 (12, Part 2): 87–9.

Waltzman SB, Cohen N, Shapiro W (1995a) Effects of cochlear implantation on the young deaf child. Advances in Oto-Rhino-Laryngology 50: 125–8.

Waltzman SB, Fisher SG, Niparko JK et al. (1995b) Predictors of postoperative performance with cochlear implants. Annals of Otology, Rhinology and Laryngology (suppl.) 165: 15–18.

Waltzman SB, Cohen NL, Gomolin RH et al. (1997) Open-set speech perception in congenitally deaf children using cochlear implants. American Journal of Otology 18(3): 342–9.

Watson SM, Henggeler SW, Whelan JP (1990) Family functioning and the social adaptation of hearing impaired youths. Journal of Abnormal Psychology 18: 143–63.

West RE, Stucky J (1995) Cochlear implantation outcomes: experience with the Nucleus 22 implant. Annals of Otology, Rhinology and Laryngology 166: 447–9.

Wever CC (2002) Parenting deaf children in the era of cochlear implantation: a narrative-ethical analysis. Nijmegen, The Netherlands: thesis, University of Nijmegen.

Wyatt JR, Niparko JK, Rothman ML et al. (1995) Cost-effectiveness of the multi-channel cochlear implant. Annals of Otology, Rhinology and Laryngology 104(9): 248–50.

# CHAPTER 8

# Medical and surgical considerations

JOHN M. GRAHAM

## Introduction

Since the first edition of this book in 1991, many of the factors that had been thought to exclude patients from receiving cochlear implants are now acceptable. There are no absolute restrictions in terms of age or general health, and many of the surgical problems that may have seemed a bar to cochlear implantation in the past have now been solved.

This chapter will deal with medical considerations and then surgical ones. Children and adults will be dealt with in separate sections, since different factors seem to apply. A third section will deal with those factors that are common to both children and adults.

## Children

### Age

There seems to be no minimum age for implanting a child. For congenitally deaf children there is a period during which the audiological assessment will need to be completed before a decision about implantation is taken. Most children who currently receive implants at, say, the age of six months do so because they have been deafened by meningitis, with a risk of ossification.

### Medical conditions

Children may have to have their cochlear implant surgery postponed if they are found, on admission, to be suffering from upper respiratory infections, especially associated with fever, or other childhood illnesses that make anaesthesia inadvisable.

*Jervell and Lange-Nielsen Syndrome*

Children with this hereditary condition have a congenital sensorineural deafness caused by a potassium channel abnormality, which leads to increased levels of potassium both in the myocardium and in the cochlea. The myocardial defect leads to a prolonged QTc interval, a delay in the electrical cycle of the electrocardiogram (ECG). The dangerous feature of this syndrome is that when the heart is challenged by an increase in sympathetic activity, for example during exercise or anaesthetic, it develops a particular type of ventricular tachycardia called 'Torsade des Pointes' which can lead to ventricular fibrillation. Identification of this syndrome should occur during the normal investigation of any case of congenital sensorineural deafness, and diagnosed with the 12-lead ECG. It should also be suspected in any child with congenital deafness who gets drop attacks or 'fainting fits' with exercise or excited behaviour. Once identified, Jervell and Lange-Nielsen Syndrome should not give rise to problems, since treatment by beta blockade prevents problems during anaesthetic. However some children may require some form of pacing or a pacer-defibrillator.

Apart from this, there are very few general medical conditions associated with sensorineural deafness in children that make general anaesthesia hazardous. In theory, a premature baby with poor lung function and oxygen dependence could also have sensorineural deafness and need a cochlear implant. It must be stressed that, for a small child having a cochlear implant anaesthesia by an experienced paediatric anaesthetist is mandatory, together with proper paediatric nursing facilities.

*Acute Otitis Media (AOM)*

This is relatively common in children. In reported series, however, this does not seem to be associated with a risk of infection of the device itself. There is anecdotal evidence to suggest that the cortical mastoidectomy performed during implant surgery reduces the incidence of AOM in implanted children. The soft tissue barrier placed around the electrode array as it enters the cochleostomy has been shown experimentally (Jackler et al., 1986) and in a post-mortem study (Nadol and Eddington, 2004) to resist the invasion of the cochlea by bacteria, should AOM occur.

*Otitis media with effusion (OME)*

There is no evidence to provide clear guidance about the management of OME or glue ear when this is found in children before cochlear implant surgery. Some teams advise the insertion of a grommet in advance of cochlear implant surgery, then either leaving the grommet in place during implantation or removing it and sealing the resulting perforation. The author's own preference is to ignore the presence of OME during surgery. The risks of increased middle ear infection with the presence of OME are probably balanced by the risk of infection reaching the middle ear from the external ear through a grommet. Grommets may, however, have already been inserted earlier in children with OME to allow the cochlear implant team to more accurately assess the severity of an underlying sensorineural deafness and the child's use of hearing, once hearing aids are fitted. In theory, adenoidectomy should reduce the risk of OME but the benefit of adenoidectomy has mainly been demonstrated in children over the age of three-and-a-half. In any case, adenoidectomy would tend to delay implant surgery.

## Meningitis

This has been described in patients, including children, with cochlear implants. This does not necessarily mean that the presence of the implant has led to meningitis; in the UK series reported by Summerfield et al. (2004) no cases of meningitis were attributed to the presence of a cochlear implant. Some patients who were deafened in the first instance by meningitis had a second attack after implantation, while others were shown to have other routes of entry of the infecting organisms into the central nervous system, separate from the cochlea. In theory, however, bacteria could reach the cerebrospinal fluid (CSF) by way of the cochlea. For this reason current public health advice is for all patients to have preoperative vaccination against the common strains of pneumococcus that have been implicated in some cases of meningitis in cochlear implant users.

## Surgical considerations

### Skull thickness

It is well recognized that the thin skull of a young child may make it necessary to expose the dura while preparing the bed for the implant package. In many cases, it is possible to leave a small island of bone that can then be depressed gently after sweeping the dura away from the edge of the surrounding skull. It is also necessary to protect the dura if holes need to be drilled for retaining sutures.

If a small incision is used, there may be some difficulty exposing the area where the bed for the package must be prepared. Manual retraction is usually necessary, although the author's own scalp elevator (Obholzer and Graham, 2003, 2004) allows good direct vision while using a small incision.

Damage to the dura is possible and should a CSF leak occur (the dura seems to be more robust in a young child than it is in an elderly person) it must be properly sealed. There is also a theoretical risk of postoperative extra-dural haematoma, so haemostasis should be particularly thorough over the dura.

### Congenital malformations of the external and middle ear

Microtia is a relatively uncommon problem in cochlear implant surgery. In the foetus the external and middle ears develop at a different time from the cochlea. It is therefore relatively uncommon for microtia to be associated with a degree of sensorineural deafness profound enough for a child to need a cochlear implant. Theoretically, the most likely situations when this could occur are in Goldenhar Syndrome, Treacher Collins Syndrome and the Klippel Feil deformity (Graham et al., 2000).

In the middle ear, there is a risk of the facial nerve taking an abnormal course in cases of congenital malformation of the inner ear. This is one reason for including a CT scan in the preoperative imaging in such cases, since this shows the course of the facial nerve in the temporal bone better than an MRI scan.

## Congenital malformations of the cochlea

These range from the relatively minor widening of the vestibular aqueduct through mild Mondini malformations, with incomplete partition, to more severe Mondini malformations, common cavities, smaller, hypoplastic common cavities and total aplasia of the cochlea (Michel deformity). X-linked deformity is also of relevance in cochlear implant surgery, since it commonly gives rise to a surgical 'gusher' (see below). Congenital malformations are normally not suspected until imaging takes place and they are generally better defined by CT than by MRI. Should a malformation be identified by MRI in the first instance, this is an indication for obtaining a CT if this has not already been performed. An additional benefit of the CT, as mentioned above, is that it helps to define an abnormal course of the facial nerve.

An abnormally wide vestibular aqueduct (WVA) may be linked to Pendred's Syndrome (Phelps et al., 1998) and the child should be referred to an appropriate paediatrician when WVA is identified on CT or MRI.

The relevance of these malformations to cochlear implantation consists of the following factors:

(a) 'Surgical gusher'. In a proportion of all the malformations described above (apart from the aplastic cochlea), performing a cochleostomy releases a gush of clear fluid that continues to pour out of the cochleostomy for a considerable time. It is likely that in all these cases, including the WVA, a gusher is the result of an abnormal communication between the perilymph in the cochlear vestibule and CSF in the internal auditory canal. In some cases, this defect can be identified by imaging, and in other cases the defect is likely to be present but too small to be detectable by current imaging techniques. There does not seem to be a consistent relationship between the severity of the congenital malformation and the presence or absence of a gusher (Graham et al., 2000). Gushers have been reported to be either present or absent in all degrees of congenital malformation. In the X-linked deformity, however, gushers are generally present; historically, this accounts for the loss of all hearing when surgeons attempted to perform stapedectomy in children with the fixed stapes that is part of the X-linked deformity. In a small proportion of cases of cochlear malformation, a spontaneous gusher may have been present before surgery, with perilymph and CSF entering the middle ear through a defect in the footplate of the stapes, through a patent *fissula ante fenestram*, or other abnormal communications between the cochlea and the middle ear. In some cases this problem may have been dealt with already, either by sealing the gusher or, in some cases, by obliteration of the middle ear and mastoid with lateral closure of the external ear canal. It will then be up to the surgeon to work out a way of gaining access to the cochlea, taking into account the particular circumstances of the individual case. The detailed surgical management of cases of congenital malformation is dealt with in Chapter 10. A few general principles will, however, be included in this discussion. The author's own strategy for dealing with a gusher is as follows.

- Tilt the head of the operating table upwards to reduce the pressure of CSF.
- Perform a cochleostomy that is approximately twice the diameter of the electrode array to be used.
- Prevent the middle ear filling with fluid, and so help the insertion of the electrode, by placing the sucker tip on the rim of the cochleostomy.
- Having inserted the electrode, place a large plug of muscle, in several pieces if necessary, around the electrode as it passes into the cochleostomy, allowing approximately two-thirds of the bulk of this soft tissue plug to lie within the lumen of the cochlea itself. The relatively wide cochleostomy allows enough space for the muscle to lie completely surrounding the electrode array as it enters the cochlea. A further layer of muscle can be 'basted' onto the outside of the cochleostomy with or without tissue glue.
- Carefully secure the electrode cable in the attic or mastoid to eliminate the risk of the cable being pulled out of the cochlea and dislodging the soft tissue plug, with recurrence of the gusher and risk of meningitis.

(b) In cases of Mondini malformation, there may normally be enough spiral ganglion tissue in the incomplete modiolus to justify using a 'pre-coiled' electrode with inward-facing terminals. In the common cavity and in severe forms of the Mondini malformation, the neural tissue is likely to be lying on the walls of the cavity, making a straight electrode a theoretically more sensible strategy, since this is likely to expand against the walls of the cochlea once inserted; a banded electrode array may provide more certain contact between the electrode terminals and the wall of the cavity.

(c) Passage of the electrode, particularly a straight electrode, through a common cavity and into the internal auditory canal through the defect mentioned earlier has been described (Tucci et al., 1995). The electrode tip can simply pass from the cochlear vestibule into the internal auditory meatus (IAM) or a 'knuckle' of electrode-bearing cable may take the same route. One implant company has produced a straight electrode ending in a silicone extension, allowing it to be inserted as a loop and less likely to protrude into the IAM (Beltrame et al., 2000). It will therefore be up to the surgeon to weigh up the relative theoretical risks and advantages of various electrode designs. In all cases, however, a preoperative plain X-ray seems a safe strategy to adopt after the electrode has been inserted.

(d) In some cases of hypoplastic common cavity, the normal bulge of the promontory in the middle ear may be absent and the medial wall of the middle ear appears concave, making direct access to the common cavity difficult or impossible through the promontory. There is also an increased risk in such cases of the facial nerve lying below the oval window at precisely the point where a cochleostomy would normally be made. In such cases, insertion of the electrode array through the lateral semi-circular canal (the 'transmastoid' approach described by McElveen et al., 1997) is simple, since the dimensions of the canal are wide enough to admit an electrode easily. The electrode can be inserted in the normal fashion or a longer 'letter box' slot can be drilled along the axis of the lateral canal to allow an electrode, for example the extended design described by Beltrame et al. (2000), to be bent back on itself to form a loop, as described above, which can then be inserted through the fenestration in the lateral semi-circular canal towards the common cavity. This also avoids the risk of penetration into the IAM. The risk of temporary postoperative vertigo is, in the author's experience, higher with lateral semi-circular canal insertion.

(e) The outcomes after cochlear implantation in cases of congenital cochlear malformation are reported to be within the same range of outcomes achieved in children with normal-shaped cochleas (Graham et al., 2000). It is possible, however, that the mean levels of performance may be towards the lower end of this range.

## Absent or attenuated vestibulocochlear nerves

An absent or attenuated vestibulocochlear nerve commonly occurs when the internal auditory canal is abnormally narrow (less than 3 mm in diameter). However, attenuation of the nerves may also be found in the presence of a normal-sized IAM; this fact is emerging with the increasing resolution of MRI scanners. If a CT has already been performed and shows either a narrow IAM or a congenital malformation of the cochlea, MRI including parasagittal views should be mandatory. Figure 8.1 shows a sagittal oblique MRI with the normal four nerves lying in the CSF of a normal-sized internal auditory canal (IAC). As in this picture, the cochlear nerve is normally the largest of the four nerves. Figure 8.2 is an axial MRI showing the facial and vestibulocochlear nerves crossing the CSF of the cerebello-pontine angle; again, the facial nerve is relatively narrow. In

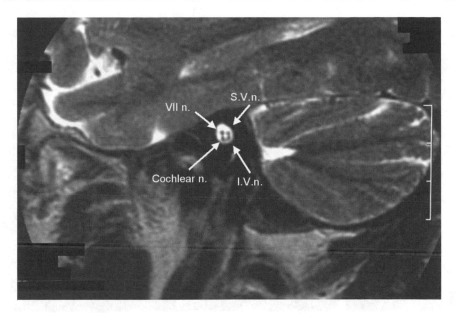

**Figure 8.1** T2 weighted sagittal oblique MRI. Normal appearance. Four nerves are clearly visible in cross section as darker 'dots' against the pale CSF in the internal auditory canal. Clockwise, from the top left, these are the facial (VII n.) nerve, the superior vestibular nerve (S.V.n.), inferior vestibular nerve (I.V.n.) and cochlear nerve.

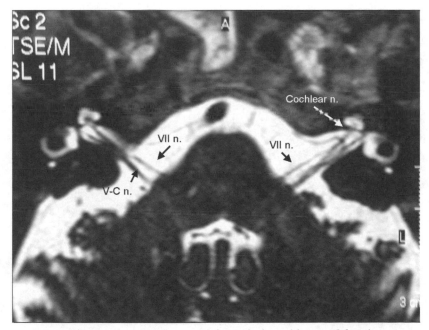

**Figure 8.2** Axial MRI, showing the normal vestibulocochlear and facial nerves crossing the CSF of the cerebellopontine angle. The vestibulocochlear nerve (V-C n) is clearly seen to be thicker than the facial nerve. A vascular loop is also seen in the left cerebellopontine angle.

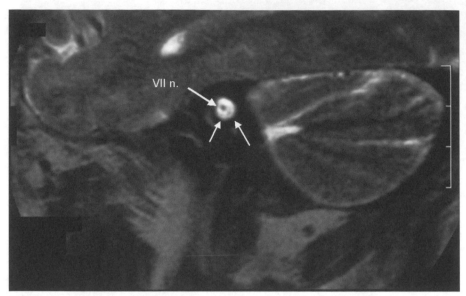

**Figure 8.3** T2 weighted sagittal oblique MRI. The IAC containing CSF is normal in width as in Figure 8.1. However, in this child, only the facial nerve is normal. Two rather thin and indistinct nerves, probably the cochlear and inferior vestibular, are seen below the facial nerve in the IAC.

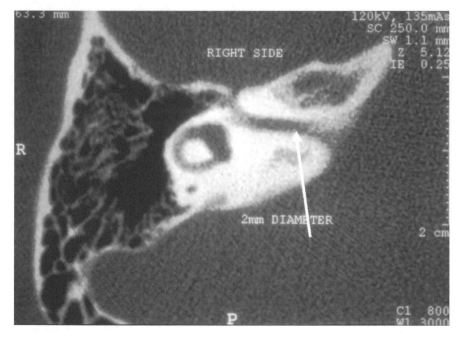

**Figure 8.4** Axial CT scan showing an abnormally narrow IAC, about 2 mm in diameter. The normal width is greater than 3 mm.

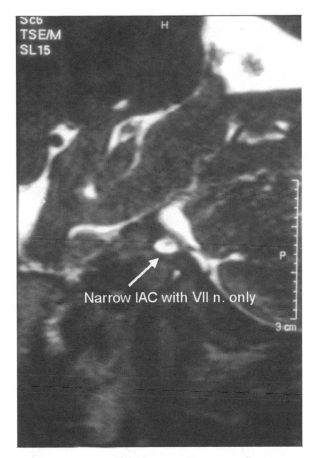

**Figure 8.5** T2 weighted sagittal oblique MRI of the IAC of the patient illustrated in Figure 8.4. The CSF-filled IAC is narrower than normal and only the facial nerve can be identified.

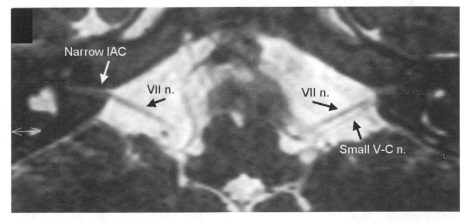

**Figure 8.6** Axial MRI of the case shown in Figures 8.4 and 8.5. Both facial nerves are clearly visible and normal. A cochleovestibular nerve, much narrower than normal, is just visible on the left side only.

Figure 8.3 the IAC is normal in width, but only the facial nerve is clearly visible, with two 'ghost-like' nerves, much thinner than normal, lying inferiorly, and probably representing the cochlear nerve and one of the vestibular branches. Figure 8.4 is a CT, showing a narrow IAC. Figure 8.5 is a sagittal oblique MRI of a narrow IAC, with only the facial nerve visible. Figure 8.6 is an axial MRI in which, in contrast to Figure 8.2, only the facial nerves are of normal size, and the right IAC can be seen to be abnormally narrow.

Cases have been reported (Jackler et al., 1987; Gray et al., 1993; Maxwell et al., 1999) in which cochlear implantation in the presence of a narrow IAM did not provide any sensation of sound for the child; these children had to be explanted. Current techniques of imaging are not sufficiently precise, however, always to allow a clear decision to be made about whether the nerves are absent or simply attenuated. At present, therefore, the most reliable way of establishing whether or not a cochlear nerve is present is by careful observation of the child's response to sound with hearing aids. If it is clear that, with the most powerful available hearing aids, the child is failing to obtain anything but vibro-tactile stimuli, then it is unlikely that any cochlear nerve fibres are present. If, however, with the imaging shown in Figures 8.3, 8.4, 8.5 and 8.6, clear aided responses to sound are present, albeit with thresholds that place the child within the criteria for a cochlear implant, then cochlear nerve tissue must be present and a cochlear implant is likely to provide a degree of benefit for that child. The outcome from the cochlear implant may, however, be less satisfactory than in a conventional case. The experience of our team (J. Bradley, personal communication of seven cases) has been that such cases show good initial responses to sound but, presumably because of the reduced amount of cochlear nerve and spiral ganglion tissue, six of these seven children seemed to 'plateau' early in their use of sound, with a corresponding limitation of their development of speech discrimination and spoken language. Such children need to be observed very carefully and, if necessary, a degree of signing input retained. An unresolved question is whether in such a child the second, contra-lateral implant could improve the outcome by doubling the amount of peripheral neural tissue serving the central auditory pathways.

## Aplasia of the cochlea (Michel deformity)

In these cases, there is clearly no likelihood that a cochlear implant would either be possible or helpful. A possible strategy is to use an auditory brainstem implant. Some early results have been published by Colletti et al. (2002).

## Postoperative factors

Although AOM does not appear to be a major problem in implanted children, episodes must be treated extremely vigorously. The policy of our programme is to instruct parents of all children who develop AOM to contact the implant team on the morning of the first working day after the attack begins, even if treatment has already been initiated by the general practitioner or emergency doctors. OME does not affect the function of the cochlear implant, but should retraction of the postero-superior quadrant of the tympanic membrane develop, it may be necessary to consider reinforcing the posterior half of the tympanic membrane with a composite cartilage graft. Where a perilymph gusher has been found at operation, there is value in obtaining a post-operative Stenver's view X-ray (see Chapter 9, Figure 9.11). This will allow the team to obtain a repeat X-ray for comparison if there is any suspicion that the electrode may partly have extruded, with the risks of the loss of the soft tissue seal and of meningitis. There are two possible strategies for assessing the depth of insertion of an electrode. A plain X-ray consisting of a reverse Stenver view should show the superior semicircular canal as a straight, vertical line, dropping at right angles to the vestibule, allowing the number of electrodes beyond this line to be considered to be inside the cochlea. Alternatively, the circular appearance of the electrode shown on a plain X-ray allows the degrees of rotation of the electrode array within the cochlea to be measured.

# Adults

### General fitness for surgery

There are relatively few cardiovascular or respiratory contra-indications for cochlear implant surgery in adults, since local anaesthetic is a perfectly feasible alternative to general anaesthetic (Toner et al., 1997). A degree of sedation, however, is necessary in performing cochlear implant surgery under local anaesthesia to alleviate the discomfort associated with having to lie on an operating table with a fixed rotation of the neck for one or more hours.

When a patient with known health problems is accepted for implantation, the surgeon or anaesthetist should contact the medical team involved for advice. In an apparently healthy patient of over 50 the author's team routinely arrange blood pressure measurement and an ECG.

Immuno-suppression, diabetes, vasculitis and other conditions that may impair normal healing or reduce the blood perfusion of the scalp over the implanted device should be detected during preoperative assessment of the patient. To this list can be added elderly patients, particularly women, with rather thin and fragile scalps. In these cases, there is an increased risk that the scalp over the implant could break down. Special care must be taken to choose an appropriate magnet for the external coil, to avoid excessive localized pressure on the scalp. In patients with this group of conditions, the surgeon may decide that a period of postoperative antibiotic cover is justified. More regular, prolonged surgical review of such cases also seems sensible.

The medical conditions of superficial siderosis (Irving and Graham, 1996) (see Chapter 9, Figure 9.8) and MELAS syndrome (Hill et al., 2001) result in deafness as well as other health problems, but should not prevent cochlear implantation.

### Patients with reduced life expectancy

The author's own view is that this is not an absolute contra-indication. There naturally needs to be sufficient time available for the patient to complete rehabilitation and to have some months of good use of the implant. This time should not be likely to be interrupted by prolonged medical treatment that would make the patient too ill to communicate, and also unable to attend rehabilitation sessions. Otherwise, the restoration of hearing for 100% of the patient's remaining lifespan seems a worthwhile goal. Where there is reasonable certainty that survival will extend for a number of months past the time when the maximum benefit from the implant should have been obtained, our team's own preference is to offer a cochlear implant but with the minimum of delay before surgery.

## Surgical, ear-related considerations

### Otitis externa

This should be cleared up before implantation because of a risk of postoperative infection. Otitis externa in patients with profound hearing loss may be related to hearing aid use. Hearing aid use may therefore need to be discontinued to allow the ears to stabilize while the patient is waiting for surgery.

### Middle ear

Previous stapedectomy is not normally a problem, although it is sensible to remove a metal prosthesis from the oval window area and, if necessary, to seal the defect in the footplate. The question of cochlear otospongiosis will be dealt with later.

### Chronic suppurative otitis media (CSOM)

Simple perforations of the tympanic membrane need to be repaired successfully before cochlear implantation can take place. In all but the most minimal of perforations it is safer to perform the myringoplasty as a separate procedure, allowing time for the new tympanic membrane to heal, rather than repairing the perforation at the time of cochlear implant surgery. Where bilateral perforations are present, these can be repaired simultaneously, breaking the normal rule, since there is no risk of causing additional sensorineural deafness.

*Active cholesteatoma and chronic middle ear and tympano-mastoid infection*

If these situations are present in an ear being considered for a cochlear implant, appropriate surgical treatment must be completed and the ear stabilized before cochlear implant surgery can go ahead. Open mastoid cavities can be dealt with in one of two ways. If the cavity is unstable, either infected or prone to regular infections, the quickest and safest strategy is to strip the cavity of its lining completely, remove all remaining air cells, obliterate the dead space with fat and perform lateral closure of the external ear canal. In the case of the dry cavity with a stable lining (this also applies to stable fenestration cavities), it may be possible to carefully elevate the lining of the cavity, insert the electrode and protect the cable with soft tissue reinforced by cartilage, possibly with an additional temporalis and pericranial flap. The use of fat alone to protect the cable carries a risk that, in time, the lining of the cavity will come to lie directly on the electrode cable, with a significant risk of exposure of the cable. When implantation takes place after a first stage in which the cavity is obliterated, with lateral closure of the external ear canal it is convenient to have left a disc of coloured silicone rubber over the promontory as a guide. Careful exploration of the cavity should take place before implantation to make sure that no epithelium has been trapped, with a risk of cholesteatoma. El-Kashan et al. (2002) suggest that leaving air, rather than fat in the cavity behind a lateral closure of the external canal, provides a natural contrast medium to detect any developing cholesteatoma.

Where there is atelectasis of the posterior quadrant of the tympanic membrane, this area can be reinforced by a composite graft of cartilage and perichondrium at the time of implantation to reduce the risk of a retraction pocket coming into contact with the cable, or deepening into the antrum. The strategy of reinforcing an atelectatic tympanic membrane with a cartilage graft is also a sensible precaution should a retraction pocket be seen to be developing at any stage after implantation.

*Acoustic neuroma*

In patients with Neurofibromatosis 2 (NF2), there may be bilateral sensorineural deafness either in the presence of untreated vestibular Schwannomas or after one or both tumours have already been removed. If bilateral tumour removal has taken place with sacrifice of the cochlear nerves, then an auditory brain stem implant is the only option available to restore hearing. If, however, the neuroma has been removed with the apparent preservation of the nerve but with a dead ear, either before or after surgery, then a conventional cochlear implant may well be effective if the nerve is truly intact. The presence of an intact nerve can be confirmed by the electrical stimulation of the cochlea, either through a promontory needle electrode or a round window electrode placed temporarily under local anaesthetic. If the nerve fibres are intact, the patient will report a sensation of sound with electrical stimulation by either of these two methods. Cases may arise in which a patient with a neuroma has a dead ear, but promontory stimulation is positive, suggesting that the deafness is cochlear rather than neural in origin. If a 'wait and see' policy is to be pursued for the neuroma, then a conventional cochlear implant will provide restoration of hearing, at least until surgery becomes advisable for the tumour, or for the indefinite future if the tumour fails to grow. The same applies if radiotherapy is to be used to treat the neuroma. In patients with NF2 regular MRI will probably be needed to monitor the behaviour of all intracerebral and upper spinal tumours. This will influence the choice of cochlear implant device to be used. The main factor is the magnet in the implant itself. There is a choice between using a magnet-free implant, with some sacrifice of stability of the external coil, using a device with a removable magnet, with the need to gain access to the magnet through the scalp (the number of times this is practical may be limited), and choosing a device that has compatibility with some strengths of MRI. Further developments in this field are likely. An editorial and two invited comments in *Cochlear Implants International* in 2001 (Hochmair et al.; Downing and Boyle, 2001; Leigh, 2001) provide an overview of the situation.

*Otospongiosis*

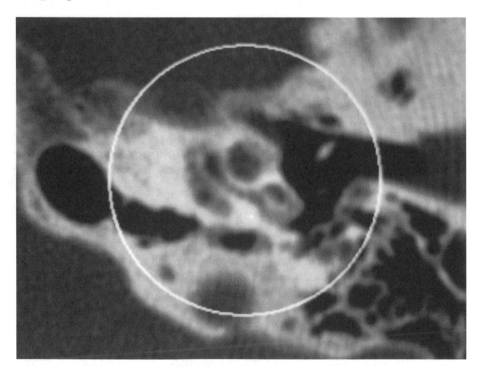

**Figure 8.7** Axial CT, showing demineralization, by otospongiosis of the temporal bone containing the cochlea making it hard to detect whether or not the cochlea is patent.

This is encountered either in patients who are known to have otosclerosis, usually with a family history of the disease, or as an unexpected finding in patients with profound progressive deafness of previously undiagnosed cause, since CT does not necessarily form part of the routine investigation of such patients. In patients with the typical CT appearance of otospongiosis (Figure 8.7) the cochlea is very poorly defined, because the demineralized bone surrounding it fails to provide the normally clear distinction between solid temporal bone and the fluid-containing spaces within it. In most cases, however, MRI will demonstrate a fully patent cochlea, and cochleostomy and insertion of the electrode array are straightforward. However, Ramsden et al. (1997) describe a case where the electrode left the lumen of the anterior end of the basal turn of the scala tympani, and entered an adjacent cystic otospongiotic space. In cases where MRI is the only form of imaging used, otospongiosis may not be recognized at all.

## Paget's disease

There has been one report of successful implantation in Paget's disease (Bacciu et al., 2004). This was of a 77- year-old man, in whom a full insertion of an electrode array was followed by excellent sentence and word recognition scores, around 100%, with no facial nerve stimulation, although there is a theoretical risk of this occurring. As in otospongiosis, the cochlea is obscured in CT scans of Paget's disease because of the diffuse changes throughout the temporal bone.

## Demineralization of the temporal bone

In otospongiosis and generalized osteoporosis, as well as in patients with old fractures of the temporal bone, the lack of electrical insulation normally provided by the solid temporal bone and presence of fluid with saline-like electrical conducting properties makes unwanted stimulation of the facial nerve more likely to occur. It is sensible to counsel patients in whom demineralization has been recognized that they may have problems with such non-auditory effects after implantation and that these effects may need to be controlled by 'turning off' some of the electrodes.

Gold et al. (1998) describe a successful attempt to treat this complication in two implanted patients with otospongiosis, by administering oral sodium fluoride. Both patients developed facial nerve stimulation from their implants at intervals of four years and two weeks respectively after switch-on. In both cases deactivation of the relevant electrodes led to a significant loss of performance. After three months of Fluoride treatment, using doses comparable to those commonly used in the treatment of otospongiosis, the facial nerve stimulation stopped, allowing the deactivated electrodes to be reintroduced. In one patient the problem returned on stopping therapy, and disappeared again when fluoride was reintroduced. In the other case no long-term follow-up was reported.

*Balance*

In the experience of most cochlear implant teams, it is relatively uncommon for implantation itself to provoke a severe and prolonged disorder of balance where no such disorder previously existed. It is quite common to have a temporary mild disturbance of balance, but this generally settles within two weeks of surgery. On the other hand, in patients who have had more severe problems with their balance associated with the underlying lesion that produced their deafness, the balance problem tends to persist after implantation, and the team must therefore be prepared to deal with the individual patient's balance disorder when necessary. Buchman et al. (2004) report the absence of significant changes in a subjective questionnaire (the Dizziness handicap inventory) and in dynamic posturography in a group of patients studied prospectively after unilateral cochlear implantation, in spite of reduction in response to bithermal caloric testing in two of five ears that had had caloric responses before they received an implant. The policy of the author's team is therefore not to perform caloric tests or other tests of balance routinely if the patient has no obvious derangement of their balance, but to reserve these tests for patients who have existing symptoms related to balance.

**Tinnitus**

Although there is a risk that tinnitus could be provoked by cochlear implantation, or existing tinnitus could be made worse, this is relatively rare. Quaranta et al. (2004), in a literature review, identify reports that between 66% and 86% of cochlear implant recipients had tinnitus before implantation. The presence of an implant, but without activation, is reported to produce complete suppression of tinnitus in between 4.3% and 31% of cochlear implant users and partial suppression in 33% to 54%. The reported incidence of tinnitus appearing for the first time after device insertion was between 0% and 4% in three studies, but 26% in another study of 23 patients. With the devices switched on, in 13 studies it was reported that 100%, 81%, 83%, 61%, 71%, 83%, 57%, 92%, 83%, 46%, 69% 95% and 42% of patients had partial or total suppression of their tinnitus; in two of these studies 2% and 4% of patients reported a worsening of tinnitus with their devices switched on. In two studies 42% and 71% of patients noticed a partial or total suppression of tinnitus in the ear opposite to their implanted ear. Although tinnitus does occur in congenitally deaf children, it seems commoner in those with moderate or severe levels of deafness than in the profoundly deaf (Graham, 1995). Tinnitus has not, so far, been studied systematically in congenitally deaf children with cochlear implants.

# Factors affecting children and adults

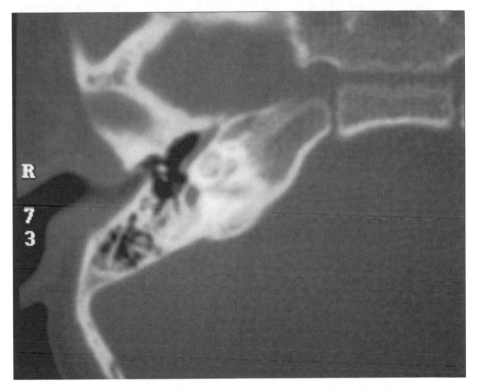

**Figure 8.8** Axial T2 weighted MRI showing obliteration of the lumen of the cochlea by osteoneogencsis from meningitis.

Obliteration of the lumen of the cochlea by osteoneogenesis (Figure 8.8) may occur after bacterial meningitis, in some cases of otosclerosis, in cases of autoimmune deafness, such as Cogan's Syndrome, after previous posterior fossa surgery, or after temporal bone fractures in which blood entered the labyrinth. Although the final stages of ossification with mineralized bone lining the cochlea are easily identified on CT, MRI is a more sensitive indicator of cochlear obstruction, particularly when the obstruction is not from mineralized mature bone. The time of onset and time course of ossification of the cochlea is extremely variable. It is important to obtain an MRI as quickly as possible should a patient with any of the above conditions be referred to a cochlear implant programme. Ossification tends to begin in the basal turn in the scala tympani since bacteria from CSF normally reach the scala tympani in the basal turn via the cochlear aqueduct.

In early cases of cochlear infiltration after meningitis, a CT may appear normal but an MRI shows a diffuse reduction in the brightness of the signal from the cochlea, either on both sides or, more easy to identify, on one side only. In Figure 8.9 the T2 weighted MRI of the right membranous labyrinth

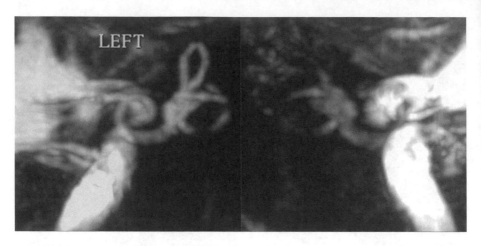

**Figure 8.9** Axial T2 weighted MRI in a teenage girl, five weeks after bacterial meningitis. The cochlea and semicircular canals on the left are normal. On the right, only a faint, ghost-like image of these structures is seen.

appears brighter than that of the left. Under these circumstances, the cochlea contains a paste-like substance which may be penetrated by a cochlear implant, particularly one which has any degree of stiffness either in its general construction or from a temporary wire stylet used during insertion. In some cases, ossification extends only along the first 3 or 4 mm of the basal turn, either partly or completely obstructing it, but with a clear cochlea if the first few millimetres of obstruction can be removed by drilling or excavation. As would be expected, in some cases the scala tympani is obstructed but the scala vestibuli is clear. In other cases ossification is more extensive, and no cochlear lumen is present. It is important for the surgeon to have a clear and up-to-date impression of the likely state of the cochlea from MRI, and to be familiar with a repertoire both of strategies and of electrodes. The strategy will range from insertion of the electrode through the paste-like material that is found in the earliest stages of ossification, to the clearing of a short obstruction occupying the first few millimetres of the scala tympani of the basal turn, to scala vestibuli insertion, and to more radical surgical approaches such as that described by Bredberg et al. (1997) for a split electrode array in the presence of extensive ossification. Further details of these techniques will be found in the chapter on surgery for cochlear implants. It must be stressed that a preoperative MRI is mandatory in such cases.

## Conclusion

This chapter has attempted to cover a range of medical and surgical considerations that might have a bearing on the selection of a patient for implantation and the selection of surgical strategies, medical management and device selection. In the 13 years since the first edition of this book, decision-making in many of these areas has become more straightforward, especially for an experienced cochlear implant team. It must be stressed, however, that in this field many of the conditions described remain relatively uncommon. Randomized controlled trials are unlikely to be available in the field of selection of patients for implantation, and much of the data presently available about outcomes in uncommon conditions arise from rather small series. In complex cases, therefore, there is still a need for better-informed decisions in individual patients. This can only be provided by the continuing collaboration and pooling of information between implant programmes.

## Acknowledgements

I am most grateful to Debbie Sadd, who kindly typed the manuscript, to Dr Tim Beale, consultant radiologist at the Royal National Throat, Nose and Ear Hospital, for advice on a number of radiology questions and for kindly providing most of the illustrations, also to the Cochlear Implant Team at the Royal National Throat, Nose and Ear Hospital for help and advice in preparing this chapter.

# References

Bacciu A, Pasanisi E, Vincenti V et al. (2004) Paget's disease and cochlear implantation. Journal of Laryngology and Otology 118: 810–13.

Beltrame MA, Bonfioli F, Frau GN (2000) Cochlear implant in inner ear malformation: double posterior labyrinthotomy approach to common cavity. Advances in Otorhinolaryngology 57: 113–19.

Bredberg G, Lindstrom B, Lopponen H et al. (1997) Electrodes for ossified cochleas. American Journal of Otology 18: 42–3.

Buchman CA, Joy J, Hodges A et al. (2004) Vestibular effects of cochlear implantation. Laryngoscope 114 (October 2004 supplement): 1–10.

Colletti V, Carner M, Fiorini F et al. (2002) Hearing restoration with auditory brainstem implant in three children with cochlear nerve aplasia. Otology and Neurotology 23: 682–93.

Downing M, Boyle P (2001) Comment. Cochlear Implants International 2(2): 111–13.

El-Kashlan HK, Arts HA, Telian SA (2002) Cochlear implantation in chronic suppurative otitis media. Otology and Neurotology 23: 53–5.

Gold SR, Miller V, Kamerer DB et al. (1998) Fluoride treatment for facial nerve stimulation caused by cochlear implants in otosclerosis. Otolaryngology, Head and Neck Surgery 119(5): 521–3.

Graham JM (1995) Tinnitus in children with hearing loss. In JA Vernon, AR Møller (eds), Mechanisms of Tinnitus. Needham Heights MA: Allyn and Bacon, pp. 51–6.

Graham JM, Phelps PD, Michaels L (2000) Congenital malformations of the ear and cochlear implantation in children: review and temporal bone report of common cavity. Journal of Laryngology and Otology (suppl. 25): 1–14.

Gray RF, Ray J, Baguley DM et al. (1993) Cochlear implant failure due to unexpected absent eighth nerve – a cautionary tale. Journal of Otology and Laryngology 112: 646–9.

Hill D, Wintersgill S, Stott L et al. (2001) Cochlear implantation in a profoundly deaf patient with MELAS syndrome. Journal of Neurology, Neurosurgery and Psychiatry 71(2): 281.

Hochmair ES (2001) Invited editorial: MRI safety of Med-El C40/C40+ cochlear implants. Cochlear Implants International 2(2): 98–111.

Irving RM, Graham JM (1996) Cochlear implantation in superficial siderosis. Journal of Laryngology and Otology 110(12): 1151–3.

Jackler RK, O'Donoghue GM, Schindler R (1986) Strategies to protect the implanted cochlea from middle ear infection. Annals of Otology, Rhinology and Laryngology 95: 66–70.

Jackler RK, Luxford WM, House WF (1987) Sound detection with the cochlear implant in five ears of four children with congenital malformations of the cochlea. Laryngoscope 97(suppl. 4): 15–17.

Leigh R (2001) Comment. Cochlear Implants International 2(2): 113–14.

McElveen JT, Carrasco VN, Miyamoto RT (1997) Cochlear implantation in common cavity malformations using a transmastoid labyrinthotomy approach. Laryngoscope 107: 1032–6.

Maxwell AP, Mason SM, O'Donoghue GM (1999) Cochlear nerve aplasia: its importance in cochlear implantation. American Journal of Otology 20: 335–7.

Nadol JB, Eddington D (2004) Histologic evaluation of the tissue seal and biologic response around cochlear implant electrodes in the human. Otology and Neurotology 25: 257–62.

Obholzer RJ, Graham JM (2003) A novel retractor for use in cochlear implantation. Otology and Neurotology 24: 749–50.

Obholzer RJ, Graham JM (2004) Erratum: a novel retractor for use in Cochlear Implantation. Otology and Neurotology 25: 83–5.

Phelps PD, Coffey RA, Trembath RC et al. (1998) Clinical Radiology 53: 268–73.

Quaranta N, Wagstaff S, Baguley DM (2004) Tinnitus and Cochlear Implantation. International Journal of Audiology 43: 245–51.

Ramsden R, Bance M, Giles E et al. (1997) Cochlear implantation in otosclerosis: a unique positioning and programming problem. Journal of Laryngology and Otology 111: 262–5.

Summerfield AQ, Cirstea SE, Roberts KL et al. (2005) Incidence of meningitis and of death from all causes among users of cochlear implants in the United Kingdom. Journal of Public Health 27(1): 55–61.

Toner JG, John G, McNaboe EJ (1997) Cochlear implantation under local anaesthesia: the Belfast experience. Journal of Laryngology and Otology 112: 533–6.

Tucci DL, Telian SA, Zimmerman-Phillips S et al. (1995) Cochlear implantation in patients with cochlear malformations. Archives of Otolaryngology: Head and Neck Surgery 121: 833–8.

# CHAPTER 9

# Radiological evaluation in cochlear implantation

COLIN L.W. DRISCOLL AND MICHAEL B. GLUTH

Modern radiological imaging techniques provide members of the cochlear implant team information that may be critical to proper implant candidate selection, surgical implantation and continued device function. Accordingly, it is important to be familiar with all current imaging modalities as they pertain to various preoperative, intraoperative and postoperative clinical scenarios (Marsot-Dupuch and Meyer, 2001; Witte et al., 2003).

## Preoperative assessment

An in-depth radiological evaluation is necessary prior to declaring any person a suitable candidate for cochlear implantation. Not only will a proper preoperative radiological evaluation identify patients with anatomic contraindications to implantation, but also it will aid in identifying certain anatomical features that have consequences in selecting the specific device and which ear is more appropriate for surgery. Furthermore, preoperative imaging may also allow the surgical team to anticipate aberrant anatomy and thus reduce the risk of surgical complications.

Preoperative imaging will ideally address several basic anatomical considerations.

### 1. Mastoid and middle ear

An assessment of the degree of mastoid pneumatization can help predict the ease of the surgical approach. A low-lying tegmen or otherwise sclerotic and contracted mastoid cavity might result in a higher risk of injury to adjacent structures. Further consideration should be given as to the presence of mastoid inflammation or cholesteatoma. When present, implantation is ideally delayed until after these conditions are dealt with in the conventional manner. Some patients have had prior surgery, and imaging helps to delineate existing anatomy. Assessing for semicircular canal dehiscence, facial nerve exposure, residual disease, tegmen dehiscence, tympanic membrane retraction, presence of grafts or prosthesis is helpful in planning surgery.

## 2. Facial nerve

The entire course of the facial nerve should be routinely evaluated for abnormal complexities. Attention to this is particularly essential when other labyrinthine anatomical anomalies are known to be present. Imaging may also identify points of nerve dehiscence.

## 3. Vascular anatomy

The orientation and course of all key vascular structures should be accounted for. These include the carotid artery, sigmoid sinus, jugular bulb, persistent stapedial artery and mastoid emmisary vein. In particular, a dehiscent jugular bulb may cause difficulty when attempting to access the usual location of electrode insertion at the promontory adjacent to the round window.

## 4. Otic capsule

The otic capsule should be inspected for evidence of abnormal bone density or other pathologic process. When present, either cochlear otosclerosis or Paget's disease may predict a higher incidence of unwanted implant electrode stimulation of the facial nerve.

## 5. Internal auditory canal (IAC)

Evaluation of the size and contents of the IAC is critical to confirm the presence of the cochlear nerve, and to rule out any other pathologic process. When the cochlear nerve is absent, cochlear implantation is contraindicated on that side. A narrowed IAC (< 3 mm) is associated with a significant risk of an underlying hypoplastic or absent cochlear nerve. With modern techniques, sagittal or oblique sagittal views will provide further details regarding the size and orientation of each nerve within the IAC.

## 6. Cochlea

The presence of a cochlea must be confirmed, since the Michel anomaly (cochlear agenesis) is a contraindication to implantation. A small modiolus (< 4 mm$^2$) should also be scrutinized and considered a risk factor for the presence of an associated absent or hypoplastic cochlear nerve.

Furthermore, a detailed inspection for evidence of cochlear ossification or membranous fibrosis is critical (Figure 9.1). This is encountered most frequently when deafness is the result of an infectious (usually meningitis) or autoimmune process. When cochlear ossification is present, the scala tympani at the basal turn is the most common site of involvement. If membranous fibrosis is evident, an attempt can be made to determine whether active inflammation and proliferation is present, thus potentially prompting heightened urgency in the timing of implantation. If the patient has some residual hearing and is undergoing a hearing aid trial, serial scans can be obtained to assess for progressive fibrosis or ossification. If ossification is noted, it may be reasonable to implant even if the opposite ear is outside typical audiometric criteria.

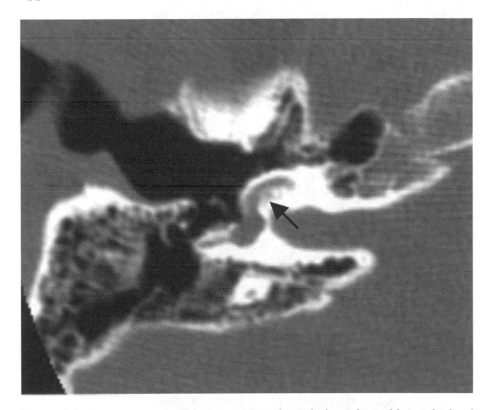

**Figure 9.1** Non-contrasted axial CT image cut through the right cochlea at the level of the basal turn demonstrates calcification and narrowing consistent with post-inflammatory changes.

## 7. Other congenital abnormalities

Various other congenital abnormalities may be present and should be accounted for. Some of the more frequently encountered anomalies are the Mondini deformity (small cochlea with reduced coiling), an enlarged vestibular aqueduct (aqueduct size measured greater than 1.5 mm in diameter) (Figures 9.2 and 9.3) or a common cavity deformity (no partition between cochlea and vestibule). The Mondini congenital labyrinthine anomalies are associated with a higher risk of intraoperative cerebrospinal fluid leak.

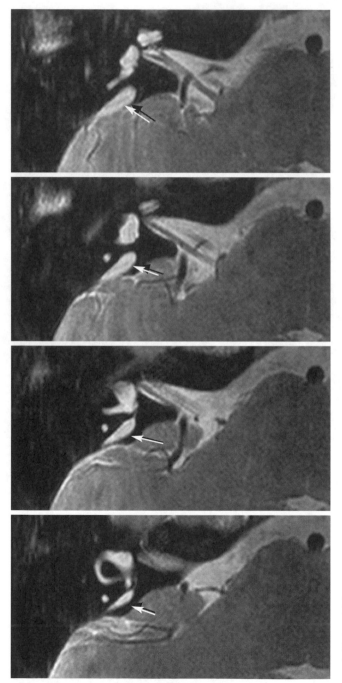

**Figure 9.2** A series of T2 weighted axial cut MRI images demonstrate an enlarged vestibular aqueduct (white arrows).

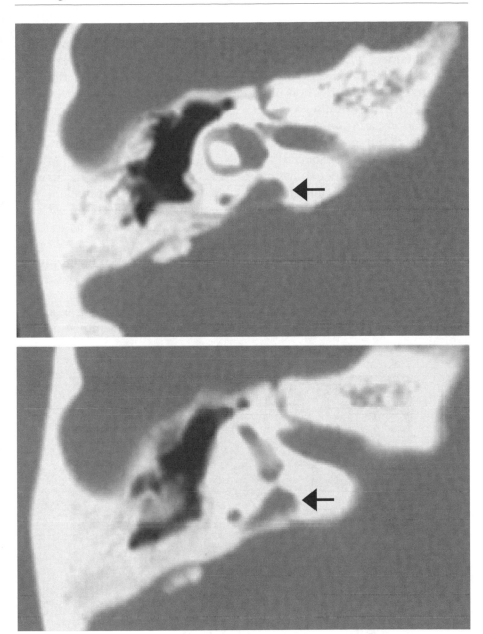

**Figure 9.3** Axial-cut CT images reveal an enlarged vestibular aqueduct (black arrows).

## Computed tomography (CT)

High-resolution thin-section computed tomography (HRCT) has been widely accepted as the imaging modality of choice for preoperative radiological assessment of cochlear implant candidates for many years. Many clinicians use HRCT as the first-line (and often the only) radiological

assessment in the preoperative evaluation. Modern HRCT affords evaluation in fine detail of most of the pertinent temporal bone anatomy and is
often obtained with relative ease at an acceptable financial expense.
Generally, axial sections 0.5–1.0 mm in thickness with bone window settings are most helpful. When obtained, axial orientation may be set in an
angled plane to avoid the ocular lenses so that potential long-term visual
complications are minimized. Intravenous contrast agents are generally
not utilized but may be beneficial if retrocochlear disease such as an
acoustic neuroma is suspected and/or the patient cannot tolerate MRI.

HRCT provides an exquisitely detailed image of all bony anatomy
including the mastoid, middle ear, cochlea, tegmen, otic capsule and pertinent vascular structures. Accurate measurements of the bony IAC will
provide information regarding the likelihood of an underlying cochlear
nerve abnormality. Compromise of cochlear patency in the form of
labyrinthitis ossificans should be evident with HRCT, yet membranous
fibrosis may not be as reliably apparent. The course of the facial nerve,
even when complex or atypical, is usually well delineated (including evidence of dehiscence). Furthermore, vascular anomalies such as a high
jugular bulb or aberrant carotid artery are usually clearly demonstrated by
HRCT.

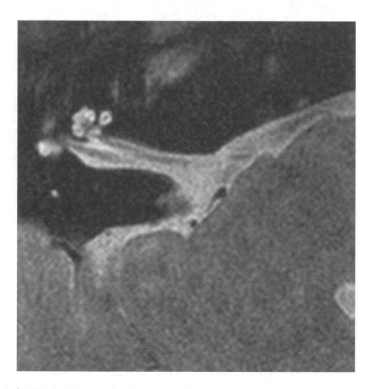

**Figure 9.4** 3-Tesla T2 weighted MRI axial cut through a normal IAC and cochlea
acquired using a hybrid phased array coil. Note the detailed view of the intracochlear
fluid partition as well as the signal void created by the cochlear nerve.

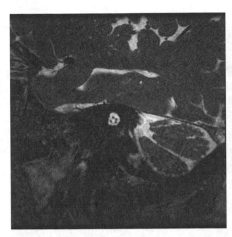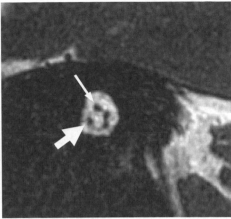

**Figure 9.5** CISS sequence MRI through the internal auditory canal demonstrating normal nerve anatomy. In the magnified image, note the cochlear nerve (large white arrow) situated in the anterior inferior quadrant. The calibre of the cochlear nerve appears roughly equivalent to that of the facial nerve (small white arrow). Also note the superior and inferior vestibular nerves in the posterior aspect of the canal.

## Magnetic resonance imaging (MRI)

MRI may currently be used to evaluate the membranous labyrinth, internal auditory canal contents and other pertinent structures of interest within the temporal bone by providing images with exceptional soft tissue detail (Figure 9.4). Recently, advances in technology pertaining to MRI have compelled some cochlear implant teams to obtain routine MRI scans on all implant candidates (Baumgartner et al., 2001; Sennaroglu et al., 2002; Gleeson et al., 2003). In fact, some centers now use MRI as the primary means of radiological assessment while reserving HRCT for those patients with congenital abnormalities and/or suspected complexities in the course of the facial nerve (Ellul et al., 2000). One advantage of MRI as compared with HRCT is a superior efficacy in identifying abnormalities in cochlear patency. In particular, fibrosis of the membranous labyrinth, not evident on HRCT, may be clearly apparent as a filling defect on T2 weighted MRI images. Multiple cases of membranous cochlear obstruction that were missed with HRCT but discovered with MRI have been reported (Klein et al., 1992; Arriaga and Carrier, 1996).

The recent availability of T2 weighted sagittal fast-spin echo (FSE) sequences and/or CISS (constructive interference of steady state) sequences also affords MRI the advantage of providing very detailed images of the IAC (Lane et al., 2004). These sequences utilize the enhancing characteristics of cerebrospinal fluid (CSF) on T2 weighted images as a functional contrast agent within the IAC. Thus, the cochlear, facial and vestibular nerves can be seen as distinct voids in CSF enhancement

(Figure 9.5). Since absent and hypoplastic cochlear nerves have been encountered in persons with normal IAC dimensions, this new technology can help avoid implanting an ear with an absent nerve or steer the implant team towards implantation on the side with a non-hypoplastic nerve (Figure 9.6). This is done by comparing the relative caliber of the cochlear nerve to that of the facial nerve. Such a consideration may be particularly important since the size of the cochlear nerve may correlate with the number of underlying spiral ganglion cells and therefore perhaps a better chance of a good hearing result. Preliminary data suggest that calculations of the ratio of cochlear nerve to facial nerve volume within the IAC might yet assist in identifying certain patients with a higher risk of a poor hearing outcome after implantation.

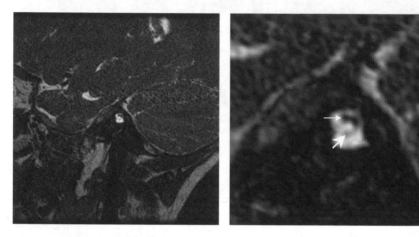

**Figure 9.6** CISS sequence MRI through the internal auditory canal. The magnified view (B) demonstrates an atretic cochlear nerve (large white arrow). Note the marked difference in size and signal void as compared to the facial nerve (small white arrow).

Finally, although there is still some debate regarding the absolute contraindication to MRI scanning after cochlear implantation, some clinicians feel that the preoperative period is the last 'best chance' to obtain detailed images of intracranial soft tissues that might provide some insight as to the underlying cause of deafness. In particular, some clinicians may desire a preoperative MRI to assess for intracanalicular pathology such as an occult vestibular schwannoma or for evidence of a pathologic process involving the central auditory pathway (Figure 9.7, 9.8 and 9.9).

Despite its recent heightened popularity, MRI scanning does have some distinct disadvantages. Most children and many adults undergoing MRI will require some level of sedation and, in many instances, general anesthesia. In contrast, nearly every patient, including children, can undergo a CT scan without sedation. Furthermore, the cost of an HRCT without contrast is significantly less than that of a head MRI with Gadolinium that includes high-resolution images through the temporal bone. Yet, when

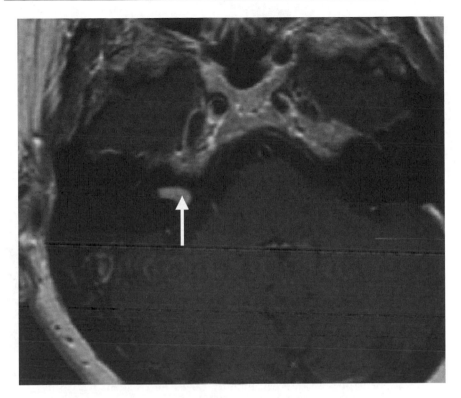

**Figure 9.7** T2 weighted axial MRI of a small intracanalicular vestibular schwannoma (white arrow) with minimal protrusion from the porus acousticus.

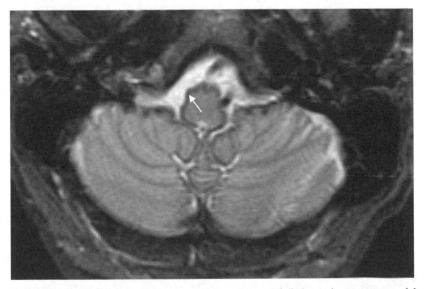

**Figure 9.8** T2 weighted axial cut MRI in a patient with bilateral sensorineural hearing loss attributed to superficial siderosis. Note the classic hypointense rim surrounding the brainstem (white arrow) and involving the cerebellar folia. This hypointensity is attributed to the ferromagnetic effect of iron-rich hemosiderin deposits.

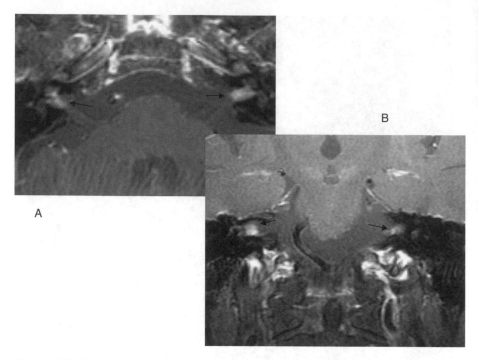

**Figure 9.9** T2 weighted axial (A) and coronal (B) MRIs demonstrate abnormal contrast enhancement in both internal auditory canals of a patient with progressive bilateral sensorineural hearing loss. This patient was found to have leptomeningeal carcinomatosis derived from a primary breast adenocarcinoma.

MRI scanning is limited to 'focused' or 'screening' fast-spin echo (FSE) or constructive interference of steady state (CISS) sequences of the temporal bone, this added cost may be minimized (Ellul et al., 2000).

Obtaining high-quality images without artifacts requires a thorough understanding of the relationship and interactions between various head coils and imaging sequences. Knowledgeable radiologists and technicians are critical to obtaining consistent, high-quality images.

**Functional MRI**

Functional MRI attempts to provide an objective assessment of neural activity within the auditory cortex during artificial electrical stimulation of the cochlea. This technique is generally performed by acquiring radiofrequency spoiled fast low-angle shot (FLASH) MRI sequences before and during transpromontory electrode stimulation of the cochlea. In theory, functional MRI may provide valuable information regarding activity along the central auditory pathway that could potentially provide prognostic information or help in selecting the ideal side for implantation (Berthezene et al., 1997). At present, the role and value of functional MRI in the preoperative assessment of cochlear implant candidates is yet undetermined.

# Intraoperative assessment

In rare cases, intraoperative assessment of the cochlear implant electrode array may be beneficial when an unpredictable pattern of electrode insertion is anticipated. Specific examples of this include cases of known severe congenital labyrinthine abnormalities or cases of extensive labyrinthitis ossificans. Also, intraoperative images may be helpful when new and/or unusual electrodes, such as those with a double array, are used. When indicated, real-time intraoperative fluoroscopy has been recommended as a safe, relatively inexpensive and easily obtainable imaging modality (Fishman et al., 2003). This is the preferred method for placing the electrode array in the case of severely malformed cochlea. Visualization during insertion will prevent placing the electrode into the internal auditory canal and allow for optimal device placement in these difficult cases (Figure 9.10).

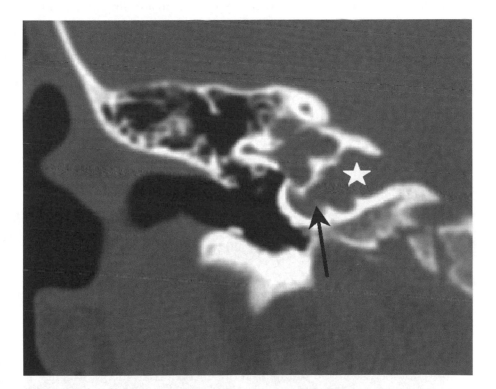

**Figure 9.10** Coronal cut CT image of a patient with a major inner ear malformation. Note the patulous communication between the cochlea (black arrow) and the internal auditory canal (star). Intraoperative fluoroscopy might be helpful during surgical implantation of a patient such as this.

# Postoperative assessment

## X-ray

Postoperative confirmation of proper electrode orientation in routine cases may be obtained with plain films. The view recommended by each implant manufacturer has some variation. The Cochlear Corporation recommends a modified Stenver's view (Fig 9.11) of the Nucleus device that will display the electrode array and petromastoid anatomy without distortion. The Stenver's view is obtained with the patient lying supine with the head slightly flexed and rotated toward the side opposite the implanted ear. The X-ray beam is angulated 15° caudad. This view affords a central ray axis that is parallel to the modiolar axis – thereby affording a view of electrode array that does not overlap itself. The Advanced Bionics Corporation advises the acquisition of a simple anterior-posterior projection (Figure 9.12). The Med-El Corporation does not have specific recommendations, yet it has been shown that the Stenver's view is most helpful in assessing the degree of electrode insertion with the Combi 40+ electrode array (Wendell and Ball, 2004). Precise positioning in the immediate postoperative period may not be possible due to pain and mental status changes associated with emergence from anesthesia.

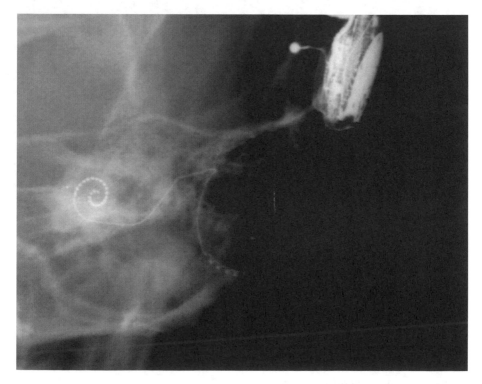

**Figure 9.11** Postoperative Stenver's view X-ray of the Nucleus Contour device electrode array.

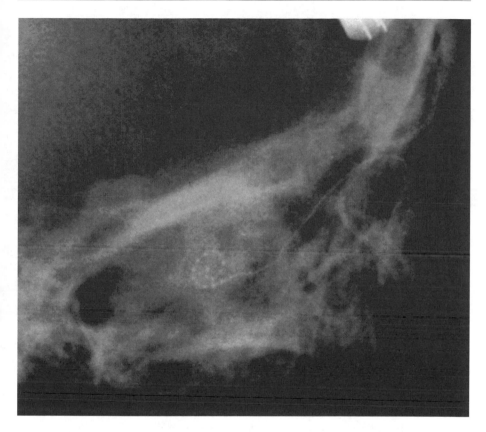

**Figure 9.12** Postoperative anterior-posterior X-ray projection of a Clarion CII device electrode array.

## CT

In the case of suspected postoperative complication such as electrode migration or infection, CT is the imaging modality of choice (Jain and Mukherji, 2003). Although some degree of signal distortion from the metal will be present, CT generally gives a clear view of the electrode array and adjacent temporal bone anatomy (Figure 9.13). When infection or other inflammatory complication is suspected, the addition of an intra venous contrast agent may provide benefit.

## MRI

In general, the presence of a cochlear implant has been considered a contraindication to MRI scanning. Multiple studies to evaluate the risk of obtaining MRI scans of cochlear implant recipients have been undertaken with somewhat consistent results that imply a very low risk of complications (Teissl et al., 1999; Schmerber et al., 2003). In general, the chief concern has pertained to the presence of the in-dwelling magnet that is

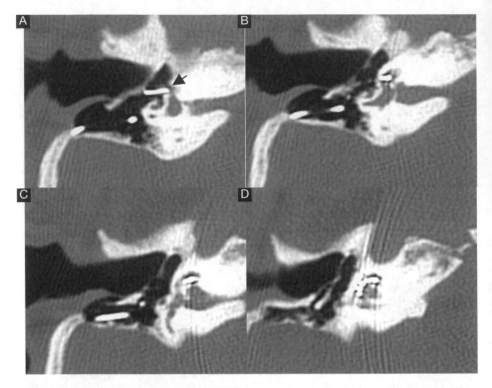

**Figure 9.13** Axial non-contrasted CT image series exhibits the entrance (A) of the electrode array through the cochleostomy site (black arrow) into the cochlea at the basal turn. (B, C, D) The electrode courses through the cochlea within the scala tympani in the proper position. Some metallic signal artifact is noted.

used to hold the external transmitting coil over the internal receiver stimulator. The potential for movement of this magnet and theoretic risk of complications has led implant manufactures to design newer hardware having magnets that can be removed with a simple surgical procedure. Yet, for those patients with implants that do not have removable magnets, the actual risk of complications is questionable. Case series have been published that describe the safe acquisition of MRI scans in implant recipients involving most implant designs at 1.0 T and 1.5 T without device malfunction, migration or heating. Furthermore, biophysical studies of MRI/cochlear implant magnet interactions as they relate to adjacent implant bed anatomy suggest that 1.5 T MRI is not capable of creating sufficient force to fracture surrounding bone or otherwise displace a cochlear implant (Sonnenburg et al., 2002). Accordingly, if a sound medical indication is present, an MRI scan can be obtained with a reasonable expectation of safety. Yet, with a theoretic risk present, routine MRI scanning might be best withheld.

If an implanted patient is to undergo MRI scanning, it is important to follow current recommendations for scanning technique. The device will create a shadow and image distortion (Figure 9.14). Altering the standard pulse sequences can reduce the extent of shadow dramatically. Factors to consider include magnet strength, patient positioning, length of time since surgery, presence or absence of bone between device and dura and presence of tie-down suture. An adult with a secured device, thick bone under the device and placed in the proper position during scanning would present a very low risk of complication. A child that has a device recessed to the dura may be at greater risk.

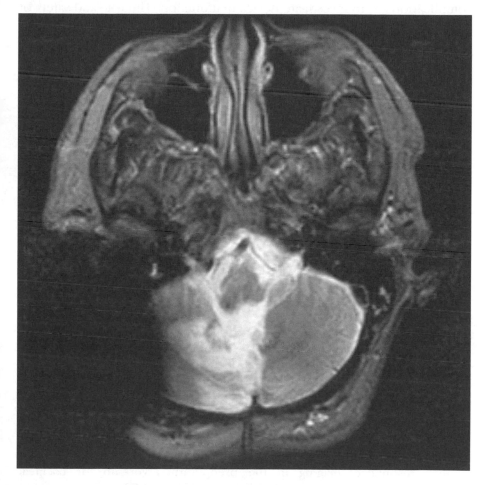

**Figure 9.14** Axial cut T2 weighted MRI demonstrates an approximate 6 cm right-sided signal void attributed to a receiver-stimulator.

## Conclusion

In summary, radiological assessment has a prominent value in modern cochlear implant assessment and management. In the preoperative period, radiological evaluation of all pertinent anatomy of the ear and temporal bone may be achieved with HRCT and MRI scanning. Newer MRI technology, such as FSE sequences, have recently enhanced the potential to clearly visualize the auditory nerve and other anatomical features within the internal auditory canal and within the cochlea. This capability, along with other emerging techniques such as functional MRI, may yet improve the ability of an implant team to choose the side of implantation most likely to result in a favorable hearing outcome. In the postoperative period, HRCT is the primary tool used to evaluate potential complications or to investigate device malfunction. The role and safety of MRI after cochlear implantation are under ongoing investigation. As advances in technology continue to emerge at a rapid pace, one might expect radiological assessment to continue to play an ever more prominent role in cochlear implantation.

# References

Arriaga MA, Carrier D (1996) MRI and clinical decisions in cochlear implantation. American Journal of Otology 17(4): 547–53.

Baumgartner WD, Youssefzadeh S, Hamzavi J et al. (2001) Clinical application of magnetic resonance imaging in 30 cochlear implant patients. Otology and Neurotology 22(6): 818–22.

Berthezene Y, Truy E, Morgon A et al. (1997) Auditory cortex activation in deaf subjects during cochlear electrical stimulation: evaluation by functional magnetic resonance imaging. Investigative Radiology 32(5): 297–301.

Ellul S, Shelton C, Davidson HC et al. (2000) Preoperative cochlear implant imaging: is magnetic resonance imaging enough?' American Journal of Otology 21(4): 528–33.

Fishman AJ, Roland JT Jr, Alexiades G et al. (2003) Fluoroscopically assisted cochlear implantation. Otology and Neurotology 24(6): 882–6.

Gleeson TG, Lacy PD, Bresnihan M et al. (2003) High resolution computed tomography and magnetic resonance imaging in the pre-operative assessment of cochlear implant patients. Journal of Laryngology and Otology 117(9): 692–5.

Jain R, Mukherji SK (2003) Cochlear implant failure: imaging evaluation of the electrode course. Clinical Radiology 58(4): 288–93.

Klein HM, Bohndorf K, Hermes H et al. (1992) Computed tomography and magnetic resonance imaging in the preoperative work-up for cochlear implantation. European Journal of Radiology 15(1): 89–92.

Lane JI, Ward H, Witte RJ et al. (2004) 3-T imaging of the cochlear nerve and labyrinth in cochlear-implant candidates: 3D fast recovery fast spin-echo versus 3D constructive interference in the steady state techniques. American Journal of Neuroradiology 25(4): 618–22.

Marsot-Dupuch K, Meyer B (2001) Cochlear implant assessment: imaging issues. European Journal of Radiology 40(2): 119–32.

Schmerber S, Reyt E, Lavieille JP (2003) Is magnetic resonance imaging still a contraindication in cochlear-implanted patients? European Archives of Oto-Rhino-Laryngology 260(6): 293–4.

Sennaroglu L, Saatci I, Aralasmak A et al. (2002) Magnetic resonance imaging versus computed tomography in pre-operative evaluation of cochlear implant candidates with congenital hearing loss. Journal of Laryngology and Otology 116(10): 804–10.

Sonnenburg RE, Wackym PA, Yoganandan N et al. (2002) Biophysics of cochlear implant/MRI interactions emphasizing bone biomechanical properties. Laryngoscope 112(10): 1720–5.

Teissl C, Kremser C, Hochmair ES et al. (1999) Magnetic resonance imaging and cochlear implants: compatibility and safety aspects. Journal of Magnetic Resonance Imaging 9(1): 26–38.

Wendell TN, Ball TI (2004) Interobserver agreement of coiling of Med-El cochlear implant: plain X-ray studies. Otology and Neurotology 25(3): 271–4.

Witte RJ, Lane JI, Driscoll CL et al. (2003) Pediatric and adult cochlear implantation. Radiographics 23(5): 1185–1200.

## CHAPTER 10
# Cochlear implant surgery

RICHARD T. RAMSDEN

## Introduction

The operation to insert the auditory prosthesis has been described by a non-surgical member of a well-known implant team somewhat cynically as the least important part of the whole cochlear implant process. That process starts with prompt referral and meticulous assessment, and goes on to a long and labour-intensive programme of mapping and rehabilitation. The hour and a half of the surgery may well be perceived in the general scheme of things to be rather insignificant. It is, however, self-evidently essential, and it is vital that the surgery is performed meticulously and in accordance with a number of well-defined surgical principles. Surgeons have long recognized the potential hazards that may accompany the insertion of a foreign body into human tissues. The foreign material may be recognized as such by the body and rejected. Infection is the arch-enemy of the implant surgeon, and scrupulous attention to asepsis is essential. The infected foreign body is a disaster and nearly always leads to the explantation of the expensive device. Furthermore, although most cochlear implant operations are straightforward, and well within the capability of a competent otologist, there are cases in which the resources of the surgeon may be taxed to the limit. A badly performed operation can therefore ruin the whole implant process by failing to ensure a favourable placement of the device, by causing damage to the remaining cochlear structures or by causing the patient unacceptable complications.

All contemporary cochlear implant systems comprise internal and external components. The internal or implanted part of the system is made up of a series of electrodes mounted on a single carrier that is threaded into the cochlear lumen, usually the scala tympani. There are some variations from this design that have been developed to deal with certain unique surgical problems, such as cochlear dysplasia and obliteration, and these will be dealt with in detail later. Extracochlear electrodes are hardly ever used these days. The electrode array is connected to the electronic package that comprises the receiver system for picking up the signal from the external component and a microchip that is responsible for determining which electrode or combination of electrodes should be stimulated at any moment. It also determines the rate of stimulation of the electrodes in accordance with the software program housed in the external speech processor. The surgeon has to deal with the problems of locating the package in the correct position on the side of the skull. He also has to gain access to the cochlea. This is usually done through a transmastoid approach, with an approach to the promontory through a posterior tympanotomy. Although some surgeons may still enter the cochlea through the round window, the majority prefer a separate cochleostomy. Stabilization of the device to prevent displacement or migration is essential. The external component is an ear-level or body-worn speech processor linked to the internal component by a magnet. The position of the external component is thus determined by the position of the implanted component. Planning is essential to ensure the best position.

## Transmastoid facial recess approach

### Surgical technique

In the following section the 'straightforward' cochlear implant operation will be described. Further special cases will then be highlighted including implantation in the very young child, the obliterated postmeningitic cochlea, the dysplastic cochlea and the problems of implantation in the presence of chronic suppurative otitis media.

The patient is positioned in the supine position with the head turned to the opposite side as for any routine mastoid procedure. The use of the facial nerve monitor should be routine and the anaesthetist should therefore avoid the use of muscle relaxants. Before the operation commences, it is important to plan the positioning of the implant. The receiver package must not be so close to the pinna that the external coil prevents the comfortable fitting of the ear-level processor. A good guide as to the height of the package is the posterior projection of the zygomatic arch (see Figure 10.1). The package should be above that line. In addition, the surgeon should use the template for the speech processor provided by the implant company to ensure that there is no contact between the processor and the coil.

### Skin incision

Meticulous skin preparation is essential to minimize the risk of infection. In the early days of cochlear implantation, surgeons employed very large

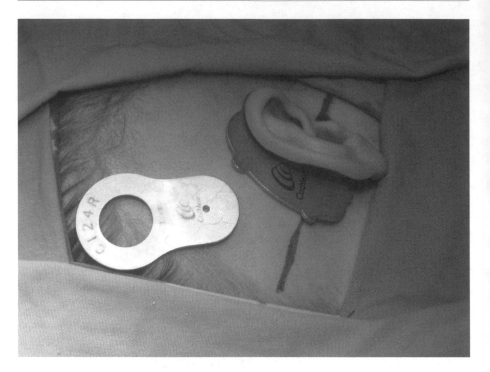

**Figure 10.1** Planning where to site the receiver stimulator. A horizontal line is projected backwards from the zygomatic arch. The receiver stimulator should be above this line and far enough back to avoid contact with the speech processor.

incisions and skin flaps. Typical of these was the extended endaural incision, curving upwards and backwards towards the occiput and favoured by the Hannover school and its disciples. It gave excellent access to the outer table of the skull for fixation of the package, but was cosmetically unacceptable, especially in children, and left a permanent linear loss of hair which could be very obvious. Furthermore, it presented a very large area of vascular scalp from which there could be a not inconsiderable loss of blood, especially in a young child. These large incisions have now been abandoned by most surgeons in favour of a modified postauricular incision as suggested by Gibson et al. (1995) and by O'Donoghue and Nikolopoulos (2002). If there have been previous operations on the ear, e.g. for chronic suppurative otitis media, the skin incision may have to be modified to make allowance for the previous incisions. The incision may be carried right down to bone, though the periosteum or the periostial layer may be preserved and a separate flap elevated.

## Preparation of the bed for the receiver stimulator

A submusculo-periostial tunnel is developed above and behind the pinna underneath the temporalis muscle. Although the profile of the implant package has become much less over the last two decades with refinements

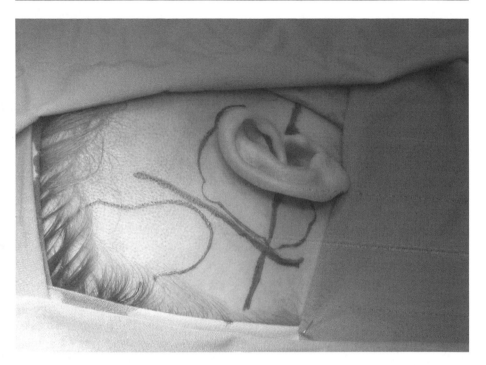

**Figure 10.2** The incision is sited between the receiver-stimulator and the speech processor.

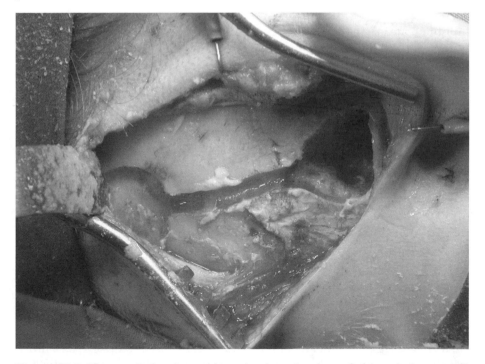

**Figure 10.3** The recess for the receiver-stimulator has been fashioned, the cortical mastoidectomy has been performed and a groove for the electrode lead has been cut.

in design, it must nevertheless be recessed into the skull in order to provide stability and protection. The surgeon rechecks the optimal position for the bony recess by inserting a dummy implant under the flap and ensuring that it does not make contact with the ear-level template. Once he or she is sure of the correct position, the surgeon drills a shallow well in the outer table of the skull that will house the package. The use of a special dummy template helps to get a really snug fit of the package in the well. Some surgeons like to secure the package with non-absorbable ties and if that is the intention tie holes have to be drilled. Care must be taken not to damage the underlying dura mater when these holes are being drilled. Access through this small incision can be a little cramped and the view under the skin/musculo-periostial flap may be improved, if the surgeon comes round to the opposite side of the operating table.

**Cortical mastoidectomy**

The requirements of the cortical mastoidectomy in cochlear implant surgery are not the same as when one is operating for infection. Widespread eradication of all the mastoid air cells is unnecessary; the aim is to provide adequate access to the fossa incudis to allow one to open the facial recess safely. It is not necessary to exenterate the mastoid tip or to remove air cells up to the middle fossa dura. In fact, it is desirable to retain some bony irregularities in the cavity for stabilization of the electrode lead. The antrum is opened and the prominence of the lateral semicircular canal identified and then the short process of the incus. The posterior bony wall of the external meatus must be thinned to ensure an adequate view of the fossa incudis. Preoperative examination should have given the surgeon a good impression of the shape and curvature of the external meatus, and it should not be necessary to elevate the skin of the external meatus. The fossa incudis is an essential landmark that must be clearly identified before one can proceed to the next stage of the operation. Some surgeons make a point of identifying the vertical portion of the facial nerve while still retaining a bony covering over it. Others (including the author) do not feel that this step is necessary and prefer to identify the level of the horizontal portion of the nerve by looking past the incus and the lateral semicircular canal into the middle ear. Finally, a gutter is drilled from the front of the well for the receiver-stimulator at the postero-superior aspect of the mastoidectomy to accommodate the electrode lead.

**Posterior tympanotomy**

The facial recess must be opened sufficiently to allow a good view of the round window. The short process of the incus is a useful landmark. It is customary but by no means essential to create the posterior tympanotomy with the incus in place. The posterior tympanotomy is commenced at the level of the tip of the short process using a 3 mm bur centred on the tip of the short process. The author likes to use a coarse diamond bur, which allows easy bone removal while avoiding the overheating of the facial nerve that may occur with a smooth diamond. Medial to the drill is the facial nerve and lateral to it the fibrous anulus of the tympanic membrane and the medial end of the bony meatus. Drilling in this area may lead very quickly into the top end of the facial recess especially if there is an extension of the air cell system into the buttress of bone, the so-called 'sentinel cells'. Drilling inferiorly in the facial recess, the opening gets progressively narrower and it is necessary to change over to a 2 mm bur. The chorda tympani will nearly always be encountered but it is usually possible to stay above it and avoid damage. On occasion if the take-off point of the chorda is very high it is possible to enter the facial recess below rather than above the chorda. Preservation of the chorda is of particular importance if one is planning bilateral implantation.

As the facial recess is entered, a view of the long process of the incus and the incudostapedial joint is usually obtained, and below it the round window niche. There is, in fact, quite considerable variation in the shape of the facial recess and its relationship to the oval and round windows and the ossicular chain. In some ears there is an immediate and unimpeded view of the incus and stapes but in others the incudostapedial joint is tucked deep into the facial recess and cannot be clearly seen. At other

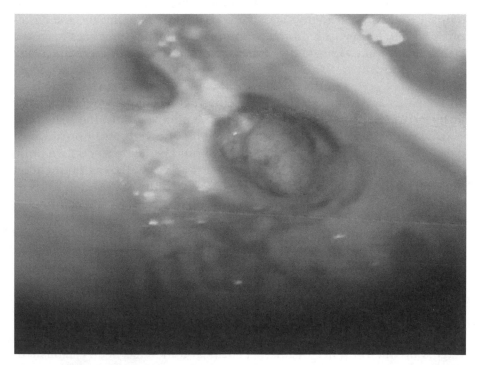

**Figure 10.4** The posterior tympanotomy has been created and through it the promontory is clearly seen.

times it may seem to be very high. Access into the facial recess may be aided by removing as much bone over the anterior aspect of the vertical portion of the facial nerve and by thinning out the posterior bony meatal wall. The visual angle can be further improved by drilling away the most lateral 2 mm of the bony ear canal. The bony buttress at the fossa incudis can also be thinned and partially removed. In an ear with a very deep facial recess a view of the round window may be obtained by filling the middle ear with saline and utilizing the phenomenon of refraction to allow the surgeon to see 'round the corner'. Just occasionally the author has had to resort to elevating a tympanomeatal flap in order to obtain secure identification of the round window. The surgeon must be certain that he or she has identified the round window niche and not a hypotympanic air cell.

## Creation of the cochleostomy

The location of the cochleostomy and the surgical technique are of critical importance if trauma to the cochlea is to be kept to a minimum. The scala tympani is preferred for several reasons. It is wider than the scala vestibuli, the stapes does not have to be removed and it is on the non-vestibular side of the cochlear duct and should in theory have less risk of causing balance problems. It should be opened just in front of and just below the midpoint of the round window niche in such a way as to avoid damage to the basilar membrane, the osseous spiral lamina and the modiolus. A 1 mm bur is used for the procedure. Drilling commences just over 2 mm below the stapes at a point just in front of the inferior lip of the round window niche. This is slightly below the centre of the scala tympani, but it is better to start a little low and work upwards than start too high and risk damage to the basilar membrane. The promontory is flattened a little and a hole is then drilled down to the endosteum of the scala tympani which shines through as a white membrane with an impression of dark fluid on the other side. Every effort should be made to remove bone dust and to retain the endosteum intact at this stage. Entry of bone dust into the cochlear lumen and excessive damage to the endosteum leads to deposition of new bone in the scala tympani. So-called 'soft surgical techniques' as described by Lehnhardt (1993) aim to minimize this risk. Further protection of the cochlea may be provided by covering the intact endostium with Hyaluronic Acid (Healon™) and creating the actual opening through the endostium through the Healon with a special microknife. The Healon prevents the entry of blood or bone dust. The use of the sucker should be kept to a minimum once the scala tympani is open. If the scala has been opened in the correct place, the gelatinous basilar membrane may be seen above the upper edge of the cochleostomy. At this stage, once the presence of a patent cochlear lumen has been established, the surgeon and scrub nurse change their gloves and the implant is carefully removed from its wrapping.

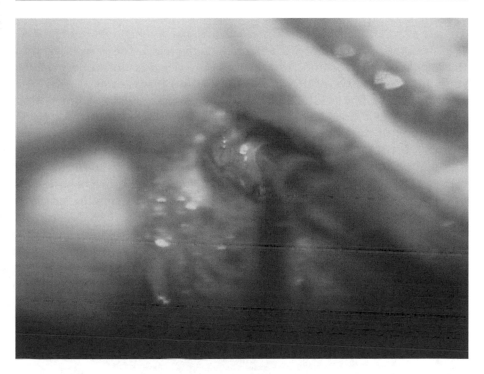

**Figure 10.5** A microdrill is used to create the cochleostomy in front of and below the round window.

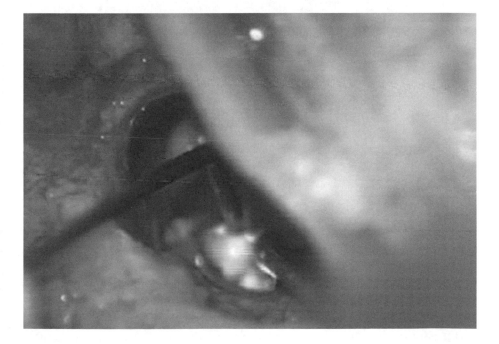

**Figure 10.6** Healon has been placed over the cochleostomy.

**Insertion of implant**

It is a matter of importance whether the active electrode is inserted into the cochlea before or after the receiver-stimulator is positioned against the skull. In the days of the large skin incision it was easy to insert the electrode array first while holding the receiver-stimulator in the other hand and facilitating the insertion by minor adjustments or twisting movements of the whole package. This was a great help with the early Nucleus devices, the CI22M and the CI24M. They had a rigid electrode that tended to impact traumatically against the anterior wall of the basal turn of the cochlea and could at times be difficult to advance beyond that point. With the new small incision and new electrode design the situation has changed. The 'modiolus hugging' Nucleus Contour device features a fine-wire stylet that holds the electrode array straight during insertion into the cochlea (see Figures 10.7a and 10.7b). Once the electrode is in position, the stylet is removed and the electrode array then curls round the modiolus.

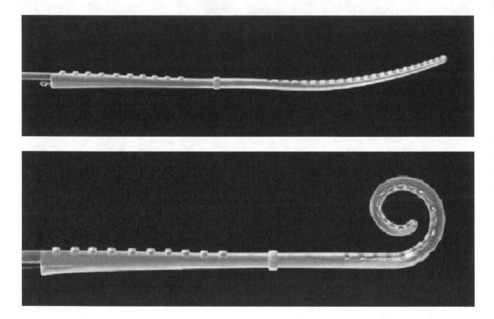

**Figure 10.7** The Cochlear 'modiolous hugging' electrode; (a) with the stylet in position, and (b) with the stylet removed.

If the electrode is inadvertently removed from the cochlea after the stylet has been removed, it cannot be reinserted and the expensive device is unusable. This could happen if the receiver package has to be manoeuvred into position after the stylet has been removed. The removal of the stylet should therefore be almost the last move in the whole operation. The receiver stimulator and coil is slipped under the musculo-periosteal flap and bedded down in the bony well. If ties are to be used, they should be inserted at this stage. In fact, most surgeons feel that ties are unnecessary as the musculo-periosteal flap itself provides considerable stability to the package. The reference electrode if present is tunnelled under the

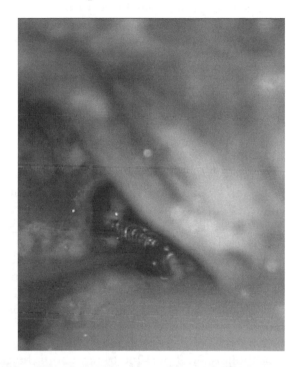

→ **Figure 10.8** The electrode array is advanced through the posterior tympanotomy towards the cochlcostomy.

↓**Figure 10.9** Full insertion of the electrode has been achieved.

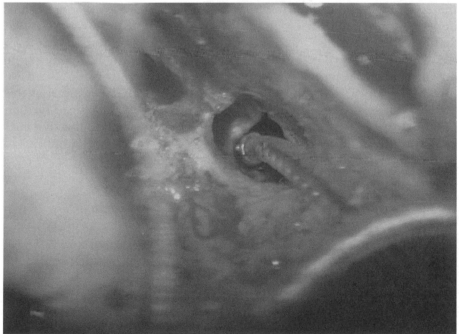

temporalis muscle. Finally, the active electrode array is advanced towards the cochleostomy. It can be held freehand or held lightly in a pair of crocodile forceps and guided with a special claw through the posterior tympanotomy. The actual insertion of the new, less rigid, electrodes into the scala tympani is usually very easy if the cochleostomy has been made wide enough. The initial direction of insertion should be downwards to avoid damage to the basilar membrane and the spiral lamina. Resistance should not be met in a patent cochlea, and, if it is, the edges of the cochloeostomy should be checked to make sure they are not catching the electrode.

Individual systems have their own specific design features. The Nucleus Contour device has semicircular electrodes on the array and they have to face the modiolus. The electrode carrier has a series of ridges in the silicone proximal to the active electrodes and are visible after complete insertion of the array. If these are pointing towards the modiolus, the surgeon knows that the array is correctly orientated within the cochlea. The electrode lead is then laid into the mastoid bowl and stabilized, usually just by positioning but some surgeons like to use a small blob of cement for added stability.

The stylet can now be removed. This can be a tricky little manoeuvre. The array must be stabilized close to the cochleostomy using a claw-like instrument. The end of the stylet is then held with a pair of crocodile forceps and gently withdrawn. The counterpressure at the cochleostomy must be sufficient to prevent withdrawal of the whole electrode and not too much to prevent withdrawal of the stylet. Unfortunately, at high magnification it is not possible to have both the cochleostomy and the end of the stylet in focus at the same time and the surgeon is to some extent dependent on haptic or somatosensory feedback. The most recent design feature of the Nucleus Contour device is a small white mark 8 mm from the tip of the array. When that mark is at the cochleostomy, the tip of the array is just about to come in contact with the anterior wall of the basal turn at a point where damage to the cochlea is likely to occur. If at this point stylet removal is commenced while the array is introduced further, the tip of array will start to curl around the modiolus without making contact with the anterior cochlear wall. This is known as the 'Advance Off Stylet' (AOS) technique.

### Closure

Recent reports concerning the possible association between cochlear implantation and the subsequent development of meningitis have drawn attention to the need for a secure soft tissue seal at the cochleostomy (Arnold et al., 2002). Small fragments of muscle or periosteum are gently packed round the electrode at the cochleostomy while taking supreme care not to disturb the position of the electrode. Another larger piece of muscle may be inserted into the posterior tympanotomy for

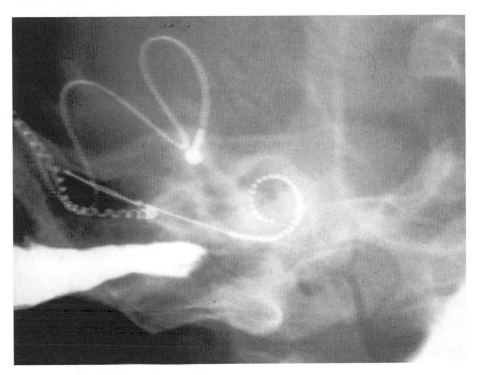

**Figure 10.10** Postoperative plain X-ray confirms satisfactory position of the electrode.

added stability. If a separate periosteal flap was preserved, this should be stitched down, providing support and protection for the device. The skin is usually closed in two layers. In children an absorbent subcuticular suture or tissue glue are more acceptable than removable stitches. A firm dressing overnight is preferable to a pressure dressing. A postoperative plain X-ray is taken to confirm the correct position of the electrode.

# The suprameatal approach (SMA)

A number of surgeons have advocated this less invasive approach (Kronenberg et al. 2004) in which a narrow tunnel is drilled from the cortex down to the attico-antral area and the middle ear is opened by elevating a tympanomeatal flap. The cochleostomy is drilled permeatally and the electrode is threaded down to the cochleostomy lateral to the incus. Among a number of advantages claimed for the technique are avoidance of risk to the facial nerve and chorda tympani, secure identification of the round window and thus location of the cochleostomy and a more natural line of entry of the electrode into the scala tympani. Some surgeons trained in transmastoid facial recess surgery might regard this approach as strange and unnecessarily cramped, but for those implant surgeons who lack the confidence or training to carry out posterior tympanotomy this approach might well be safer, although care must be taken to avoid damage to the middle fossa dura, the level of which must be checked preoperatively on a coronal CT scan.

# Special surgical situations

# The very young child

There are a number of reasons why implant teams are now implanting younger and younger children. These include the increasing availability of universal neonatal screening with very early diagnosis of deafness, more awareness on the part of referrers and of parents and a realization that the younger child is implanted, the more likely he or she is to acquire speech and language and be educated in a mainstream environment (Govaerts et al., 2002). Many teams are regularly implanting children aged 2 years or less and there have been a number implanted during the first year of life, usually for post-meningitic deafness. There are certain issues surrounding the surgery of these very small children.

*Anaesthetic issues*

Little children are not just very small adults. Their physiology is uniquely different from that of adults. Their homeostatic mechanisms are more unstable than adults, their reaction to anaesthetic agents and other drugs may be capricious, they are usually anaemic and handle the blood loss of surgery less well than adults and they often have pulmonary problems. In particular, children born prematurely who spend time in the Special Care Baby Unit (SCBU) may have multiple coexisting pathologies that make general anaesthesia difficult and, indeed, risky. Comorbidity associated with deafness includes cardiac problems in the Jervell–Lange–Nielsen Syndrome and the CHARGE Association, and renal problems in the Otorenobranchial Syndrome. It is therefore imperative that such children are managed by a paediatric anaesthetist supported by a specialist team. The surgeon must also be aware that very young children may be deaf because of a failure of organogenesis and that various degrees of dysplasia may be present, some of which can be a real surgical challenge (see below).

*Surgical issues*

A number of factors have to be considered in carrying out cochlear implant surgery in the very young child. Some relate to the different anatomy in the small ear, and others to pathophysiological changes that are common in the middle ears of small children. The middle and inner ears of the child are of adult size at birth. The mastoid process, however, is poorly developed so that the surgeon may have fairly cramped access.

Furthermore, the bone may be diploeic and thus more likely to bleed. In children under the age of 2 years the facial nerve is relatively superficial in its descending portion and is thus vulnerable to damage from the drill. Recurrent acute otitis media and chronic otitis media with effusion are frequently encountered, and there may be long-term inflammatory changes in the middle ear mucosa which make it difficult for the surgeon to see clearly what he or she is doing. The swollen mucosa is often very vascular which adds to the problem of visibility and even the most experienced implant surgeon can find it difficult to progress with safety and confidence.

In this situation it is often a good idea to remove the incus and increase access to the facial recess and mesotympanum. More room is thus created to allow one to remove swollen mucosa from the field of vision, and, by angling the line of vision from above, the surgeon can see the round window area without having to create a large posterior tympanotomy, thus reducing risk to the facial nerve. If glue is known to be present, most surgeons would choose to treat this by conventional means such as adenoidectomy and ventilation tubes. If glue is found by chance at the time of cochlear implant surgery, the operation can, however, proceed. If ventilation tubes have been inserted previously, they should, in the view of the author, be removed and the drum allowed to heal before implant surgery is performed, although some surgeons are happy to remove the tube at the time of implant surgery and place a fat graft in the drum defect. This is probably satisfactory most of the time but in the occasional case that does not heal, the subsequent operation of myringoplasty in a 2-year-old ear with an implant in place is one to test the nerve of the surgeon.

The other part of the operation that requires particular care in the young child is the preparation of the well for the receiver-stimulator on the side of the skull. The skull of the 1- to 2-year-old is very thin, perhaps no more than 2 mm and the dura is inevitably exposed during this step. That in itself is no great problem provided the surgeon takes care not to penetrate the dura with the drill when cutting either the well itself or adjacent tie holes. It is also important to be meticulous to achieve total haemostasis and avoid the risk of an extradural collection. One possible technique involves the preservation of a central island of bone over the dura that can be depressed when the package is inserted. Even if all the bone in the bottom of the recess is removed, it will often regrow rapidly and provide a bony covering for the dura.

## Chronic suppurative otitis media

Several studies have confirmed that chronic otitis media is no bar to implantation (Axon et al., 1997; Incesulu et al., 2004) as long as certain rules are followed. The condition may occur in active or inactive forms and may or may not be associated with cholesteatoma. There may have been previous surgery and there may or may not be a mastoid cavity. If there is active infection or cholesteatoma present, it is mandatory to perform a two-stage procedure.

At the first stage, all the cells in the mastoid bone and middle ear must be opened. If there is a simple perforation, this may be grafted, but certainly if cholesteatoma is present an open cavity must be created with blind sac closure of the external auditory canal to provide isolation from the environment. The procedure is completed with closure of the Eustachian tube and cavity obliteration for which the preferred material is autologous abdominal fat, which is readily available and remarkably resistant to necrosis.

At the second stage operation some 3 to 6 months later, it is an easy matter to elevate the fat from the promontory and identify the round window niche, and of course it allows the surgeon the opportunity to check for residual disease. The cochleostomy is created in the usual manner, and in fact access to the cochleostomy site is much easier in an open cavity than in a closed middle ear. Olgun et al. (2003) suggest that in an open cavity the sinus tympani should be opened from behind and that the electrode be inserted medial to the vertical portion of the facial nerve for added stability. Total familiarity with the anatomy of the facial nerve is essential and the technique is not recommended unless the surgeon is totally confident in his or her ability to perform this approach.

After insertion the fat is replaced over the electrode lead and, in fact, provides excellent protection for the device. In the presence of a preexisting mastoid cavity the surgeon must decide between a one-stage and two-stage procedure, but whichever policy is adopted the essential step is obliteration of the cavity. Failure to do so will lead to extrusion of the implant into the ear canal. If there is any suggestion of active disease in the cavity, a two-stage procedure is recommended, with eradication of disease, blind sac closure, obliteration of the Eustachian tube and an abdominal fat graft. Recently, El-Kashlan et al. (2003) recommended meatal closure and cochlear implantation in a one-stage procedure for the cases with a healthy mastoid cavity. In cases where there is doubt it is best to play safe and do a two-stage procedure.

Whatever the technique, the most important step is elevation of the fibro-epithelial lining of the mastoid. It can be preserved or discarded, but the surgeon should be in no doubt that all squamous epithelium has been removed to minimize the risk of recurrence. It is also important to take note of any previous skin incisions and to try to incorporate them into the new incision, rather than risk creating areas of skin of precarious vitality. Furthermore, some of these patients have had many operations and the skin behind the ear may be thin and have a poor blood supply. It may be necessary to provide extra protection for the receiver-stimulator and for the electrode lead to prevent extrusion by swinging down local temporalis muscle flaps.

Recently, Colletti et al. (1998) described their technique of basal turn cochleostomy via the middle fossa route for implantation in the presence of chronic otitis or a mastoid cavity. They argue that this technique avoids the need for a two-stage operation in infected ears and minimizes the risk of meningitis. It also prevents the possibility of entrapment of squamous epithelium in an obliterated cavity. They also claim that inserting the electrode where they do allows greater access to the middle and apical turns of the cochlea where there is greater survival of fibres suitable for electrical stimulation. It has to be said that this claim is not universally supported – the counterclaim is that because the spiral ganglion does not reach to the apical turn there is little point in inserting the electrode that far into the cochlea. Regardless of these theoretical arguments, the technique is interesting. A small temporal craniotomy approximately 3 cm × 3 cm is cut above the external meatus (two-thirds in front, one-third behind). After elevation of the dura and identification of the greater superficial petrosal nerve, drilling is commenced in the triangle between that nerve and the labyrinthine portion of the facial nerve. The distal basal turn of the cochlea is encountered and the bone over it thinned. A cochleostomy is created in the most superficial part of the turn.

## The obliterated cochlea

Obliteration of the cochlea is most frequently encountered after meningitis, although it also occurs in otosclerosis, autoimmune inner ear disease, following skull base fracture and in association with suppurative middle ear disease. In meningitis there is an endosteal reaction which may be confined to the region in the scala tympani where the cochlear aqueduct enters, or may extend much further along the scala tympani as far as or beyond the anterior basal turn while still sparing more apical parts of the scala tympani and the scala vestibuli. In extreme cases there may be complete obliteration of both scalae. The extent of neo-ossification can be predicted with a considerable degree of accuracy on state-of-the-art imaging such as 3D Surface Rendered T2 MRI described by Hans et al. (1999, 2003). If obliteration is confined to the most basal part of the scala tympani, limited additional drilling in front of the cochleostomy leads one into a patent lumen, and a good insertion will be assured perhaps utilizing a special compressed electrode (see below).

The new bone is usually soft and friable and is whiter than the surrounding otic capsule. It is usually easy to remove using the microdrill, picks or rasps. The tissue may in fact be a mixture of new bone, calcified osteoid and fibrous tissue. New bone can be removed right up to the anterior basal turn. As the basal turn starts to turn upwards and medially, it becomes increasingly difficult to drill round the bend. Care must be taken at this point to avoid the intrapetrous carotid artery, which is just in front of the basal turn. There are a number of options at this stage if a patent lumen has not been encountered. Gantz et al. (1988) and Balkany et al. (1998) describe techniques both of which involve the creation of a C-shaped perimodiolar gutter on the promontory into which the electrode is laid. These operations require the creation of an open cavity for access, blind sac closure of the external meatus and obliteration of the cavity with fat harvested from the abdomen. Apart from the fact that this is a much greater operation than the usual facial recess approach, there can be problems with poor fixation of the electrode array and lateral displacement of the array from its gutter. These techniques are rarely employed these days.

## Partial insertion

This solution was described by Cohen and Waltzman (1993) who proposed a short insertion tunnel technique, drilling an enclosed tunnel forwards from the cochleostomy a distance of 8 mm towards the anterior end of the cochlea and inserting a compressed electrode array on which there is a higher concentration of electrodes than on a conventional carrier. The anterior limit of the drill out is the carotid artery. This still remains a useful technique, although the scala vestibuli insertion and/or the split electrode technique are possibly preferred options. A compressed electrode can also be employed in cases in which a patent cochlear lumen is encountered at the anterior basal turn after drilling forwards through new bone from the cochleostomy site.

## Scala vestibuli insertion (Steenerson et al., 1990)

The cochlear aqueduct is the usual route of infection from the subarachnoid space into the inner ear and enters the scala tympani, and so the scala vestibuli may remain patent even in the face of quite severe scala tympani obliteration. A scala vestibuli insertion is an acceptable alternative if the scala tympani cannot be entered. The incus and stapes are removed and gentle drilling at the anterior-inferior aspect of the oval window leads one into the scala vestibuli of the basal turn. Although the scala vestibuli is narrower than the normal scala tympani, it is usually easy to insert the electrode. Results with the scala vestibuli insertion are usually every bit as good as with a scala tympani insertion. There is a theoretical possibility of postoperative vertigo because the electrode is inserted on the vestibular side of the cochlear partition, but this rarely seems to be the case.

## Split electrode insertion

Bredberg et al. (1997) came up with this solution to the problem of total cochlear obliteration. They propose the creation of two parallel gutters, one along the line of the basal turn and the other along the line of the middle turn of the cochlea. Into these are inserted two short electrode

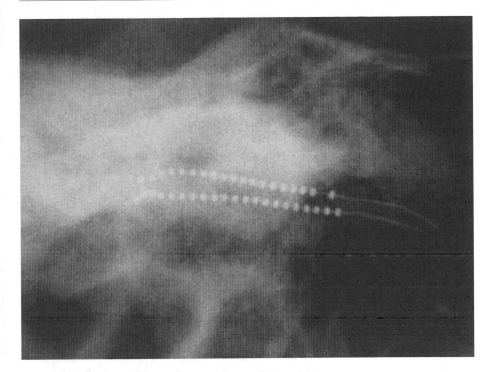

**Figure 10.11** Split electrode in a case of cochlear obliteration.

arrays with the electrodes divided between them (see Figure 10.11). The lower channel is drilled from the standard cochleostomy anteriorly towards the anterior limit of the basal turn. The upper channel is drilled parallel to the lower channel starting from a point just below the processus cochleariformis. The incus has to be removed for access, which is usually adequate. Occasionally, it is necessary to remove the posterior wall of the external auditory canal in order to gain access and carry out a blind sac closure of the external meatus with obliteration of the middle ear cleft. The technique is also described in some detail by Lenarz et al. (2001).

## The dysplastic cochlea

There is a wide spectrum of developmental abnormalities of the inner ear depending upon the stage in organogenesis at which development is arrested or modified. The reader is referred to the excellent paper by Sennaroglu and Saatci (2002) for a detailed account of current classification. Some of these abnormalities have no real impact on the operation to insert the cochlear implant. Others are of major significance. Minor degrees of dysplasia of the vestibule or of the lateral semicircular canal are common and although visible on high-quality imaging are not always apparent to the surgeon. One of the commonest dysplasias is the Large Vestibular Aqueduct Syndrome (LVAS) often seen as a feature of Pendred's Syndrome. It may occur in isolation or in association with other dysplasias such as the Mondini dysplasia. The only abnormality that the surgeon may be aware of is of transmitted pulsation of the cochlear fluids as he or she opens the scala tympani. This reflects pressure changes in the posterior cranial fossa transmitted to the scala media through the large aqueduct. There is, however, no gush of fluid into the middle ear, because it should be a closed system. If there is, it implies that there must be another coexisting malformation that allows communication between the subarachnoid space and the cochlea, such as failure of formation of the bony partition at the lateral end of the internal auditory meatus. The typical abnormality in Mondini's dysplasia is a failure of partitioning of the middle and apical cochlear turn so that they form a common turn. The basal turn is normal. The Mondini dysplasia may occur in isolation or with absence of the lateral wall of the internal auditory canal. LVAS and the Mondini dysplasia are not contraindications to implantation using a conventional electrode, and usually the surgery is uncomplicated (Miyamoto et al., 1986; Temple et al., 1999).

The common cavity represents arrest of development at an earlier stage of organogenesis. There is total or partial failure of separation of the primitive inner ear into its anterior (cochlear) and posterior (labyrinthine) components. Such a cavity will nearly always contain some neural elements in its outer wall, although the exact location and extent may be unpredictable. It may also have an associated failure of formation of the party wall between the internal meatus and the common cavity with direct communication between the subarachnoid space and the cavity. There are thus major problems if one tries to insert a conventional electrode, especially a 'modiolus hugger' in which the electrodes point away from the outer wall of the cavity and the neural elements. Special electrodes have been developed by the companies to provide for this situation.

The special risks in this type of case are insertion of the electrode through an absent lateral meatal wall into the posterior fossa, and a CSF gusher from the posterior fossa through the unpartitioned internal meatus/inner ear. In dealing with a dysplastic inner ear, the surgeon must also be aware that there may be coexisting abnormalities of the facial nerve, such as a widely dehiscent nerve, or an ectopic nerve, or a nerve that splits and passes on both sides of the stapes with the lower division crossing the promontory. Hoffman et al. (1997) found the facial nerve to have an anomalous position in 16% of ears with cochlear dysplasia. The facial nerve monitor, regarded by the author as an essential in all cochlear implant surgery, is mandatory when there is preoperative knowledge of dysplasia. Other surprises for the surgeon include persistence of the stapedial artery, which may cross the promontory just where one wants to create the cochleostomy.

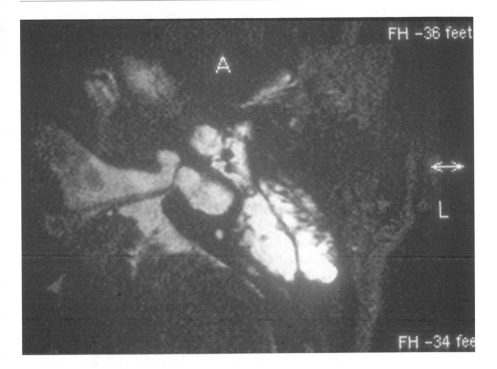

**Figure 10.12** Severe inner ear dysplasia with failure of the cochlea to develop, absence of the bony wall between the inner ear and the internal meatus, but a demonstrable cochlear nerve.

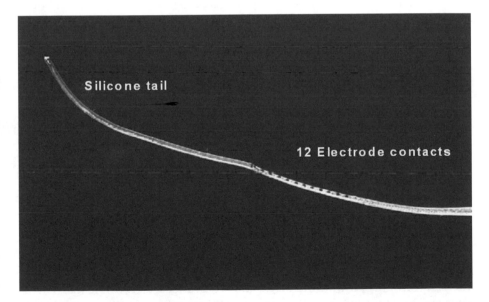

**Figure 10.13** Special electrode designed for the so-called common cavity by the Med-El company.

# Revision of cochlear implant surgery

There are a number of reasons why an implant may have to be removed and replaced. These are:

1. device failure;
2. infection;
3. non-auditory stimulation;
4. technical upgrade.

Device failure is relatively rare but may be spontaneous or related to an identifiable episode of trauma. Spontaneous failure is usually due to a manufacturing problem rather than the implant 'wearing out'. It is thus more likely to occur in the first year or two after implantation. Thereafter the cumulative survival of implanted systems seems to be in the region of 97%, and all the implant companies guarantee their products against failure for a period of 10 years. Of course, we cannot know what the long-term survival of cochlear implants will turn out to be but so far they seem to be reliable well beyond the 10-year warranty period. Environmental hazards are an ever-present threat to a cochlear implant, and direct trauma especially in children will always account for a certain number of failures each year. Sudden electrostatic effects may also be a hazard, such as the child in the author's series whose implant failed with a loud crack as he was careering down a plastic slide. Despite our best efforts, the occasional device will become infected and threaten to extrude through the skin. In all probability the device will still be functioning normally and it is a difficult decision for the clinician to remove an expensive functioning implant in order to control the infection. The fact is that once the package has been colonized by bacteria the only solution is the radical step of explantation and subsequent re-implantation. Technical upgrade is rarely a reason for removing a functioning device. If a multichannel device is functioning well, it should not be removed simply to upgrade the hardware. Early single-channel extracochlear devices may, however, be removed and be replaced with multichannel intracochlear systems, which perform very much better.

The implanted device gives rise to a number of reactions in the tissue with which it is in contact. Very soon after implantation there is an inflammatory reaction around the silicone casing that produces a smooth avascular fibrous sheath round the receiver stimulator and the electrode lead as it runs through the mastoid. A similar reaction has been shown to occur within the cochlear lumen. This reaction has the beneficial effect of stabilizing the system and minimizing the risk of displacement.

The other reaction that one frequently encounters is osteogenesis in the mastoid and around the active and reference electrode leads. This is especially but not exclusively seen in children who exhibit a marked tendency to remodelling after any mastoid operation.

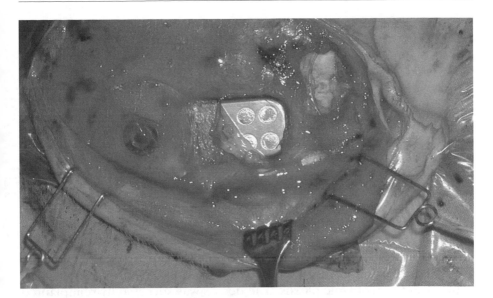

**Figure 10.14** Cochlear explantation. There is a firm connective tissue capsule round the implanted device.

During revision surgery for device failure, the surgeon wants to remove the old system and insert a new implant as expeditiously as possible at the same operation. It should be done with as little damage to the explanted device as possible so that when it is returned for analysis by the manufacturer the extent of the damage has not been exaggerated by the trauma of the removal. In this situation there are certain rules to follow. The electrode array should be removed from the cochlea at the last possible moment so that the fibrous sheath does not have time to close down and make reinsertion difficult. Before that stage is reached, the receiver-stimulator must be freed up from its bony well. This may require a considerable amount of drilling if there has been extensive remodelling of bone. The leads for the active electrode array and for the reference electrode must be carefully dissected out from the enveloping sheath of fibrous tissue under high magnification to avoid damage. It is not uncommon to find that leads which were originally on the surface of the temporal bone have become surrounded by bone, and careful drilling with a smooth diamond bur is necessary in order to free them up. Once the package has been mobilized, it should be turned forward and stabilized by an assistant. It may be necessary to carry out further modifications to the shape of the mastoid and to the bed for the receiver-stimulator, especially if the new device is a different model from the explant. The new device is removed from its packaging ready for implantation. It is only at this stage that the old implant is removed from the cochlea and the new device is inserted as quickly as possible. It usually enters the cochlea without a problem.

The steps are different if explantation is necessary in order to control infection. In these unfortunate cases the infection is nearly always confined to the superficial subcutaneous layers in the region of the receiver package. It is uncommon for it to extend into the mastoid or middle ear. The aim of surgery is just to remove the receiver-stimulator. If the whole device is removed with the intracochlear electrode, the cochlear lumen will rapidly obliterate making later re-implantation very difficult if not impossible. The active electrode should therefore be cut off the receiver-stimulator and left in place. The surgeon should avoid dissecting down to the cochleostomy because of the risk of encouraging the spread of infection. The electrode will keep the cochlear lumen patent until such time as re-implantation is contemplated, usually some 3 months after the infection has settled.

Maas et al. (1996) describe the explantation of a functioning multi-channel device from a patient who had uncontrollable non-auditory stimulation. His deafness occurred as a result of bilateral skull base fracture, a condition in which current may spread out of the cochlea through the fracture line and cause unwanted stimulation of sensory nerves, particularly in the tympanic plexus. The device was successfully reimplanted in the contralateral ear at the same sitting. It is clearly essential to avoid any damage to the device during removal if such a strategy is to be successful.

# Complications of cochlear implant surgery

No surgical procedure is without some risk. Cochlear implantation is relatively free from complications. They are usually described as being 'major' if the complication necessitates a further operation, e.g. the removal of the implant or thinning of the scalp flap, or 'minor' if they can be successfully resolved by simple conservative means. The incidence of major complications in the literature is between 3% and 13 % (Hoffman and Cohen, 1995; Aschendorff et al., 1997; Collins et al., 1997; Proops et al., 1999). A recent series from Green et al. (2004), the largest UK series reported, quotes an incidence of 6% of which implant extrusion and sepsis were the most serious. There was no case of permanent facial weakness. One thick skin flap had to be thinned, and there was one case of non-auditory stimulation that could not be programmed out and the implant had to be removed. Fayad et al. (2003) review 705 patients over a 22-year period and note an incidence of postoperative facial weakness of 0.7%. All cases were delayed in onset and all recovered completely. Minor complications are not uncommon with a quoted incidence between 7% and 37% (Cohen et al., 1988; Webb et al., 1991; Summerfield and Marshall, 1995). By far the most common is non-auditory stimulation (22%) by a small number of channels but such is the redundancy in the system that the rogue electrodes can usually be removed from the map without any adverse effect on performance.

Non-auditory effects are most commonly seen in cases of otosclerosis and skull base fracture when current may escape from the cochlea through a line of low electrical resistance and stimulate either the facial nerve or the sensory nerves of the tympanic plexus (Broomfield et al., 2000). Fina et al. (2003) report an incidence of post-implantation vertigo in 39% subjects, a figure very much higher than the 8% quoted by Green et al. (2004), most of whom in the experience of the latter authors got better with time. Fina et al. (2003), however, point out that many of their cases experienced delayed episodic symptoms that were possibly due to delayed hydrops rather than direct surgical intervention. Worsening of tinnitus is seen in around 1% and minor degrees of scalp or flap infection in 2%. Taste disturbance is commented upon by under 1%. Gillett et al. (2002) report the unusual occurrence of pneumocephalus following cochlear implantation, but intracranial complications from cochlear implantation are excessively rare.

## The auditory brainstem implant (ABI)

The successful employment of a cochlear implant demands the presence of an intact cochlear nerve and an implantable cochlea. There are a number of conditions in which the cochlear nerves are absent or the cochlea is so dysplastic that a cochlear implant cannot be inserted. In these cases electrical stimulation of the auditory pathways may be considered at a more central site. The ABI was developed to deal with this situation, originally for the condition of Neurofibromatosis Type 2 (NF2). The hallmark of this condition is the presence of bilateral vestibular schwannomas (acoustic neuromas), benign tumours that arise on the audiovestibular nerves. As a result of the tumours themselves and/or the surgery to remove them, the majority of these patients end up totally deaf, and nearly always without functioning auditory nerves.

The ABI stimulates the auditory pathway at the level of the cochlear nucleus complex, which is located in the pons in the lateral recess of the fourth ventricle. The device has a modified electrode with a carrier paddle with 21 disc electrodes (see Figure 10.15). Technically, insertion of the electrode is not easy, as surgical landmarks are not always obvious. Following the removal of the vestibular schwannoma either via the translabyrinthine or retrosigmoid route, the opening of the lateral recess of the fourth ventricle is explored, the so-called foramen of Luschka. This is found at the ponto-medullary junction by following the stump of the auditory nerve inferiorly and the glossopharyngeal nerve superiorly. The choroid plexus will usually be seen coming out of the foramen of Luschka and cerebrospinal fluid will be seen to emerge from it, especially if the anaesthetist raises the intracranial pressure. Arachnoid adhesions may have to be broken down in order to gain access to the foramen, and it is usual to have to deal with a plexus of veins or even to have to move an arterial loop in order to do so.

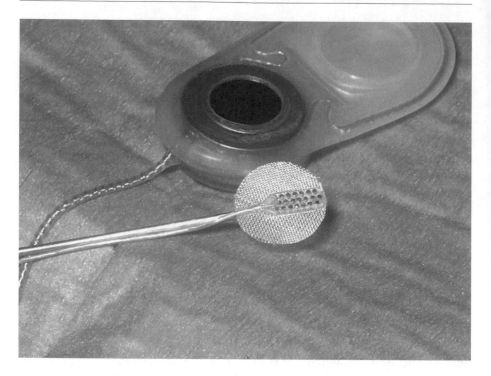

**Figure 10.15** Auditory brainstem implant. The electrode array comprises three parallel rows of contacts that are placed on the cochlear nucleus.

The walls of the lateral recess are recognized by their smooth white appearance. The electrode paddle is slipped into the lateral recess with the electrode discs pointing upwards to make contact with the dorsal cochlear nucleus. The correct position of the implant is verified by eliciting the electrically evoked auditory brainstem response (EABR). Adjacent cranial nerves (facial, glossopharyngeal, accessory and trigeminal) are monitored to minimize the risk of non-auditory stimulation. From the point of view of neuro-anatomy, there is a major problem with the frequency maps, or tonotopicity, of the cochlear nucleus compared with the cochlea. A surface electrode will function most effectively if the frequency map is distributed across the surface of the nucleus. In the cochlear nucleus, the map is disposed obliquely through the depths of the nucleus, and to take advantage of this arrangement a penetrating electrode has been developed, but as yet it has not been used in clinical trials. Relatively few ABIs have been performed worldwide, but most users have environmental awareness and assistance with lipreading. A small number are able to score well on open-set BKB sentences. A realistic comparison is with the performance that one used to see with single-channel cochlear implants.

Other possible indications for the ABI are a congenital absence of the cochlear nerve and total obstruction of the cochlea. Colletti et al. (2002)

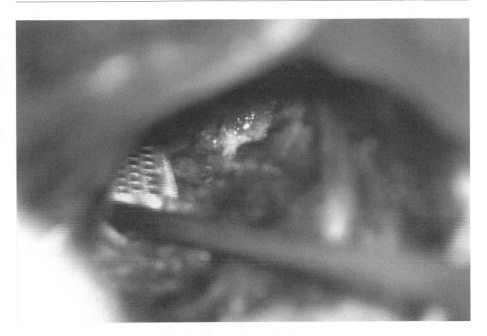

**Figure 10.16** The electrode array is placed on the brainstem.

reported three such cases, all congenitally deaf children on whom he operated without mishap. It is too early yet to state with confidence if these children will be able to use their implants to gain access to speech. Grayeli et al. (2003) describe the use of the ABI in the case of a man deafened postlingually from meningitis who had bilateral totally ossified cochleas. After 2 years of implant use, he achieved 50% of disyllabic word scores and 60% of sentence scores using the implant alone. There is a real possibility that a non-tumour patient who receives an ABI should do better than one whose cochlear nucleus has been damaged by pressure from a large tumour and surgical attempts to remove it.

## Conclusion

The operation to insert a cochlear implant is not particularly difficult for the experienced otologist. It does, however, demand meticulous attention to detail to avoid infection and to ensure the correct location of both the receiver-stimulator and the electrode array. As patients with more and more residual hearing are now being considered for implantation, the importance of atraumatic insertion, 'soft surgery', places greater demands on surgical technique. In congenitally abnormal ears, the surgical problems can be challenging and these cases must be handled by surgeons with considerable experience in the middle ear. For these reasons, it is essential that cochlear implantation is carried out by teams with a high annual throughput of cases.

The auditory brainstem implant is unlikely to be a commonly performed operation, but there are exciting possibilities in non-tumour cases and as yet poorly explored opportunities for children born without cochlear nerves.

# References

Arnold W, Bredberg G, Gstöttner W et al. (2002) Meningitis following cochlear implantation: pathomechanisms, clinical symptoms, conservative and surgical treatments. Journal for Oto-Rhino-Laryngology and its Related Specialities 64: 382–9.

Aschendorff A, Marangos N, Laszig R (1997) Complications and reimplantation. Advances in Otorhinolaryngology 52: 167–70.

Axon PR, Mawman DJ, Upile T et al. (1997) Cochlear implantation in the presence of chronic suppurative otitis media. Journal of Laryngology and Otology 111: 228–32.

Balkany T, Bird PA, Hodges AV et al. (1998) Surgical technique for implantation of the totally ossified cochlea. Laryngoscope 108: 988–92.

Bredberg G, Lindstom B, Lopponen H et al. (1997) Electrodes for ossified cochleas. American Journal of Otology 18: 42–3.

Broomfield S, Mawman D, Woolford TJ et al. (2000) Non-auditory stimulation in adult cochlear implant users. Cochlear Implants International 1(1): 55–66.

Cohen N, Waltzman SB (1993) Partial insertion of the Nucleus multichannel cochlear implant: technique and results. American Journal of Otology 14: 357–61.

Cohen NL, Hoffman RA, Stroschein M (1988) Medical or surgical complications related to the Nucleus multichannel cochlear implant. Annals of Otology, Rhinology and Laryngology (suppl. 135): 8–13.

Colletti V, Fiorino FG, Carner M et al. (1998) Basal turn cochleostomy via the middle fossa route for cochlear implant insertion. American Journal of Otology 19: 778–84.

Colletti V, Carner M, Fiorino F, Sacchetto L, Miorelli V, Orsi A, Cilurzo F, Pacini L (2002) Hearing restoration with auditory brainstem implants in three children with cochlear nerve aplasia. Otology and Neurotology 23(5): 682–93.

Collins MM, Hawthorne MH, el Hmd K (1997) Cochlear implantation in a district general hospital: problems and complications in the first five years. Journal of Laryngology and Otology 111: 325–32.

El-Kashlan HK, Arts HA, Telian SA (2003) External auditory canal closure in cochlear implant surgery. Otology and Neurotology 24(3): 404–8.

Fayad JN, Wanna GB, Micheletto JN et al. (2003) Facial nerve paralysis following cochlear implant surgery. Laryngoscope 113(8): 1344–6.

Fina M, Skinner M, Goebel JA et al. (2003) Vestibular dysfunction after cochlear implantation. Otology and Neurotology 24(2): 234–42.

Gantz BJ, McCabe BF, Tyler RS (1988) Use of multichannel cochlear implants in obstructed and obliterated cochleas. Otolaryngology: Head and Neck Surgery 98: 72–81.

Gibson WPR, Harrison HC, Prowse C (1995) A new incision for cochlear implants. Journal of Laryngology and Otology 109: 821–5.

Gillett D, Almeyda J, Whinney D et al. (2002) Pneumocephalus: an unreported risk of Valsalva's manoeuvre after cochlear implantation. Cochlear Implants International 3(1): 68–74.

Govaerts PJ, De Beukelaer C, Daemers K et al. (2002) Outcome of cochlear implantation at different ages from 0 to 6 years. Otology and Neurotogy 23: 885–90.

Grayeli AB, Bouccara D, Kalamarides M et al. (2003) Auditory brainstem implant in bilateral and completely ossified cochleae. Otology and Neurotology 24(1): 79–82.

Green KMJ, Bhatt YM, Saeed SR et al. (2004) Complications following adult cochlear implantation: experience from Manchester. Journal of Laryngology and Otology 118: 417–20.

Hans P, Grant AJ, Laitt RD et al. (1999) Comparison of 3D visualization techniques for demonstration of scala vestibuli and scala tympani of the cochlea by using high-resolution MR imaging. American Journal of Neuroradiology 20: 1197–1206.

Hans P, Jackson A, Gillespie JE et al. (2003) Virtual reality modelling language: freely available cross-platform visualisation for 3D visualisation of the inner ear. Journal of Laryngology and Otology 117: 766–74.

Hoffman RA, Cohen NL (1995) Complications of cochlear implant surgery. Ann. Otol. Rhinol. Laryngol. (suppl. 166): 420–2.

Hoffman RA, Downey LL, Waltzman SB ct al. (1997) Cochlear implantation in children with congenital malformations. American Journal of Otology 18: 184–7.

Incesulu A, Kocaturk S, Vural M (2004) Cochlear implantation in chronic otitis media. Journal of Laryngology and Otology 118: 3–7.

Kronenberg J, Baumgartner W, Migirov L et al. (2004) The suprameatal approach: an alternative surgical approach to cochlear implantation. Otology and Neurotology 25(1): 41–5.

Lehnhardt E (1993) Intracochleare Plazierung der Cochlear-Implant – Electroden in Soft Surgery Technique. HNO 41: 356–9.

Lenarz T, Lesinski-Schiedat A, Weber BP et al. (2001) The Nucleus double array cochlea implant: a new concept for the obliterated cochlea. Otology and Neurotology 22: 24–32.

Maas S, Bance M, O'Driscoll M et al. (1996) Explantation of a Nucleus multi-channel cochlear implant with reimplantation into the contralateral ear: case report of a new strategy. Journal of Laryngology and Otology 110: 881–3.

Miyamoto RT, McConkey-Robins AJ, Myres WA et al. (1986) American Journal of Otology 7: 258–61.

O'Donoghue GM, Nikolopoulos TP (2002) Minimal access surgery for cochlear implantation. Otology and Neurotology 23: 891–4.

Olgun L (2003) Paper presented to 50th Annual meeting of the Slovakian Society of Otolaryngology, Bratislava, October 2003.

Proops DW, Stoddart RL, Donaldson I (1999) Medical, surgical and audiological complications of the first 100 adult cochlear implant patients in Birmingham. Journal of Laryngology and Otology (suppl. 24): 14–17.

Sennaroglu L, Saatci (2002) A new classification for cochleovestibular malformations. Laryngoscope 112: 2230–41.

Steenerson RL, Gray LB, Wynens MS (1990) Scala vestibuli cochlear implantation for labyrinthine ossification. American Journal of Otology 11: 360–3.

Summerfield AQ, Marshall DH (1995) Cochlear Implantation in the UK
    1990–1994. Report by the MRC Institute of Hearing Research on the evaluation
    of the national cochlear implant programme. London: HMSO.
Temple RH, Ramsden RT, Axon PR et al. (1999) The large vestibular aqueduct syn-
    drome: the role of cochlear implantation in its management. Clinical
    Otolaryngology 24: 301–6.
Webb RL, Lehnhardt E, Clark GM et al. (1991) Surgical complications with the
    cochlear multiple-channel intracochlear implant: experience at Hannover and
    Melbourne. Annals of Otology Rhinology and Laryngology 100: 131–6.

# CHAPTER 11

# Utility of electrically evoked potentials in cochlear implant users

PAUL J. ABBAS AND CAROLYN J. BROWN

## Introduction

Over the course of the last two decades, a significant body of research has been published that describes the role that objective measures can play in the management of patients with cochlear implants (e.g. Cullington, 2003). Methods for measuring a range of different neural responses to electrical stimulation have been reported. These include the electrically evoked compound action potential (Brown et al., 1990), the electrically evoked brainstem response (van den Honert and Stypulkowski, 1986; Abbas and Brown, 1991), the electrically evoked middle latency response (Kileny and Kemink, 1987; Shallop et al., 1990), electrically evoked measures of the mismatch negativity potential (Kraus et al., 1993; Ponton and Don, 1995; Kileny et al., 1997), as well as electrically evoked versions of long latency potentials (Kaga et al., 1991; Micco et al., 1995; Kileny et al., 1997). There have also been a number of studies that describe potential applications for the electrically evoked stapedial reflex threshold in cochlear implant recipients (Battmer et al., 1990; Stephan et al., 1991; Spivak and Chute, 1994; Shallop and Ash, 1996; Hodges et al., 1997, 2003).

In general, all of these electrically evoked potentials have characteristics that are very similar to their acoustically evoked counterparts. The similarity between the electrically and acoustically evoked responses is apparent both for postlingually deafened adults as well as for children with congenital deafness. On a very global level this suggests that the basic organization of the auditory system is intact in both groups of cochlear implant users. On closer examination, however, there are some significant differences between electrically and acoustically evoked neural responses. These differences are primarily due to the fact that electrical stimulation bypasses the normal mechanical transduction mechanisms in the cochlea and stimulates the auditory nerve fibers directly. As a result, the response of the auditory nerve to electrical stimulation has a shorter latency, greater synchrony and steeper growth characteristics compared with single-fiber responses evoked using acoustic stimulation (Kiang and Moxon, 1972). It is not possible to measure single-fiber responses from the auditory nerve in humans; however, these differences in the mode of stimulation observed at the single-fiber level in animal preparations are also observed in the short latency gross potentials that can be measured non-invasively in implant patients. Specifically, the response latencies of early potentials such as the electrically evoked compound action potential (ECAP) and the electrically evoked auditory brainstem response (EABR) tend to be shorter, amplitudes tend to be greater and the growth of response with stimulation level tends to be steeper for electrical stimulation than is typically observed with acoustic stimulation (van den Honert and Stypulkowski, 1986; Brown et al., 1990).

In the early years of cochlear implant research the possibility of using objective measures before implantation in order to predict eventual performance with the implant was investigated using promontory stimulation (Smith and Simmons, 1983). However, the limitations of this technique were quickly apparent and have constrained the use of such measures (van den Honert and Stypulkowski, 1986). In contrast, stimulation through the implant either at the time of surgery or post-operatively has proven to be feasible and a number of possible applications for such measures have been and continue to be investigated.

The next section describes the general methodology used to measure electrically evoked neural responses as well as issues and stimulation paradigms relevant to the measurement of specific neural responses. The final section describes several potential applications for objective measures with cochlear implant users.

# Recording electrically evoked potentials

## 1. General considerations

Several early studies have investigated the possibility of recording electrically evoked neural potentials using extracochlear promontory stimulation. More recent research has focused on measuring responses evoked via intracochlear stimulation (through the implant). The techniques for recording electrically evoked potentials are dependent on whether direct intracochlear or extracochlear stimulation is used and to some extent on when these responses are recorded (pre-, peri- or post-operatively).

### Recording evoked potentials using extracochlear stimulation

The basic technique for pre-implant stimulation is to place an electrode in the middle ear, either on the promontory or the round window niche. This can be accomplished with a needle electrode through the tympanic membrane or using a ball electrode visually placed through a flap opening in the tympanic membrane. The stimulator used to elicit the neural response should be a wide-band current source capable of producing biphasic, charge-balanced current pulses with phase durations of less than 100 microseconds. If the frequency response of the current source is sufficiently broad, it will adequately reproduce the pulse waveform and minimize ringing. The biphasic nature of the pulses is important to provide charge-balanced stimuli to the cochlea.

In order to successfully measure neural potentials evoked using promontory stimulation, two particular issues should be considered. The first is the need to eliminate or substantially reduce the relatively large stimulus artifact that results when electrical stimulation is used. When extracochlear stimulation is used, the stimulation levels needed to excite the auditory nerve can be substantially higher than those required when intracochlear stimulation is used. As a result, contamination of the recording by stimulus artifact can be particularly problematic. A number of techniques have been used to eliminate or minimize stimulus artifact contamination. For example, the position of the stimulating and recording electrodes is known to affect the amplitude of the stimulus artifact that is recorded (Gardi, 1985). Bipolar stimulating electrodes coupled with a contralateral recording electrode montage generally results in relatively small artifact compared to monopolar stimulation coupled with an ipsilateral recording electrode montage. This is because the EABR is typically recorded using differential amplification and, when bipolar stimulation is applied to a site that is distant from either of the two recording electrodes, each recording electrode picks up a similar potential. Consequently, the electrical stimulus artifact is minimized. Also if the stimulus duration is short and if the recordings are made using relatively wide-band filtering, the spread of the artifact in the time domain can be minimized. Additionally, many researchers have also used some type of blanking circuit to minimize input to the recording amplifier during the period of stimulus presentation. This reduces the possibility of recording amplifier saturation. Prolonged recovery from saturation can significantly distort and/or mask the response. Finally, alternating polarity stimulation can also be used to minimize stimulus artifact because opposite phase stimuli will sum in the averaged response leaving the evoked neural potential largely unaffected. All of these techniques can help to minimize the spread of the stimulus artifact in the time domain and consequently reduce the overlap of stimulus artifact and the neural response.

In addition to stimulus artifact problems, a second factor that needs to be taken into consideration is the source of the response. When promontory stimulation is used, it is possible that the recorded potential results from, electrical stimulation of structures outside of the auditory pathway (e.g. the vestibular nerve and/or the facial nerve). It is therefore particularly important to be sure that responses have the appropriate morphology and dependence on stimulus level in order to distinguish auditory responses from those of other systems (van den Honert and Stypulkowski, 1986).

### Recording evoked potentials using intracochlear stimulation

Once the implant is in place, it is possible to stimulate the auditory system electrically using the cochlear implant itself. The main advantage afforded by the use of intracochlear rather than extracochlear stimulation is that the site of stimulation is much closer to the auditory nerve. This in turn leads to lower response thresholds and less stimulus artifact. However, contamination of recorded neural response by electrical stimulus artifact is still possible and many of the techniques described in the previous section for separating the neural response from the recorded stimulus artifact can be used to minimize artifact contamination in responses recorded post-operatively using intracochlear stimulation.

The procedure for stimulation is somewhat simpler than with extracochlear stimulation since the electrodes for stimulation are already implanted. One simply needs to access those electrodes to present a stimulus. This can be accomplished by acoustic stimulation through the cochlear implant speech processor. However, this method can result in considerable stimulus artifact that can interfere with recording neural responses. Therefore, it is often necessary to bypass the speech processor and to stimulate individual electrodes within the implant directly with short duration electrical pulses. The major cochlear implant manufacturers provide software to stimulate the auditory nerve with single-pulse stimuli and an external trigger stimulus that can be used to initiate averaging on a separate evoked potential recording system. In this way, short duration, pulsatile stimuli on specific electrode combinations with correspondingly short stimulus artifact can be used to evoke a response. Artifact cancellation procedures discussed in the previous section can be used to minimize artifact contamination and to isolate the neural response. In addition to these techniques, because the implant systems use RF transmission to activate the internal electronics, careful RF shielding at the electrode input to the averaging system is needed to avoid contamination of the evoked potential by artifact caused by demodulation of the RF signal used to activate the internal electronics of the cochlear implant.

### Intra- vs post-operative measures

From a clinical perspective, there are many reasons why intra-operative measures of the response of the auditory system to electrical stimulation might be preferred over post-operative measures. Intra-operative assessment of the neural response to electrical stimulation can provide valuable information to the surgeon as well as the patient's family concerning the functioning of the implant and the peripheral auditory system at the time of surgery and can be obtained with no concern about the potential for overstimulation. Sensitivity across different electrodes within the implant can be evaluated and potentially malfunctioning electrodes as well as electrodes that may result in facial nerve stimulation can be identified. Such information can be useful during the initial programming sessions.

Unfortunately, however, not all of the electrically evoked auditory potentials can be recorded reliably in the operating room. For example, the electrically evoked stapedial reflex, as well as most of the middle and long latency responses, is adversely affected by anesthetic agents. Even measures of the peripheral auditory system (ECAP and EABR) might be better recorded during the post-operative period. For example, intra-operative measures of the EABR, and to a lesser extent the ECAP, can be adversely affected by the fact that the operating room is typically a very noisy environment and the time available for making these measures is typically quite limited. Additionally, the response measured initially may be different than those measured at the time of hook-up or at a later post-operative visit (Brown et al., 1994; Hughes et al., 2001). In contrast, post-implant measures can be obtained on the day of initial stimulation or at any time following that, and those measures have proven to be fairly stable over time (Brown et al., 1995; Hughes et al., 2001) and therefore may be preferable in many respects to similar measures made intra-operatively.

## 2. Electrically evoked auditory brainstem response

The first descriptions of the EABR were published in the late seventies and early to mid-1980s (Starr and Brackmann, 1979; Dobie and Kimm, 1980; Black et al., 1983; van den Honert and Stypulkowski, 1986). Figure 11.1 shows a series of EABRs recorded for a range of stimulation levels in a Nucleus CI24M cochlear implant user. As described in the literature and as illustrated in this figure, the EABR consists of a series of vertex positive peaks occurring within the first 6–8 ms following electrical stimulation of the auditory nerve. The responses in Figure 11.1 were recorded using a 25 $\mu$s/phase biphasic current pulse and standard filtering and recording electrode montages.

The general morphology of the EABR is similar to its acoustic counterpart, and the most prominent peak of the EABR is typically labeled with Roman numeral V. The primary difference between the EABR and its acoustically evoked counterpart is that the EABR is recorded with significantly shorter peak latencies. Typically, wave V of the EABR has a latency of 4–5 ms, while at high stimulation levels wave V of the auditory brainstem response (ABR) has a latency of 5–6 ms. At high stimulation levels a series of earlier peaks analogous to waves II–IV of the acoustically evoked ABR are also often recorded. The earliest peaks of the EABR are generally obscured in the averaged response by uncancelled stimulus artifact. The amplitude of wave V of the EABR is often larger than the amplitude of wave V of the ABR, presumably reflecting greater neural synchrony associated with electrical as opposed to acoustic stimulation of the auditory system. Additionally, the amplitude of the peaks in the EABR grow relatively rapidly

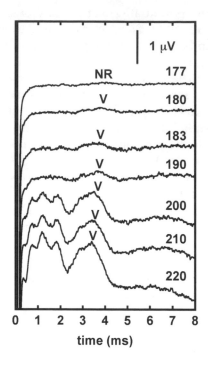

**Figure 11.1** EABR waveforms recorded from a Nucleus 24 implant user are plotted as function of time after stimulus onset. In each case the stimulus is a 25 μs/phase biphasic pulse. Current levels (in clinical units) are indicated for each trace. Wave V peak is indicated on each trace.

with increases in current level, compared to similar growth measures obtained using acoustic stimuli.

Another major difference between the EABR and the ABR is that the latency of the individual peaks of the EABR changes very little with stimulation level (see Figure 11.1). The lack of a change in latency is probably because electrical stimulation bypasses normal cochlear mechanics and activates the nerve fibers directly (Abbas and Brown, 1988). As latency does not change with stimulation level, analysis of the EABR depends on measuring wave V amplitude versus intensity rather than latency versus intensity functions that are used more commonly for general clinical purposes. As such, control of noise in the EABR recordings is critical.

While the EABR is an appropriate tool to use in pediatric applications, it is a small amplitude response that is susceptible to contamination by both electrical noise and muscle artifact and as such requires a sleeping or sedated subject and careful control of the electrical environment. While there is some evidence that the latency of wave V may show developmental effects during the early post-implant period (Gordon et al., 2002b), the fact that the EABR can be recorded intra-operatively in congenitally deaf children with little or no previous auditory stimulation

(Abbas and Brown, 1991; Mason et al., 2001; Shallop et al., 1990) suggests that the major neural pathways through the auditory system are not dependent on intact auditory periphery.

## 3. Electrically evoked compound action potential

In the mid-1990s Cochlear Corporation introduced the Nucleus CI24 cochlear implant system. This device contained the electronic circuitry necessary to use intracochlear electrodes as recording rather than stimulating electrodes and for the first time it was possible to measure the ECAP in children and individuals who used a cochlear implant system without a percutaneous connection. Cochlear Corporation named the hardware and software used to record the ECAP Neural Response Telemetry (NRT). In 2001, Advanced Bionic Corporation followed suit, introducing the Clarion CII cochlear implant system. This device was also equipped with neural telemetry capabilities. The hardware and software used to record the ECAP with the Advanced Bionics system is called Neural Response Imaging (NRI). The development of telemetry measures for recording the ECAP provide additional advantages of the ECAP relative to EABR measures in that no additional instrumentation or recording electrodes are needed to acquire neural responses. Introduction of the NRT/NRI technology meant that for the first time it was possible to include evoked potential testing as part of the routine testing of patients.

The ECAP is a gross potential that reflects the synchronous firing of a large number of electrically stimulated auditory nerve fibers. Figure 11.2 shows a series of ECAPs recorded from two cochlear implant users, one with a Nucleus CI24 implant and the other with a Clarion CII implant. In each case, response waveforms are plotted over a range of stimulus levels from below ECAP threshold up to a maximum comfortable level. The ECAP is characterized by a single negative peak with a latency of approximately 0.2 ms for both subjects. Like the EABR, latency of the ECAP changes very little with stimulation level. As shown in Figure 11.2, however, the amplitude of the ECAP can be several hundred times larger than the amplitude of the EABR.

While difficult or impossible to record pre-operatively, the ECAP has several advantages over the EABR or other auditory evoked potentials. For example, it is recorded from an electrode inside the cochlea rather than from surface electrodes. Therefore, the ECAP is much larger than the EABR, is not adversely affected by muscle activity, requires less averaging than the EABR and, as a result, the subject is not required to sit still during ECAP recording sessions. Additionally, because the ECAP is a peripherally generated auditory response, it is not affected by development, anesthesia, attention or sedation. All of these factors make the ECAP ideal for many pediatric applications.

On the other hand, since the ECAP is a peripheral response, it does not reflect differences among subjects in central processing nor can it be used

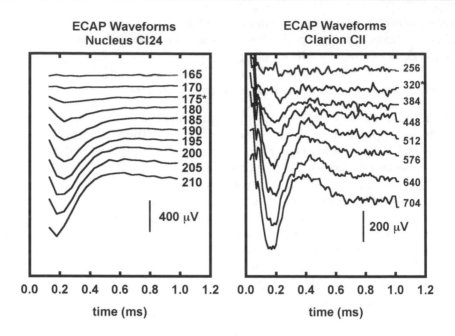

**Figure 11.2** ECAP waveforms recorded from a Nucleus CI24 implant user and a Clarion CII user are plotted as a function of time after stimulus onset. In each case the stimulus is a 25 μs/phase biphasic pulse. Current levels (in clinical units for Nucleus 24 and μA for Calrion CII) are indicated for each trace. Threshold response level is indicated by the asterisk.

to assess developmental changes in the central nervous system (CNS) in children. Also, since the latency of the response is relatively short and the stimulating and recording electrodes are in such close proximity to each other, difficulties with stimulus artifact contamination are much greater for the ECAP than for other evoked potential measures.

While stimulus artifact reduction techniques such as stimulus alternation can be used in some instances to record the ECAP (Wilson et al., 1997b), the use of a two-pulse subtraction technique that takes advantage of the neuron's refractory properties has proven to be a more reliable recording method. The first recordings using this technique were obtained from individuals who used the Ineraid cochlear implant system. This device allowed for direct access to intracochlear electrodes through a transcutaneous pedestal (Brown et al., 1990). Typically, one measures the response to a probe pulse with and without a masker pulse preceding it. The theory behind the subtraction method is that if the masker pulse is high enough in level the auditory nerve fibers will fire in response to the masker pulse, and, if the interpulse interval (IPI) is sufficiently short, these auditory nerve fibers will be in a refractory state and therefore unable to respond to the probe. The probe-alone recording therefore should contain both probe stimulus artifact and a neural response to the probe; the masker-plus-probe recording, however, will contain only probe stimulus artifact but no neural response to the probe should be recorded. The subtraction of these two recordings will allow the probe stimulus artifact to be minimized without affecting the neural response to the probe.

## 4. Electrically evoked middle and late potentials

The latency and morphologic characteristics of both the electrically-evoked middle latency response (EMLR) and the long latency electrically evoked auditory responses are very similar to their acoustic counterparts. The EMLR is characterized by a series of slow vertex positive peaks occurring within a time window of 10–50 ms following stimulation. Electrically evoked long latency responses consist of a series of potentials occurring within a time window of approximately 50–300 ms. The EMLR reflects neural activity at the level of the auditory midbrain, and, while there are several different long latency cortical or pre-cortical responses that can be recorded from cochlear implant users, to date most of the focus recently has been on the electrically evoked N1/P2 complex (Ponton et al., 1996; Ponton and Eggermont, 2001; Sharma et al., 2002). Both the mismatched negativity (MMN) response as well as the event-related P300 potential evoked using electrical rather than acoustic stimulation have also been reported (Kileny, 1991; Kraus et al., 1993; Ponton and Don, 1995; Makhdoum et al., 1998a).

These relatively centrally generated evoked potentials have several advantages over the EABR or the ECAP. Since the latency of these responses is long, the problems with stimulus artifact reduction are not as severe as those typically encountered with EABR or ECAP. Consequently, recording procedures typically used for acoustic stimulation are adequate for recording the middle or late response to stimulation through the implant. Additionally, speech or speech-like stimuli rather than single electric pulses can be used. Finally, in some circumstances, the fact that these responses reflect higher-order processing within the auditory system can also be advantageous since they may reflect changes in processing within the central nervous system over time.

## 5. Electrically evoked stapedial reflex thresholds

In addition to the neural responses described in the previous sections, it is also possible to use electrical stimulation to activate the stapedial reflex. In order to do this, electrical stimulation is applied via the implant. Contraction of the stapedial muscle in the non-implanted ear can then be measured using standard immittance equipment. Research has shown that the threshold of the electrically evoked stapedial reflex occurs at or near the maximum levels used by the speech processor (Jerger et al., 1986; Battmer et al., 1990; Hodges et al., 1997, 2003). Intra-operative measures of stapedial reflex can also be assessed by visualizing the contraction of the stapedial muscle in the open middle ear cavity (van den

Borne et al., 1996) or by recording electromyographic (EMG) activity directly from the stapedial muscle (Almquist et al., 2000).

The ESRT has the advantage that it is recorded easily using standard audiometric equipment, is not adversely affected by electrical stimulus artifact and, unlike the ECAP or the EABR, can be recorded using the same stimulus used to program the speech processor. One disadvantage of the ESRT is that studies show that the ESRT cannot be recorded in as many as 25–35% of subjects at maximum stimulation levels (Spivak and Chute, 1994; Hodges et al., 1997) and does require some compliance on the part of the child. Intra-operative measures of the ESRT have been shown to be elevated, presumably owing to the effects of anesthesia (Makhdoum et al., 1998c), and little information is available regarding how variable this response is over time and/or how stimulation parameters, such as stimulus rate or duration, impact the estimate of stapedial reflex threshold. Still, the ESRT remains a potentially important tool for assisting with device programming in pediatric patients.

## 6. Average electrode voltages

Finally, surface recording electrodes and evoked potential recording techniques can also be used to record the effect of current delivered by the implant when the internal device is activated. This potential has been called an 'averaged electrode voltage' (AEV). This method cannot measure absolute current amplitude since the amplitude of the recorded voltage will depend on many factors such as the orientation of the stimulating electrode and the recording electrodes. Nevertheless, such measures can be useful in diagnosing malfunctions of the internal components of the cochlear implant and monitoring changes in the function of the implant over time.

Figure 11.3 shows a series of AEVs recorded using the Nucleus Crystal System. This is an evoked potential system that is designed specifically to allow for the measurement of the AEV using surface recording electrodes in Nucleus cochlear implant users. Panel A shows the response measured when electrodes 1 through 22 are stimulated sequentially in a monopolar configuration. Recording AEVs using monopolar stimulation is important because typically this is the mode that is used for stimulation through the speech processor and because this mode of stimulation results in large amplitude recordings that will be sensitive to open circuits. Panel B shows the AEVs recorded from the same electrodes with common ground stimulation. In this case the current return path is through all remaining intra-cochlear electrodes. Recording AEVs using common ground stimulation is important because this mode will allow for identification of electrodes that are short-circuited. The recorded impedance for each electrode is shown in panel C.

In the recordings shown in Figure 11.3, the recording electrode configuration is ipsilateral mastoid positive relative to contralateral mastoid

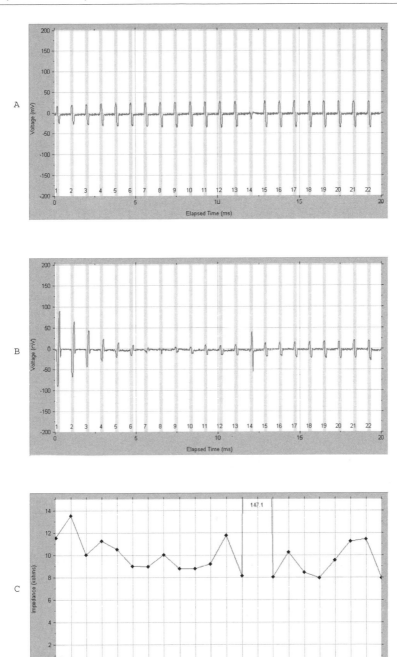

**Figure 11.3** AEVs recorded from a CI24 implant user. All recordings are made with the Nucleus Crystal System using an ipsilateral mastoid positive relative to contralateral mastoid negative recording configuration. Panel A shows the response measured for each stimulating electrode using monopolar configuration. Panel B shows response using a common ground configuration. Panel C shows the impedance values for each electrode.

negative into a differential amplifier. In a normally functioning device, the AEVs recorded using monopolar stimulation show gradually increasing response amplitude as the stimulating electrode is moved from base to apex. The AEVs recorded using common ground stimulation should be largest when stimulation is applied to the basal electrodes and should gradually decrease in amplitude, reverse polarity and then increase in amplitude again as the stimulating electrode is moved from base to apex. The AEVs shown in Figure 11.3 were obtained from a device with a known fault at electrode 14. When electrode 14 was stimulated either in monopolar or in common ground stimulation modes, abnormal AEV amplitudes and waveforms were recorded. These results are consistent with the finding of abnormally high electrode impedance for electrode 14 (see Figure 11.3, panel C).

The current generation of cochlear implants are equipped with telemetry systems that can be used to measure the integrity of the internally implanted electrodes. However, tens of thousands of individuals across the world received their cochlear implants before impedance telemetry became available. For these individuals, AEVs are the only way to monitor device function or malfunction. For individuals with current technology, the AEV recordings can be used in conjunction with the impedance measures to more fully characterize device function. There are several anecdotal reports in the literature describing abnormalities in device function diagnosed on the basis of abnormal AEVs in spite of normal electrode impedance measures.

# Applications of electrically evoked potentials in clinical practice

## 1. Decisions relative to implantation

One theory that many clinicians and researchers held during the early years of cochlear implantation was that post-implant performance might be related to the number and/or status of the surviving auditory nerve fibers. Consequently, the goal of many of the initial studies with objective measures was to find an electrically evoked auditory potential that could be recorded pre-operatively and that could be used to predict post-implant performance. For instance, one might theorize that the amplitude of the EABR would be proportional to the number of stimulated fibers in the auditory nerve. The number of stimulable auditory nerve fibers that a profoundly deaf individual had might, in turn, be related to the eventual performance with the cochlear implant. Obviously, if there are no surviving neurons in the auditory nerve, then the implant would not be effective. Studies in experimental animals and analysis of human temporal bones have demonstrated that some surviving spiral ganglion cells were present in subjects who were able to perceive sound in response to electrical stimulation through a cochlear implant (Pfingst et al., 1981; Johnsson et al., 1982; Pfingst and Sutton, 1983). In addition, early animal studies demonstrated that the number of surviving neurons in the auditory nerve could be related to performance with a cochlear implant (Pfingst et al., 1979; Clopton et al., 1980). Although there are clearly other factors that may affect performance, such as cognitive abilities or spatial distribution of surviving neurons, such considerations have motivated research investigating the relationships among evoked potentials, auditory nerve survival and performance with the implant.

There have been a number of studies using experimental animals that have investigated the relationship between the EABR and neuron survival in the spiral ganglion as determined using histological techniques. Some of these studies have used intracochlear stimulation; others have used extracochlear stimulation. Most of those studies have used animal models and have shown a relationship between response amplitude, or growth of response amplitude with level, and spiral ganglion cell survival (Smith and Simmons, 1983; Lusted et al., 1984; Shepard et al., 1983). Hall (1990) observed particularly strong correlations between nerve survival and the rate of growth of wave I (or auditory nerve component) of the EABR with increasing levels of stimulation. Modeling of the ECAP based on single-fiber response properties is consistent with the generally held theory that the number of active fibers is the primary determinant of the amplitude of the electrically evoked compound action potential (Miller et al., 1999).

Recordings of the EABR in human subjects have demonstrated a great deal of variability in the EABR threshold, amplitude and waveform morphology. While no studies have yet reported comparisons to post-mortem assessments of neural survival, a number of studies have investigated the degree to which such measures are correlated with speech perception.

Pre-implant measures would be particularly useful if they could in fact reliably predict post-implant performance. Unfortunately, most studies that have assessed correlations between EABR parameters, such as threshold or growth of response with level, have not shown a clear correlation to measures of speech perception (Meyer et al., 1984; Simmons et al., 1984; van den Honert and Stypulkowski, 1986; Game et al., 1987; Gantz et al., 1988, 1994, Fifer et al., 1991; Kileny et al., 1994; Kubo et al., 2001). A recent study by Gantz et al. (2002) used bilaterally implanted subjects to compare performance with the implant in each ear to the pre-implant EABR thresholds and amplitude growth measures obtained using promontory stimulation. No correlation was observed between those electrophysiologic measures and speech perception scores in each ear. Nikolopoulos et al. (1999, 2000) published two studies that directly explored the clinical utility of EABRs recorded using promontory stimulation. Those studies compared EABR measures obtained in a set of 30 children who were congenitally deaf with those obtained from 19 children who were deaf following meningitis. Nikolopoulos et al. (1999) found EABR responses from the children who were deaf due to meningitis had poorer morphology and smaller amplitudes than similar measures made from the children who were congenitally deaf. These children were followed post-operatively, and in 2000 they reported no significant correlation between the presence of a poor EABR measured pre-operatively and performance with the implant.

There are several possible reasons why pre-operative measures of electrically evoked potentials may not correlate with post-operative performance. One challenge associated with making evoked potential measures prior to cochlear implantation is that, when an extracochlear stimulating electrode is used, the amount of current injected to the cochlea can be quite variable. It is difficult to control or quantify the amount of current that is shunted into the middle ear and away from the auditory nerve when electrical stimulation is applied via an electrode placed either on the promontory or on the round window. In order to get around this limitation, several investigators have used post-operative measures of EABR, EMLR or late potentials to try to determine whether or not a metric such as response threshold or amplitude growth is correlated with post-operative performance. Presumably, responses to stimulation through the intracochlear electrode array would be more likely to correlate with performance since the stimulation path is the same. Makhdoum et al. (1998b) demonstrated that measures such as the amplitude, latency and/or growth of the EABR are not significantly related to post-operative performance. Firszt et al. (2002) also failed to find a strong correlation between the EABR and speech perception for 11 postlingually deafened adults who used the Clarion device. They did note, however, that the subjects without open-set word understanding tended to be those with poor response morphologies. The only significant correlations that have been reported in recent years have been between EABR measures and performance in subjects who use the Digisonic cochlear implant (Gallego et al., 1997, 1998). It is unclear why the relationship between the EABR and performance would be device-specific. More research will be needed to see if the reported correlations between word recognition and EABR threshold or growth measures will hold as the number of subjects using the Digisonic device increases.

Speech perception is a high-level cognitive function. The EABR (and the ECAP for that matter) is a measure of peripheral neural responsiveness. No correlation exists between the acoustically evoked ABR and performance on tests of speech perception. It is, therefore, not surprising that the EABR is not strongly correlated with performance with a cochlear implant. Nevertheless, several clinical centers record EABR just prior to surgery in each ear. They argue that pre- or peri-operative stimulation using an extracochlear electrode allows the clinician to determine that a particular ear is 'stimulable' (Kileny, 1991; Kileny et al., 1991). Additionally, it has been argued that comparison of the amplitude of the EABR evoked pre-operatively in the individual ears might inform the decision-making process regarding which ear to implant (Kileny et al., 1991;

Mason et al., 1997). Unfortunately, there is very little data to support either clinical application, and many cochlear implant centers have chosen to abandon pre- or peri-operative measurement of the EABR in routine cases. Nikolopoulos et al. (2000) also note that the absence of an EABR elicited using promontory stimulation has little prognostic value. Nevertheless, the presence of a measurable EABR can be significant in cases where there is cause for concern about the status of the auditory nerve (e.g. small internal auditory canal, auditory neuropathy).

## 2. Differentiating patients who fail to stimulate from patients with failed devices

Although they represent the minority of patients who receive cochlear implants, there are times when a child or adult fails to respond to electrical stimulation, fails to progress as expected with their implant or shows some evidence of a decline in performance over time. While cochlear implants are generally very reliable, all manufacturers have reported that there have been instances of failure both of specific electrodes within the electrode array and of malfunction of the entire device. For postlingually deafened adults who are good reporters of what they hear and who have used their device successfully for some period of time, diagnosing device failure is fairly straightforward. For congenitally deaf children, however, determining whether the lack of progress with an implant is due to a lack of stimulation or device malfunction is not always so straightforward. Pediatric cochlear implant recipients cannot reliably report qualitative or quantitative changes in the perception of electrical stimulation through the implant. Some go for several months before exhibiting any overt response to electrical stimulation. This can be a challenging period for both the families and for the professionals working with that child, particularly if there is some reason to question the integrity of the child's auditory nerve.

Most implants are now equipped with a telemetry system to measure current levels produced by the implant and consequently are able to directly assess the impedance of the internal electrodes in the array. The present generation of cochlear implants (Nucleus CI24, Med-El Combi 40 and the Advanced Bionics CII) all provide the ability to assess monopolar electrode impedance, so it is possible to detect open-circuit electrodes within the array. With the Med-El or Nucleus device, it is also possible to diagnose short circuits between individual electrodes within the array. Regardless of the implant type, AEVs can also be used to assess the integrity of the implanted electronics. Neither procedure requires any behavioral response from the child. Additionally, the manufacturers are typically very willing to assist the programming audiologist in confirming that the internal device is functioning as it should. The next step in these cases is to try to record a response that would be consistent with an intact auditory nerve. Evoked potential measures can be particularly useful for such assessments.

Research with both pediatric and adult cochlear implant recipients has shown that the ECAP threshold, as it is most commonly measured using low-rate stimulation, indicates a level where the high-rate stimulus train used to program the device will be audible. Therefore, in children who initially fail to respond behaviorally to electrical stimulation, ECAP thresholds can be used to guide device programming until the child is able to participate in behavioral testing.

NRT/NRI measures have also been shown to be stable over time (Hughes et al., 2001). Therefore, these neural responses coupled with AEV and electrode impedance measures can be used to assist in determining whether an apparent change in response to stimulation is due to a change in device function or a change in neural responsiveness. Obtaining baseline NRT/NRI measures on all cochlear implant recipients at some time during the first few months of stimulation and annually or even bi-annually thereafter can be useful as a baseline of comparison for future measurements. If an individual has a change in sensitivity or if a child is failing to progress at a normal rate with his/her implant, such information can be invaluable in determining the underlying cause.

In some instances, it is not possible to record an ECAP in a patient for whom the internal device is apparently functioning appropriately. Often this occurs in patients with very high stimulation thresholds who require wider pulse durations to perceive the stimulus. At high stimulation levels and long pulse durations, stimulus artifact is problematic and often causes saturation of the amplifier used to record the ECAP. In these cases, EABR measures can be used in much the same way as the ECAP. In cases where a child is not exhibiting any overt response to electrical stimulation despite indications that the internal device is functional, the presence of an EABR is a good indication that the auditory nerve is intact and that the stimulus generated by the speech processor should be audible.

## 3. Establishing appropriate programming levels

Implanting children of 12–18 months of age or younger not only presents problems in candidate identification but also in post-operative programming. Programming the speech processor generally requires establishing threshold and/or an upper level of stimulation on as many as 22 intra-cochlear electrodes. Additionally, adult cochlear implant recipients are typically asked to identify electrodes that sound unusual or distorted and to pitch rank or to balance the loudness of the electrodes across the array. For very young cochlear implant recipients, simply establishing threshold and upper levels of stimulation can be a difficult task. Often, these children do not have a clear idea of what constitutes 'comfortably loud' and minimum response levels may be significantly elevated relative to the child's 'true' threshold. Additionally, very young children have neither the language abilities nor the auditory experience necessary to pitch rank or to balance loudness across electrodes. Also they have neither the auditory experience nor communication skills necessary to identify electrodes that produce distorted or unusual sound percepts.

Electrophysiological measures of auditory function do not require a behavioral response from the subject, so they have the potential to be particularly useful in the clinical management of the pediatric cochlear implant recipients. Central to this issue is the extent to which electrophysiological thresholds correlate with behavioral threshold measures. In general, when the stimuli used for both physiologic and behavioral measures are similar, the correlation between the two measures of threshold has been shown to be strong. This finding applies to both acoustically evoked CAP and ABR as well as to their electrical counterparts, the ECAP and the EABR (Coats and Martin, 1977; Gorga et al., 1985; Abbas and Brown, 1991; Shallop et al., 1991; Brown et al., 1994; Hodges et al., 1994; Smith et al., 1994; Miller et al., 1995). Typically, however, the stimuli used to measure ECAP or EABR thresholds are very different from the stimuli used to program the speech processor. Pulse trains at rates of 30–80 Hz are generally used to measure the ECAP and/or EABR thresholds. Pulse trains of 250 Hz or greater are generally used to program the speech processor. Moreover, behavioral measures of threshold and maximum comfort will clearly reflect temporal integration, while physiologic estimates of threshold will not. As such, it is not surprising that previous

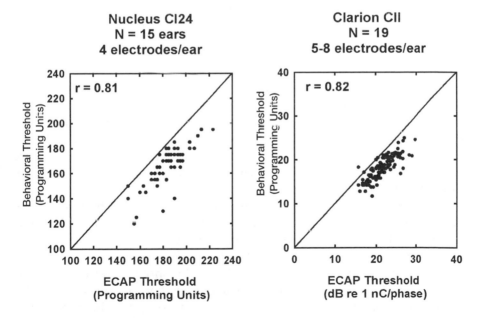

**Figure 11.4** Scatter plots show the relationship between behavioral threshold and ECAP threshold, both measured with single-pulse stimuli (25 μs/phase). Data from 15 Nucleus implant users are plotted in the left panel with current level expressed in clinical programming units. Data from 19 Clarion CII users are plotted in the right panel with current level expressed in nC/phase. The diagonal line indicates where behavioral threshold and ECAP threshold would be equal.

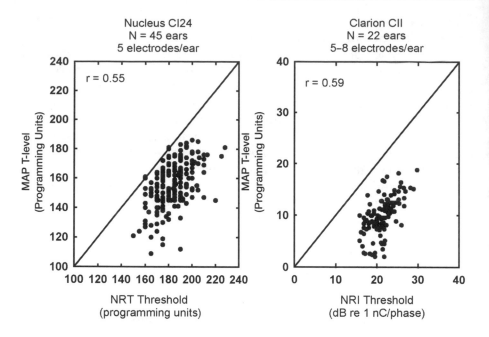

**Figure 11.5** Scatter plots show the relationship between MAP T-level (measured using pulse trains) and ECAP threshold for single-pulse stimuli. Data from 45 Nucleus implant users are plotted in the left panel with current level expressed in clinical programming units. Data from 22 Clarion CII users are plotted in the right panel with current level expressed in nC/phase. The diagonal line indicates where behavioral threshold and ECAP threshold would be equal.

research has shown the correlation between ECAP and/or EABR thresholds and behavioral MAP levels to be only moderate and to include significant cross-subject variability (Shallop et al., 1990; 1991; Mason et al., 1993, 2001; Brown et al., 1994, 2000; Cullington, 2000; Hughes et al., 2000; Thai-Van et al. 2001; Gordon et al. 2002a). That variability is, at least in part, due to differences in temporal integration among cochlear implant users (Brown et al., 1999).

These trends are illustrated in Figures 11.4 and 11.5, where measures made using the Nucleus NRT system and the Clarion NRI system are compared to behavioral threshold measures. Figure 11.4 shows a scatter plot of the behavioral threshold vs. ECAP threshold, where the rate of pulse presentation was the same (80 pps). ECAP thresholds tend to be somewhat higher than behavioral thresholds, but the correlation between the two measures is quite strong. The levels used to program the implant are typically made at a much higher pulse rate, 250 Hz or higher. As shown in Figure 11.5, when the same ECAP thresholds are compared to behavioral thresholds for the programming stimulus, the correlation is considerably weaker, suggesting that the relatively higher pulse rate affects threshold in individuals differently and, as a result, the strength of the correlation between behavioral thresholds and ECAP thresholds declines.

Similar variations in scatter plots are seen between ECAP/EABR thresholds and maximum comfort levels that are also used to program the speech processor of the cochlear implant. In some subjects the ECAP/EABR threshold is obtained at a level close to the behavioral threshold; for others the ECAP/EABR threshold indicates a point that may be at or slightly exceed the maximum comfortable stimulation level. Rarely, if ever, is the programming stimulus inaudible to the cochlear implant user when it is presented at stimulation levels that are known to elicit a threshold-level physiologic potential. Such information can facilitate the stimulus conditioning process and can provide a first order approximation of where the MAP levels should be set. Also, as mentioned in the previous section, ECAP or EABR thresholds have been shown to be stable over time (Hughes et al. 2001) and therefore can be helpful in determining whether or not changes in performance that occasionally occur for individual cochlear implant users many years after implantation are related to device failure and/or changes in the peripheral neural response to electrical stimulation.

More recently there have been several attempts to use ECAP thresholds to predict programming levels more quantitatively (Brown et al., 2000; Franck and Norton, 2001; Smoorenburg et al., 2002). All of the procedures that have been proposed involve the combination of NRT/NRI measures and a limited amount of behavioral data to determine where the MAP T- and C-levels should be set. These NRT/NRI-based MAP levels are not strongly correlated with the behaviorally determined MAP levels. Nevertheless, several investigators have reported that speech perception measures obtained using these MAPs are not significantly different from those obtained using a MAP fit using traditional behavioral programming techniques (Seyle and Brown, 2002; Smoorenburg et al., 2002).

As noted previously, cross-subject variation in temporal integration for the high-rate stimuli used for programming the implant is at least one important factor that will influence perceptual thresholds and loudness levels. Finding a way to approximate temporal integration for an individual cochlear implant user may allow us to improve the accuracy of physiologically based MAP predictions. The acoustic reflex threshold is known to demonstrate some properties of temporal integration (Korabic and Cudahy, 1984; Stephan and Welz-Muller, 1994; Rawool, 1995). Therefore the ESRT is potentially a tool that could be used to predict MAP C- or M-levels. Consistent with this is the finding that research has shown ESRT to be related to MAP levels for the Nucleus cochlear implant (Stephan et al., 1991; Spivak and Chute, 1994; Hodges et al., 1997). As noted previously, one difficulty with stapedial reflex testing is that the response is measurable typically in only approximately 65% of implant users (Spivak and Chute, 1994; Hodges et al., 1997). Therefore, while in many cases the prediction of maximum comfort level can be quite good, it may not be useful in all individuals.

The EMLR could also be used to assist with device programming (Shallop et al., 1990). The major limitation of the EMLR, however, for practical clinical applications is that it is not always reliably recorded in pediatric patients and can be adversely affected by sleep and sedation. Consequently, there has never been strong interest in the EMLR as a tool for programming the speech processor of the cochlear implant in very young children.

## 4. Choosing programming parameters

Given the variability in individual performance with cochlear implants and the increasing flexibility of cochlear implant speech processors, the issue of choosing stimulation parameters on an individual basis to maximize performance is clearly important. There is no way to evaluate even a small portion of all the possible combinations of stimulation parameters in a typical clinical setting. Identifying a set of physiologic parameters that may determine optimal speech processing parameters for an individual subject would have immense clinical significance.

There are significant differences in peripheral physiological responses (threshold, growth, spatial and temporal) among subjects and among electrodes within a subject. Parameters such as stimulation rate (Brill et al., 1997), numbers of processing channels (Fishman et al., 1997; Dorman et al., 1998; Fu et al., 1998) and choice of stimulus channels (Lawson et al., 1996) can have a significant effect on speech perception ability. It is therefore likely that the differences in both spatial and temporal properties of the neural response can have an effect on an individual's ability to encode features of the stimulus, such as frequency and fine-temporal structure. Several studies have shown relationships between physiological measures and specific psychophysical response variables, such as forward masking (Brown et al., 1996), perception of pitch (Wilson et al., 1997a) and spatial masking (Cohen et al., 2000).

Peripheral physiological measures have the ability to assess both temporal and spatial properties at the auditory periphery. For example, refractory properties of the auditory nerve have been assessed using two current pulses presented in a forward-masking paradigm (Hartmann et al., 1984; Stypulkowski and van den Honert, 1984; Brown et al., 1990; Dynes, 1995). In cochlear implant users, significant variations in refractory recovery rates have been observed with stimulus level, across electrodes within a subject, as well as across subjects (Brown and Abbas, 1990; Brown et al., 1996; Finley et al., 1997). While such experiments tell us something about temporal processing of electrical stimuli, responses to more complex stimulus patterns (such as those produced by the cochlear implant speech processor) are likely to be affected not only by refractory properties but also by other factors such as stochastic effects and long-term adaptation. Responses to pulse trains generally demonstrate an alternating pattern of ECAP amplitude in response to constant-amplitude pulse trains as well as a decrease in amplitude across the duration of the electrical pulse train (Wilson et al., 1997a; Wilson,

1997; Matsuoka et al., 2000; Javel, 1990; Vischer et al., 1997; Haenggeli et al., 1998). Experiments that more realistically simulate temporal stimulation patterns through a cochlear implant have used amplitude-modulated pulse trains (Lawson et al., 1997; Wilson et al., 1997a). The degree to which the pattern of stimulus pulse amplitudes is represented in the neural response (ECAP amplitudes) is of interest since the auditory nerve is the medium through which all auditory information is transferred centrally.

An important determinant of the performance level of a cochlear implant user may be the degree of interaction that occurs when overlapping subsets of nerve fibers are stimulated by various electrodes of a multi-channel array. Such lack of across-fiber independence in excitation is known as channel interaction and may impose significant limitations on performance in present cochlear implant designs (White et al., 1984; Fu et al., 1998). Channel interaction has been assessed psychophysically using simultaneously excited electrodes (Shannon, 1983; Abbas and Brown, 1988) as well as with a forward-masking procedure (Shannon, 1983; White et al., 1984; Boex et al., 2003). Physiological measures have demonstrated differences in the degree of interaction across subjects and with differences in electrode configuration (Abbas and Brown, 1988; Abbas et al., 2004).

ECAP and EABR data collected to date demonstrate variations in the temporal and spatial response patterns. These data suggest that there are differences in the way the peripheral auditory system is stimulated among individuals with the same implant. Knowledge of those response patterns provided by the ECAP or EABR could then be used to modify the stimulation through the implant in order to compensate for deficiencies in the neural responses. For example, one could develop a profile of physiological response characteristics analogous to our current efforts to assist in fitting protocols. In this case, decisions such as choice of electrodes, pulse rate and filtering properties could be based on that physiological profile. Such a method could be used in adults, but would be especially useful in children, for whom comparison of multiple processing strategies is clearly not feasible.

## 5. Prediction of post-implant performance using cortically evoked potentials

The preceding section focused on clinical applications of peripheral electrophysiological measures of auditory function. It is also possible to record middle and long latency auditory evoked potentials using electrical stimulation rather than acoustic stimulation. The latency of these potentials is relatively long, so they are not affected by stimulus artifact to the same degree as EABR and ECAP. They can therefore be measured using the speech processor and can be used to assess responses to complex stimuli (such as speech) as they are processed through the implant.

Higher-level auditory potentials recorded following implantation are generally evoked using stimulation paradigms (oddball) that assess discrimination and higher-level auditory function. Consequently, evoked responses such as the MMN or P-300 may be useful in indicating changes in the perception of stimulus contrasts. Generally, factors related to attention and patient age and state, such as sleep or anesthesia, will affect these measures, and so clinical utility may be limited in those populations.

Interest in electrically evoked cortical potentials has resurged in recent years. This is primarily because of work by Sharma et al. (2002) as well as by Ponton et al. (1996, 2001), who have shown that it is possible to record electrically evoked late potentials in pediatric cochlear implant users and that the latency of the P1 response to peripheral electrical stimulation is affected by the length of profound deafness. Specifically, children who were born deaf but implanted at young ages had shorter P1 response latencies than children who were born deaf but implanted later in life. Additionally, evidence has shown that the latency of the electrically evoked P1 response can change during the first few weeks or months following hook-up, presumably reflecting the plasticity of the auditory system in very young children (Sharma et al., 2002). This has significance from a clinical perspective because it suggests that this electrically evoked cortical response might be used to assess benefit from amplification pre-operatively and/or to help confirm that the speech processor of the cochlear implant is fit appropriately early in the post-implant period when the child may not yet be capable of being tested using behavioral methods. Additionally, for children with a pre-operative diagnosis of auditory neuropathy or for children with multiple developmental delays, the EMLR and the electrically evoked cortical responses may be particularly helpful in documenting the effectiveness of electrical stimulation in an individual who may never be able to participate in behavioral testing procedures.

# Summary

Objective measures of cochlear implant function have most certainly played a role in developing a better understanding of the process of electrical stimulation of the auditory nerve and the activation of the central auditory pathways. The types of measures that have been made with electrical stimulation span the range of measurements that are typical with acoustic stimulation. There are several areas in which objective measures are used in clinical situations as outlined in this chapter. An important remaining issue in further improvements with cochlear implants is the better understanding of variability across subjects and the development of methods to improve signal processing in poor performers. The measurement of electrically evoked neural activity, both peripheral and central responses, can be an important tool for accomplishing such tasks.

# References

Abbas PJ, Brown CJ (1988) Electrically evoked brainstem potentials in cochlear implant patients with multi-electrode stimulation. Hearing Research 36: 153–62.

Abbas P, Brown C (1991) Electrically evoked auditory brainstem response: growth of response with current level. Hearing Research 51: 123–38.

Abbas PJ, Hughes ML, Brown CJ et al. (2004) Channnel interaction in cochlear implant users evaluated using the electrically evoked compound action potential. Audiology and Neurotology 9: 203–23.

Almquist B, Harris S, Shallop JK (2000) Objective intraoperative method to record averaged electromyographic stapedius muscle reflexes in cochlear implant patients. Audiology 39: 146–52.

Battmer RD, Laszig R, Lehnhardt E (1990) Electrically elicited stapedius reflex in cochlear implant patients. Ear and Hearing 5: 370–4.

Black R, Clark G, Sheperd R et al. (1983) Intracochlear electrical stimulation: brainstem response audiometric and histopathological studies. Acta Oto-Laryngologica (suppl. 339): 1–18.

Boex C, Kos MI, Pelizzone M (2003) Forward masking in different cochlear implant systems. Journal of the Acoustical Society of America 114: 2058–65.

Brill SM, Gstöttner W, Helms J et al. (1997) Optimization of channel number and stimulation rates for the fast continuous interleaved sampling strategy in the Combi 40+. American Journal of Otology 18: S104–6.

Brown CJ, Abbas PJ (1990) Electrically evoked whole-nerve action potentials II. Parametric data from the cat. Journal of the Acoustical Society of America 88: 2205–10.

Brown CJ, Abbas PJ, Gantz B (1990) Electrically evoked whole-nerve action potentials I. Data from Symbion cochlear implant users. Journal of the Acoustical Society of America 88: 1385–91.

Brown CJ, Abbas PJ, Fryauf-Bertschy H et al. (1994) Intraoperative and postoperative electrically evoked auditory brainstem responses in Nucleus cochlear implant users: implications for the fitting process. Ear and Hearing 15: 168–76.

Brown CJ, Abbas PJ, Bertschy M et al. (1995) Longitudinal assessment of physiological and psychophysical measures in cochlear implant users. Ear and Hearing 16: 1–11.

Brown CJ, Abbas PJ, Borland J et al. (1996) Electrically evoked whole-nerve action potentials in Ineraid cochlear implant users: responses to different stimulating electrode configurations and comparison to psychophysical responses. Journal of Speech and Hearing Research 39: 453–67.

Brown CJ, Hughes ML, Lopez SM et al. (1999) Relationship between EABR thresholds and levels used to program the Clarion speech processor. Annals of Otology, Rhinology and Laryngology 177(suppl.): 58–63.

Brown CJ, Hughes ML, Luk B et al. (2000) The relationship between EAP and EABR thresholds and levels used to program the Nucleus CI24M speech processor: data from adults. Ear and Hearing 21: 151–63.

Clopton BM, Spelman FA, Miller JM (1980) Estimates of essential neural elements for stimulation through a cochlear prosthesis. Annals of Otology, Rhinology and Laryngology 89(suppl. 66): 5–7.

Coats AC, Martin JL (1977) Human auditory nerve action potentials and brainstem evoked responses: effects of audiogram shape and lesion location. Archives of Otolaryngology 103(10): 605–22.

Cohen LT, Saunders E, Cowan RSC (2000) The measurement of spatial spread of neural excitation using forward masking and NRT methods. 5th European Symposium on Paediatric Cochlear Implantation, Antwerp, Belgium.

Cullington HT (2000) Preliminary neural response telemetry results. British Journal of Audiology 34: 131–40.

Cullington HT (2003) Cochlear Implants: Objective Measures. London: Whurr.

Dobie RA, Kimm J (1980) Brainstem responses to electrical stimulation of cochlea. Archives of Otolaryngology 106: 573–7.

Dorman MF, Loizou PC, Fitzke J (1998) The identification of speech in noise by cochlear implant patients and normal-hearing listeners using 6-channel signal processors. Ear and Hearing 19(6): 481–4.

Dynes S (1995) Discharge characteristics of auditory nerve fibers for pulsatile electrical stimuli. PhD Thesis, MIT, Cambridge, MA.

Fifer RC, Novak, Novak MA (1991) Prediction of auditory nerve survival in humans using the electrical auditory brainstem response. American Journal of Otology 12: 350–6.

Finley CC, Wilson B, van den Honert C et al. (1997) Speech Processors for Auditory Prostheses. Sixth Quarterly Progress Report, NIH Contract NO1-DC-5-2103.

Firszt JB, Chambers RD, Kraus N (2002) Neurophysiology of cochlear implant users II: Comparison among speech perception, dynamic range, and physiological measures. Ear and Hearing 23(6): 516–31.

Fishman K, Shannon RV, Slattery WH (1997) Speech recognition as function of the number of electrodes used in the SPEAK cochlear implant processor. Journal of Speech and Hearing Research 40: 1201–15.

Franck KH, Norton SJ (2001) Estimation of psychophysical levels using the electrically evoked compound action potential measured with the neural response telemetry capabilities of Cochlear Corporation's CI24M device. Ear and Hearing 22(4): 289–99.

Fu Q, Shannon RV, Wang X (1998) Effects of noise and spectral resolution on vowel and consonant recognition: acoustic and electric hearing. Journal of the Acoustical Society of America 104: 1–11.

Gallego S, Truy E, Morgon A et al. (1997) EABRs and surface potentials with a transcutaneous multielectrode cochlear implant. Acta Oto-Laryngologica 117(2): 164–8.

Gallego S, Frachet B, Micheyl C et al. (1998) Cochlear implant performance and electrically evoked brainstem response characteristics. Electroencephalography and Clinical Neurophysiology 108(6): 521–5.

Game C, Gibson W, Pauka C (1987) Electrically evoked brainstem auditory potentials. Annals of Otology, Rhinology and Laryngology 96(suppl. 128): 94–5.

Gantz BJ, Tyler RS, Knutson JF et al. (1988) Evaluation of five different cochlear implant designs: audiologic assessment and predictors of performance. Laryngoscope 98: 1100–6.

Gantz BJ, Brown CJ, Abbas PJ (1994) Intraoperative measures of electrically evoked auditory nerve compound action potential. American Journal of Otology 15: 137–44.

Gantz BJ, Tyler RS, Rubinstein JT et al. (2002) Binaural cochlear implants: results of subjects implanted bilaterally during the same operation. Otology and Neurotology 23: 169–80.

Gardi JN (1985) Human brainstem and middle latency responses to electrical stimulation: preliminary observations. In: RA Schindler, MM Merzenich (eds), Cochlear Implants. New York: Raven Press, pp. 351–63.

Gordon KA, Ebinger KA, Gilden JE et al. (2002a) Neural response telemetry in 12- to 24-month-old children. Annals of Otology, Rhinology and Laryngology (suppl. 189): 42–8.

Gordon KA, Papsin BC, Harrison RV (2002b) Auditory brainstem and midbrain development after cochlear implantation in children. Annals of Otology, Rhinology and Laryngology (suppl. 189): 32–7.

Gorga MP, Worthington DW, Reiland JK et al. (1985) Some comparisons between auditory brainstem response threshold, latencies, and the pure-tone audiogram. Ear and Hearing 6: 105–12.

Haenggeli A, Zhang JS, Vischer MW et al. (1998) Electrically evoked compound action potential (ECAP) of the cochlear nerve in response to pulsatile electrical stimulation of the cochlea in the rat: effects of stimulation at high rates. Audiology 37: 353–71.

Hall RD (1990) Estimation of surviving spiral ganglion cells in the deaf rat using the electrically evoked auditory brainstem response. Hearing Research 45: 123–36.

Hartmann R, Topp G, Klinke R (1984) Discharge patterns of cat primary auditory fibers with electrical stimulation of the cochlea. Hearing Research 13: 47–62.

Hodges AV, Ruth RA, Lambert PR et al. (1994) Electrical auditory brainstem responses in Nucleus multichannel cochlear implant users. Archives of Otolaryngology: Head and Neck Surgery 120: 1093–9.

Hodges AV, Balkany TJ, Ruth RA et al. (1997) Electrical middle ear muscle reflex: use in cochlear implant programming. Otolaryngology: Head and Neck Surgery 117: 255–61.

Hodges AV, Butts SL, King JE (2003) Electrically evoked stapedial reflexes: utility in cochlear implant patients. In: H Cullington (ed.), Cochlear Implants: Objective Measures. London: Whurr.

Hughes ML, Brown CJ, Abbas PJ et al. (2000) The relationship between EAP and EABR thresholds and levels used to program the Nucleus CI24M speech processor: data from children. Ear and Hearing 21: 164–74.

Hughes ML, Vander Werff KR, Brown CJ et al. (2001) A longitudinal study of electrode impedance, the electrically evoked compound action potential, and behavioral measures in Nucleus 24 cochlear implant users. Ear and Hearing 22(6): 471–86.

Javel E (1990) Acoustic and electrical encoding of temporal information. In: JM Miller, FA Spelman (eds), Models of the Electrically Stimulated Cochlea. New York: Springer-Verlag.

Jerger J, Fifer R, Jenkins H et al. (1986) Stapedius reflex to electrical stimulation in a patient with a cochlear implant. Annals of Otology, Rhinology and Laryngology 95: 151–7.

Johnsson L-G, House WF, Linthicum FH Jr (1982) Otopathological findings in a patient with bilateral cochlear implants. Annals of Otology, Rhinology and Laryngology 91(suppl. 91): 74–89.

Kaga K, Kodera K, Hirota E et al. (1991) P300 responses to tones and speech sounds after cochlear implant: a case report. Laryngoscope 101: 905–7.

Kiang NYS, Moxon EC (1972) Physiological considerations in artificial stimulation of the inner ear. Annals of Otology 81: 714–30.

Kileny PR (1991) Use of electrophysiologic measures in the management of children with cochlear implants: brainstem, middle latency, and cognitive (P300) responses. American Journal of Otology (suppl. 12): 37–42.

Kileny PR, Kemink JL (1987) Electrically evoked middle latency auditory evoked potentials in cochlear implant candidates. Archives in Otolaryngology: Head and Neck Surgery 113: 1072–7.

Kileny PR, Zimmerman-Phillips S, Kemink JL et al. (1991) Effects of preoperative electrical stimulability and historical factors on performance with multichannel cochlear implants. Annals of Otology, Rhinology and Laryngology 100: 563–8.

Kileny PR, Zwolan TA, Zimmerman-Phillips S et al. (1994) A comparison of round-window and transtympanic promontory electric stimulation in cochlear implant candidates. Ear and Hearing 13: 294–9.

Kileny PR, Boerst A, Zwolan T (1997) Cognitive evoked potentials to speech and tonal stimuli in children with implants. Otolaryngology: Head and Neck Surgery 117: 161–9.

Korabic EW, Cudahy EA (1984) Acoustic reflex temporal summation measured at threshold. Ear and Hearing 5: 331–9.

Kraus N, Micco A, Koch D et al. (1993) The mismatch negativity cortical potential elicited by speech stimuli in cochlear implant patients. Hearing Research 65: 118–24.

Kubo T, Yamamoto K, Iwaki T et al. (2001) Significance of auditory evoked responses (EABR and P300) in cochlear implant subjects. Acta Otolaryngologica 121: 257–61.

Lawson DT, Wilson BS, Zerbi M et al. (1996) Speech Processors for Auditory Prostheses. Third Quarterly Progress Report, NIH Contract N01-DC-5-2103.

Lawson DT, Wilson BS, Finley CC et al. (1997) Cochlear implant studies at Research Triangle Institute and Duke University Medical Center. Scandinavian Audiology (suppl. 46): 50–64.

Lusted HS, Shelton C, Simmons FFB (1984) Comparison of electrode sites in electrical stimulation of the cochlea. Laryngoscope 94: 878–82.

Makhdoum MJ, Hinderink JB, Snik AF et al. (1998a) Can event-related potentials be evoked by extra-cochlear stimulation and used for selection purposes in cochlear implantation? Clinical Otolaryngology and Allied Sciences 23: 432–8.

Makhdoum MJ, Groenen PA, Snik AF et al. (1998b) Intra- and interindividual correlations between auditory evoked potentials and speech perception in cochlear implant users. Scandinavian Audiology 27: 13–20.

Makhdoum MJ, Snik AF, Stollman MH et al. (1998c) The influence of the concentration of volatile anesthetics on the stapedius reflex determined intraoperatively during cochlear implantation in children. American Journal of Otology 19: 598–603.

Mason SM, Sheppard S, Garnham CW et al. (1993) Application of intraoperative recordings of electrically evoked ABRs in a paediatric cochlear implant programme. Nottingham Paediatric Cochlear Implant Group. Advances in Oto-Rhino-Laryngology 48: 136–41.

Mason SM, O'Donoghue GM, Gibbin KP et al. (1997) Perioperative electrical auditory brainstem response in candidates for pediatric cochlear implantation. American Journal of Otology 18: 466–71.

Mason SM, Cope Y, Garnham J et al. (2001) Intra-operative recordings of electrically evoked auditory nerve action potentials in young children by use of neural response telemetry with the Nucleus CI24M cochlear implant. British Journal of Audiology 35(4): 225–35.

Matsuoka AJ, Abbas PJ, Rubinstein JT et al. (2000) The neuronal response to electrical constant-amplitude pulse train stimulation: evoked compound action potential recordings. Hearing Research 149: 115–28.

Meyer B, Drira M, Gegu D et al. (1984) Results of the round window electrical stimulation in 400 cases of total deafness. Acta Oto-Laryngologica (suppl. 411): 168–76.

Micco A, Kraus N, Koch D et al. (1995) Speech-evoked cognitive P300 potentials in cochlear implant recipients. American Journal of Otology 16: 514–20.

Miller CA, Woodruff KE, Pfingst BE (1995) Functional responses from guinea pigs with cochlear implants. I: electrophysiological and psychophysical measures. Hearing Research 92: 85–99.

Miller CA, Abbas PJ, Rubinstein JT (1999) An empirically based model of the electrically evoked compound action potential. Hearing Research 135: 1–18.

Nikolopoulos TP, Mason SM, O'Donoghue GM et al. (1999) Integrity of the auditory pathway in young children with congenital and postmeningitic deafness. Annals of Otology, Rhinology and Laryngology 108(4): 327 30.

Nikolopoulos TP, Mason SM, Gibbin KP et al. (2000) The prognostic value of promontory electric auditory brainstem response in pediatric cochlear implantation. Ear and Hearing 21(3):236–41.

Pfingst BE, Sutton D (1983) Relation of cochlear implant function to histopathology in monkeys. Annals of the New York Academy of Science 405: 224–39.

Pfingst BE, Donaldson JA, Miller JM et al. (1979) Psychophysical evaluation of cochlear prostheses in a monkey model. Annals of Otology, Rhinology and Laryngology 88: 613–24.

Pfingst BE, Sutton D, Miller JM et al. (1981) Relation of psychophysical data of histopathology in monkeys with cochlear implants. Acta Oto-Laryngologica 92: 1–13.

Ponton CW, Don M (1995) The mismatch negativity in cochlear implant users. Ear and Hearing 16: 131 46.

Ponton CW, Eggermont JJ (2001) Of kittens and kids: altered cortical maturation following profound deafness and cochlear implant use. Audiology and Neuro-Otology 6: 363–80.

Ponton CW, Don M, Eggermont JJ (1996) Maturation of human cortical auditory function: differences between normal-hearing children and children with cochlear implants. Ear and Hearing 17: 430–7.

Rawool VW (1995) Ipsilateral acoustic reflex thresholds at varying click rates in humans. Scandinavian Audiology 24: 199–205.

Seyle K, Brown CJ (2002) Speech perception using maps based on neural response telemetry measures. Ear and Hearing 23(1S): 72S 79S.

Shallop JK, Ash KR (1996) Relationships among comfort levels determined by cochlear implant patient's self programming, audiologist's programming, and electrical stapedius reflex thresholds. Annals of Otology, Rhinology and Laryngology 166: 175–6.

Shallop JK, Beiter AL, Goin DW et al. (1990) Electrically evoked auditory brainstem responses (EABR) and middle latency responses (EMLR) obtained from patients with the Nucleus multichannel cochlear implant. Ear and Hearing 11: 5–15.

Shallop JK, Van Dyke L, Goin DW et al. (1991) Prediction of behavioral threshold and comfort values for Nucleus 22-channel implant patients from electrical auditory brainstem response test results. Annals of Otology, Rhinology and Laryngology 100: 896–8.

Shannon RV (1983) Multichannel electrical stimulation of the auditory nerve in man. II: channel interaction. Hearing Research 12: 1–16.

Sharma A, Dorman MF, Spahr AJ (2002) A sensitive period for the development of the central auditory system in children with cochlear implants: implications of age of implantation. Ear and Hearing 23: 532–9.

Shepard RK, Clark GM, Black RC (1983) Chronic electrical stimulation of the auditory nerve in cats. Acta Oto-Laryngologica (suppl. 399): 19–31.

Simmons FB, Lusted H, Meyers T et al. (1984) Electrically induced auditory brainstem response as a clinical tool in estimating nerve survival. Annals of Otology, Rhinology and Laryngology 93 (suppl. 112): 97–100.

Smith DW, Finley CC, van den Honert C et al. (1994) Behavioral and electro-physiological responses to electrical stimulation in the cat absolute threshold. Hearing Research 81: 1–10.

Smith L, Simmons FB (1983) Estimating eighth nerve survival by electrical stimulation. Annals of Otology, Rhinology and Laryngology 92: 12–23.

Smoorenburg GF, Willeboer C, van Dijk JE (2002) Speech perception in Nucleus CI24M cochlear implant users with processor settings based on electrically evoked compound action potential thresholds. Audiology Neuro-Otology 7(6): 335–47.

Spivak LG, Chute PM (1994) The relationship between electrical acoustic reflex thresholds and behavioral comfort levels in children and adult cochlear implant patients. Ear and Hearing 15: 184–92.

Starr A, Brackmann DE (1979) Brainstem potentials evoked by electrical stimulation of the cochlea in human subjects. Annals of Otology 88: 550–60.

Stephan K, Welz-Muller K (1994) Effect of stimulus duration on stapedius reflex threshold in electrical stimulation via cochlear implant. Audiology 33: 143–51.

Stephan K, Welz-Muller K, Stiglbrunner H (1991) Acoustic reflex in patients with cochlear implants (analog stimulation). American Journal of Otology 12: 48–81.

Stypulkowski PH, van den Honert C (1984) Physiological properties of the electrically stimulated auditory nerve. I: compound action potential recordings. Hearing Research 14: 205–23.

Thai-Van H, Chanal JM, Coudert C et al. (2001) Relationship between NRT measurements and behavioral levels in children with the Nucleus 24 cochlear implant may change over time: preliminary report. International Journal of Pediatric Otorhinology 58: 153–62.

Van den Borne B, Mens LHM, Snik AFM et al. (1996) Stapedius reflex and EABR thresholds in experienced users of the Nucleus cochlear implant. Archives in Otolaryngology 114: 141–3.

van den Honert C, Stypulkowski P (1986) Characterization of the electrically evoked auditory brainstem response (EABR) in cats and humans. Hearing Research 21: 109–26.

Vischer M, Haenggeli A, Zhang J et al. (1997) Effect of high-frequency electrical stimulation of the auditory nerve in an animal model of cochlear implants. American Journal of Otology 18: S27–S29.

White MW, Merzenich MM, Gardi JN (1984) Multichannel cochlear implants. Archives in Otolaryngology 110: 493–501.

Wilson BS (1997) The future of cochlear implants. British Journal of Audiology 31: 205–25.

Wilson BS, Finley CC, Lawson DT et al. (1997a) Temporal representations with cochlear implants. American Journal of Otology 18: S30-S34.

Wilson BS, Zerbi M, Finley CC et al. (1997b) Speech Processors for Auditory Prostheses. Seventh Quarterly Progress Report, NIH Contract N01-DC-5-2103.

# CHAPTER 12

# Device programming

## LOUISE C. CRADDOCK

## Introduction

Programming of the external speech processor takes place in the first instance at the initial fitting, typically about four weeks after surgery. The initial fitting is the first appointment in a life-long process of regular programming or tuning appointments. These serve to optimize a patient's speech processor program and also as a check of device function, particularly in older generation implants without telemetry. Speech processor programming can be a lengthy procedure and is a task that has traditionally accounted for much of an audiologist's clinical time. However, it is becoming clear that this traditional approach of re-mapping processors via careful behavioural measures on each channel is no longer a feasible approach to managing our growing patient caseload and, more importantly, may not be the most effective method of long-term patient care.

Three factors are changing the nature of device programming away from the traditional behavioural approach. First of all, the implanted patient population grows steadily. Implant teams see regular numbers of new cases implanted every year, as well as all their existing implanted patients. Patients with cochlear implants in the UK are never discharged and only leave our care if they transfer to other teams or when they die. This lifetime of care involves regular review appointments and routine retunes, and audiologists can easily spend all their time reviewing implanted patients without time to assess or switch-on the new cases. Secondly, as selection criteria expand, not only are more patients receiving implants but also the types of patients being implanted are becoming more complex. These aspects are addressed in other chapters but, briefly, adult programs have patients with more residual hearing requiring ipsilateral or contralateral hearing aid fittings, bilaterally implanted patients and patients with additional disabilities. Moreover, no population is more challenging to program than very young deaf children.

Finally, in the UK, the British Cochlear Implant Group has been instrumental in maintaining a limited number of highly specialist implant teams spread across the country, as opposed to numerous small centres mushrooming all over the UK implanting just a few patients a year. This is mainly because the outcomes from cochlear implantation have a tendency to improve as the experience of the team grows (Summerfield and Marshall, 1995). This model has ensured that while patients may have to travel quite significant distances to attend appointments, they can be assured that their implant team has the benefit of a great deal of experience, based on many years of working with large numbers of cochlear implant patients. However, there remains the question as to whether it is always necessary for a patient to be seen in a specialist centre and whether certain appointments could be dealt with closer to home. The concept of local implant service centres has been considered for many years, where patients could attend a nearby centre for routine retunes and repairs. A quick and simple method of programming would be highly beneficial in centres such as these, leaving established teams freer to scc the more complex and challenging cases. The drawback of this is that it is not always possible to tell in advance how complex a problem is going to be. The risk is that the patient ends up at the specialist centre anyway, perhaps with more problems than they had in the first place. Secondly, although there are a limited number of cochlear implant manufacturers, each company supports a range of devices and speech processors and the programming software is regularly upgraded. This leaves the local centre with the responsibility to maintain a significant amount of stock and keep staff up to date with all new developments, all for a relatively small number of patients.

Whatever the pros and cons of this model are, the fact is that many of the new developments in programming have focused on reducing the time spent on tuning the processor. This has been achieved either through modified behavioural techniques or via a greater use of objective measures. Some of the newer features available in programming software are certainly quick, efficient and result in acceptable programs. Using preset and default parameters, the audiologist's job appears straightforward and easy. This clearly has benefits when time spent in programming is critical, either in a busy clinic or when working with children or adults with very limited attention spans. But when things do not go according to plan and the default parameters are inappropriate, the task of programming the speech processor can become highly complex and elaborate.

This chapter will address the steps performed in a typical and traditional behavioural method of programming the device and then look at some of the more advanced features available, including some of the new techniques in use by some of the implant companies. Some of the objective tools used to assist device programming will be reviewed, including a method we have found highly successful in Birmingham. While some of the features used by different cochlear implant manufacturers will be considered, no attempt is made to rate the relative merits of each system.

## Equipment

Most implant centres have a clinic room dedicated to programming or tuning. Larger centres may have multiple programming rooms where the computers are networked. The computer requires some interface with the clinical programming unit, which may be fixed or portable. This provides the connection to the speech processor. Each implant manufacturer provides centres with the required programming software and should ensure that each centre has the latest version of the software and the appropriate level of training.

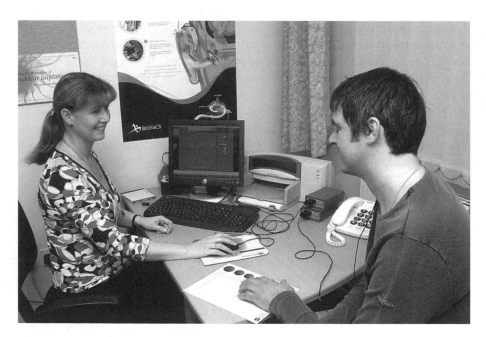

**Figure 12.1** Performing a retune in the programming room.

It is useful to have easy access to the stock of implant spares and accessories from the programming room. Care should be taken to ensure patients feel relaxed with comfortable chairs, appropriate lighting to assist with lipreading and written instructions and loudness charts available if required. Paediatric programmes should provide child-friendly environments in order to minimize the feeling of being in a hospital or clinic and make the programming room as welcoming as possible. While it is not essential that the room is sound treated, it should nevertheless be reasonably quiet so that environmental sounds do not become intrusive.

# Underlying principles

The normal ear has a wide dynamic range, with the threshold of hearing at 0 dBHL and the loudness discomfort level over 100 dBHL. Normal ears are also capable of discriminating small changes in intensity, pitch, phase and spectral information. The dynamic range of a cochlear implant is defined as the range between the threshold or T-level and the maximum comfortable loudness level, and this is typically in the range of 3–20 dB (Moore, 2003). The dynamic range of speech typically is about 30 dB for a single speaker but increases to over 60 dB for multiple talkers (Zeng et al., 2002). Moreover, most cochlear implant recipients have unilateral implants and therefore do not have any binaural advantages when listening in background noise, nor can they take advantage of many of the redundant speech cues available to the normally hearing listener.

Hence the job of the speech processor is to compress the speech signal into the narrow electrical dynamic range while ensuring that speech is still intelligible and that loud sounds are not uncomfortable. Bearing in mind that some of the quieter speech sounds may be below the level of any background noise, this is a complex task. The speech processor has to select the range of intensities in the input that will be coded, and this is known as the input dynamic range (IDR). The use of a compressed IDR ensures that most of the speech spectrum is accessible to the patients while minimizing the effects of background noise, as shown in Figure 12.2 (Cochlear Ltd, 2001). In addition, many implant systems use a second stage of compression via fast-acting modification to the pulse height and width. Information regarding spectral shape, time and pitch is dependent on the speech processing strategy, the number of available active channels and the capability of the system to represent complex tones. Nonetheless, many of the auditory cues available to normal ears, such as interaural time and intensity differences, are unavailable to implant users due to the inherent limitations in current implant design (Moore, 2003).

# Creating a program

## Telemetry

The principles of telemetry are discussed in Chapter 11, but briefly, with respect to programming, the first job for the audiologist is to check whether all electrodes are functioning appropriately and whether they are all intra-cochlear. At switch-on the audiologist must have access to the post-operative X-ray or at least a copy of the surgical report. Impedance telemetry will indicate whether the electrodes have normal impedances. Any with short or open circuits must be switched off, as must electrodes with abnormally high impedances. Since open circuits may be the result of an air bubble inside the cochlea, it is important to re-measure impedances

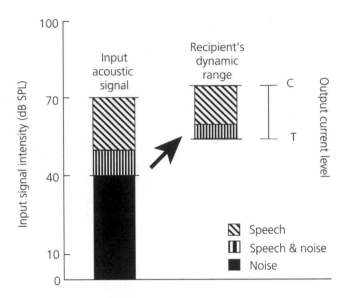

**Figure 12.2** Coding speech in noise using a 32 dB IDR. Most of the recipient's dynamic range of hearing would be available for speech. (Diagram courtesy of Cochlear Ltd.)

on several occasions as the impedances of these electrodes may return to normal after a period of stimulation. However, electrodes with short circuits will never be stimulable and must be permanently deactivated or flagged.

## Behavioural method

Processor programming is a task performed individually for each patient and usually at every review appointment. The individual programs (known as MAPs with the Nucleus system) are saved in the speech processor for use by the patient. The number of programs available for use depends on the memory capacity of the speech processor, and this varies between systems. The first program is created at the initial connection, known as 'hook-up' or 'switch-on', and the audiologist has the responsibility to select the processing strategy, the number of active channels, the rate of stimulation and the mode of stimulation – all before a stimulus has been delivered to the patient. Fortunately, most software programming systems have recommended default parameters, and although these may not provide the optimum program for every patient they are often a good point at which to start.

Processor programming must be performed repeatedly at regular review appointments since the parameters change over time, especially in children (Skinner et al., 1997; Hughes et al., 2001; Henkin et al., 2003) and performance may deteriorate if the program is not optimized. Similarly, some adults have program levels that fluctuate significantly and they too require regular review appointments.

## Selection of strategy

Speech processor strategies are described in Chapter 2 and there is an enormous amount of data published on the benefits of one strategy over another. It is not in the remit of this chapter to discuss the relative merits of each; suffice it to say that the implant systems normally have available a range of strategies that can be used, including high-rate strategies such as Advanced Combination Encoder, or ACE, Continuous Interleaved Sampling, or CIS (Wilson et al., 1993), and High Resolution from Advanced Bionics. Programming software usually allows the clinician to select the rate of stimulation, either directly or indirectly via adjustment of the pulse width, since the narrower the pulse width the faster the rate in some implant systems. There is a large amount of research that has suggested that performance is significantly improved when high-rate strategies are used (Parkinson et al., 2001; Frijns et al., 2003; Tyler et al., 2004) but there may be a minority of patients who benefit from slow-rate strategies.

It is important therefore to give the patient the opportunity to try different strategies in order to determine which provides optimum performance. The processor may be loaded with alternatives for the patients to try at home over at least six weeks. In this way the optimum strategy may be determined individually (Skinner et al., 2002b). Moreover, it has been shown that preference of a particular strategy is strongly correlated with performance. In other words, it is important to optimize parameters for each patient and then give them ample time to try each one (Holden et al., 2002; Skinner et al., 2002a). Even if a patient has had significant experience using one strategy, they may still improve with an alternative, even after several months (Tyler et al., 2004).

Selection of strategy may be affected by factors other than patient performance or preference. In cases of incomplete insertions or partial device failure, there may be a limited number of active electrodes available for stimulation. For patients with limited numbers of intra-cochlear electrodes, the CIS strategy has been shown to result in better performance and is more likely to be preferred by this group of patients (Plant et al., 2000). Even when all electrodes are stimulable, performance can be affected by the appropriate selection of the number of channels used in a program, and this too must be done individually for each patient (Frijns et al., 2003).

## Establishing a threshold level

Traditionally, the next task in processor programming is to establish the electrical dynamic range, and it is common practice to begin with the threshold (T-) level. In the Nucleus system, the stimulus is adjusted to a level at or just above the threshold of audibility (Cochlear Ltd, 2001). Various techniques may be employed to achieve this: an ascending/

descending bracketing technique or use of a loudness growth chart, where the patient points to the scale to indicate the level at which the stimulus is perceived. This may be performed by the audiologist via the keyboard or patients can set the level themselves with the patient control knob. It should be noted that these different methods result in different program levels (Skinner et al., 1995). At initial switch-on, the setting of T-levels may be harder to establish since the patient is unfamiliar with the electrical stimulation and may not respond until the stimulus is clearly audible. A larger step size is often useful in the early stages, moving to a finer step size as the patient becomes more accustomed to the task.

The setting of T-levels is also affected by the processing strategy involved. In strategies using continuous stimulation such as CIS, it is necessary to reduce the T-level to just below the level of audibility. This ensures that the patient does not hear the constant T-level stimulation, which can be perceived as a steady hum. The Med-El CIS+ system defines threshold as the highest stimulation at which no sound sensation occurs, and, again, this is to ensure that the patient does not hear the T-level stimulation even in quiet (Brickley and Boyd, 2000). T-level measurements are normally made on every active channel. In devices using bipolar modes of stimulation, this is essential as levels can differ dramatically from one channel to the next. Devices now all use monopolar stimulation, and in this mode levels are fairly consistent across the electrode array (Plant and Psarros, 2000; Sainz et al., 2003a). Occasionally, a patient can report a stimulus as just audible or very quiet over a range of current levels and this is known as a T-tail. Increases in current level do not at first produce an increase in the perceived loudness of the stimulus. Then a point is reached at which the patient reports that the stimulus does start to get louder. In strategies other than CIS, the T-level should be set to this point in order to produce a typical loudness growth function on a given channel.

Although cochlear implants have been shown to be effective in tinnitus suppression (Ruckenstein et al., 2001; Mo et al., 2002), some patients find that the task of determining program levels triggers tinnitus, which then affects their ability to perceive a low-level stimulus. This has the potential to result in raised T-levels since the stimulus has to be clearly audible in order for it to be perceived above the level of the tinnitus. Solutions to this problem include using multiple presentations of the stimulus, which is more alerting, or setting T-levels over the tinnitus and then using a global T-level reduction. Another technique is to set T-levels indirectly from a midpoint in the electrical dynamic range. In this method, loudness balancing is performed at 50% in a small group of electrodes. If one channel is perceived as louder than the others, the loudness is reduced by a reduction at T-level until all channels in the group are perceived as equally loud. Similarly, a quieter channel can be increased in loudness via an increase in T-level.

Appropriately set T-levels should ensure that speech sounds are audible and that soundfield responses are in line with manufacturer's recommendations for their device. However, there is some controversy as to whether accurate T-level measures have any significant effect on performance. For example, in one study the T-level was artificially raised above the measured T and it was found that performance was enhanced. Reportedly, these programs improved the perception of softer sounds even though the dynamic range had effectively been reduced. Moreover, all the subjects fitted with programs with raised T-levels preferred these programs (Skinner et al., 1999). Conversely, in another study programs were created with C-levels kept constant but T-levels set progressively higher and higher, again effectively reducing the dynamic range. Performance with these programs was affected very little and was not significantly different from performance with conventionally measured programs (Fu and Shannon, 2000). These two studies reached very different conclusions and raise the question as to how critical it really is to measure an accurate T-level. This will be considered later in the chapter.

## Comfort and most-comfortable levels

Once thresholds have been established on all channels, the next step is to determine the upper limit of the electrical dynamic range. This level varies according to the system used. In the Nucleus device, the level is called the C- or Comfort level and is set to the level below the maximum comfortable listening level to allow for loudness summation when all channels are active in live mode (Cochlear Ltd, 2001). Electrical stimulation is never allowed to exceed C-level and adjustments of the volume control are limited to this point. The Med-El device defines the upper limit of the electrical dynamic range as the 'maximum comfortable level', and this is the highest stimulus level at which sound is loud but still comfortable (Brickley and Boyd, 2000). In the Advanced Bionics system, the M-level is defined as the 'Most Comfortable Level'. Adjustments of the volume control are allowed to exceed the M-level to a value determined by the audiologist. In setting the volume control in live mode, care must be taken to ensure that over-stimulation does not occur at the maximum volume setting.

The setting of the M- or C-level should always be done in fine ascending steps to avoid over-stimulation. Loudness growth functions may be very steep in some patients and a small increase in current level can produce a sharp increase in loudness. Programming systems sometimes default to a fine increment step in M-level adjustment for this very reason. Again, there are various methods used in setting the upper limit of the electrical dynamic range. Loudness charts are helpful, where the patient points to a loudness scale as the stimulus is increased, indicating to the audiologist when the comfort level has been reached. It is important that multiple stimulations are given at each level, as it is very hard to make a reasonable loudness judgement on one brief stimulus.

Use of the patient control knob has also been shown to be an efficient method of setting C-levels (Shallop and Ash, 1995; Skinner et al., 1995).

Using the knob and with the stimulus set to deliver a continuous train of pulses, the patient takes control of the loudness level. The stimulus is increased until the desired level is reached and then a button is pushed to fix the C-level at this point. As the next channel is selected, the stimulus automatically drops close to the T-level to protect the patient from accidental over-stimulation. The sensitivity of the knob can be adjusted, again to ensure that over-stimulation does not occur by mistake. It is also important to give patients ample sessions to set their C-levels since the levels can vary in the early weeks and some patients require practice in making loudness judgements before their program levels become stable (Sun et al., 1999).

Variations in C- or M-levels are also dependent on the patient's own subjective rating of the loudness. There are wide individual differences in loudness tolerance, which in turn affects C-levels. Moreover, this is also dependent on the patient's understanding of the task. This is particularly pertinent in programming very young children, who may have no understanding of the concept of loudness at all. Some children demonstrate remarkable tolerance to increasing levels of stimulation before they give any indications of loudness discomfort. The challenges this presents to the audiologist are discussed later.

## Loudness balancing

Once the C- or M-level has been established on all channels, it is important to ensure equal loudness across the electrode array. This is a critical part of device programming, and studies have shown that incorrect loudness balancing can be detrimental to performance (Dawson et al., 1997; Sainz et al., 2003a). Equal loudness can be achieved via loudness balancing and sweeping. In loudness balancing, two channels are compared, one channel as the reference, the other the comparison. Adjustments are made to the comparison until both channels are perceived as equally loud. Balancing may be done between adjacent channels or channels spaced along the array. Another technique is to sweep across a group of channels, either apically to basally or in the other direction. Modifications to individual channels may be made until they are all perceived as equally loud. The most difficult part of this procedure can be in explaining the task to the patient. If the sweep is to be performed in an apical-to-base direction, the analogy of listening to notes played on a piano has proven useful, as it differentiates the task of judging loudness when the perceived pitch is changing.

## Live mode

Validation of the dynamic range must always be done in live mode in order to take into account the effect of loudness summation. When setting the upper limit of the electrical dynamic range on individual channels, the patient may rate all channels as comfortable but the overall loudness level for speech may be too loud. If this is the case, global modifications may be made to C- and T-levels. This may be done either as a percentage of the electrical dynamic range or by a defined number of stimulus units. If the patient reports that the sound quality is 'echoey', this is nearly always an indication that C-levels have been set too high and a global C-level reduction is required. If the patient can hear a constant low-level humming even in quiet with the CIS strategy, this may indicate that T-levels are too high and so the patient is picking up the constant T-level stimulation. In this case, global T-level reduction should eliminate this unwanted noise.

## Gain and frequency adjustment

Further adjustments in live mode may be made if the patient reports a poor sound quality. High-frequency gain reduction may reduce 'tinniness', low-frequency gain reduction may reduce a perception of 'boominess'. A hollow sound may be improved by the reduction of mid-frequency gains. Alteration of the frequency allocation tables may shift the overall perception of pitch range up or down, where a higher-frequency allocation results in a lower perception of pitch as the balance towards the lower frequencies changes. It is important to be aware that changes in frequency allocation may actually result in a deterioration in performance (Fu and Shannon, 2000; Henshall and McKay, 2001) and should be monitored carefully. This is because optimum speech recognition may be more likely if acoustic frequency information is mapped to the appropriate location in the cochlea (Baskent and Shannon, 2003).

## Other influences on program levels

Program levels are influenced by the mode of stimulation. Current levels of T/C-levels are higher in bipolar mode than in common ground and lowest for monopolar stimulation. Research has shown that program levels in monopolar stimulation uniformly increase from apex to base but there is no consistent pattern in bipolar programs. Moreover, the dynamic range in monopolar stimulation tends to be smaller than in other modes (Busby et al., 1994).

T- and C-levels are also affected by the rate of stimulation. In the Nucleus system, as the rate of stimulation increases, the T- and C-levels decrease, but only at current levels below 190 units. At current levels above 210 units there is little change in program levels with an increasing rate of stimulation (Skinner et al., 2000). In very high-rate strategies such as High Resolution, it has been shown that the electrical dynamic range is significantly larger and this is a result of lower T-levels (Vickers et al., 2004). The proximity of the electrode array to the modiolus also influences threshold and comfort levels. 'Modiolar-hugging' (or peri-modiolar) electrodes are designed to lie closer to the neural elements, and program levels with these devices tend to be lower (Franck et al., 2002).

### User controls

Speech processor controls enable the user to adjust the volume, the microphone sensitivity or both. As we have seen, adjustments to the volume control alter the C- or M-levels, and it is dependent on the system whether stimulation is allowed to exceed measured levels. Alterations of the sensitivity control allow the user to manipulate the range of the microphone. This also produces a change in soundfield responses that affects the processing of the speech signal. Manufacturers usually recommend specific sensitivity settings to ensure that the long-term average speech spectrum is within the dynamic range of the processor. However, some research has suggested that higher-sensitivity settings should be used with children as this has been found to enhance speech recognition (Muller-Deile, 1997).

# Further considerations

### Non-auditory stimulation

Care must be taken, when setting the upper limit of the electrical dynamic range, that non-auditory stimulation (NAS) does not occur. This usually results either from the electrical current reaching the facial or other cranial nerves at the apical portion of the array or because the basal electrodes are extra-cochlear (Stoddart and Cooper, 1995). Symptoms of NAS can include facial twitching, pain or unpleasant sensations on the face or throat. If NAS does occur on a channel, there are various options to eliminate it. The channel may be clipped in order to limit stimulation to a level below the threshold of the NAS. Psychophysical measurements may be repeated with wider pulse widths, which allow for a lower current level to be used to achieve the same percept of loudness. In some implant systems, this may in turn affect the rate of stimulation due to the inverse relationship between pulse widths and rate per channel. Once NAS has been eliminated on a particular channel, checks must always be repeated in live mode to allow for the effect's loudness summation. If NAS persists, the only option available may be to deactivate a particular channel. In this case, the frequencies assigned to that channel will be automatically reallocated to neighbouring channels. Alternatively, the channel may be left active but with the levels set to minimum; this would have the effect of eliminating the NAS but without automatic frequency reassignment, although it leaves a gap in the frequency response.

### Pitch ranking

With a normal full electrode insertion, the patient should ideally perceive the pitch moving from low to high as stimulation moves from apical to base. However, there are some cases, for example when the electrode has rolled over on itself, that the pitch ranking is abnormal. In cases such as these, it is necessary to reorder channels sequentially. This is done by balancing neighbouring channels and moving the lower-pitch ranked channel apically to the other. This is a time-consuming task; as each channel is moved one position apically, it must then be compared with its new neighbour to ensure that all channels end up in the correct order.

In any program, regardless of the number of channels, there may be channels that are indistinguishable from each other in terms of pitch. The process of determining pitch perception between channels is a lengthy one, typically a research tool only. Research is ongoing as to whether patient performance might be enhanced if the indistinguishable channels are deactivated. However, one study showed that in fact removing electrodes with non-tonotopic percepts did not enhance performance. This was probably due to the fact that when a channel is deactivated the frequency reallocation is changed so that the frequencies assigned to the deactivated channel are represented by adjacent channels. The effect of this is to shift the frequency-to-electrode relationship, and this in turn may lead to a deterioration in performance (Henshall and McKay, 2001).

**Noise reduction algorithms**

Specially designed features to assist listening in background noise are available in some systems. The Nucleus system employs an AGC autosensitivity option that can be selected for use in one of the program locations on the BTE processor or added to each program location on the body-worn processor. In addition, Adaptive Dynamic Range Optimization (ADRO) is a feature that continually adjusts the gain in each frequency band to optimize the signal (James et al., 2002). Multi-microphone technology, as in Beam-forming, can also reduce the effects of background noise, and is also now available with the Nucleus system.

# Programming young children

No population presents more of a challenge to the audiologist than the very young deaf child, and this aspect cannot be fully explored here. Briefly, the three factors that make this so are time, co-operation and understanding of the task. As addressed at the beginning of this chapter, the responsibility of determining behavioural measures of threshold and comfort level on a possible twenty-two channels is time-consuming, even with the most co-operative and reliable adult. Any small child, regardless of hearing status, has a narrow window of time in which they may concentrate on a given task. The trouble is one never knows in advance just how long this time window is. All we can do as professionals is prioritize which single piece of information is the most essential and go for that. If successful and the going is still good, then you can try for the second most essential thing and so on. The child will let you know when your time is up.

The second confounding factor is simply getting the child to co-operate with the task. This can be challenging at the best of times but even more so with profoundly deaf children, who are known to have more significant behavioural problems than their hearing peers, as shown in Chapter 7. However child-friendly a programming room may be and however skilled the professionals involved are, the fact is it still may be an intimidating environment for a child. Most clinics provide a range of toys to be utilized during programming that will interest the child and make the process as enjoyable as possible. Games that are more appealing alternatives to the 'man in the boat' game used in play audiometry can keep the child on task for a little longer so that the audiologist can determine some T-levels. Use of alerting puppets in the VRA (Visual Reinforcement Audiometry) room, child-oriented decorations, pictures and furniture all help to make the child feel more relaxed. Nonetheless, children do not always sit and perform a task required of them, or they may do so one day but not another, or for one adult but not another. Enlisting the help of parents and the local professional, such as the teacher of the deaf, can often persuade a recalcitrant child to join in after all. Giving the parents a clear and defined role to perform during programming sessions, particularly at switch-on, reduces their anxiety too (Lynch et al., 1999).

Finally, it is extremely hard to get a child to co-operate with a task if they do not know what the task is. Young deaf children will probably have spent many hours in audiology rooms and may be well conditioned to auditory or vibrotactile stimuli in VRA, VROCA (Visual Reinforcement Operant Conditioning Audiometry) or play audiometry. When presented with electrical stimulation for the first time, however, they may not associate this with hearing and, even if they do, they may not respond until the stimulus is well above threshold. More challenging still is the task of setting comfort levels on a child who has no concept of loudness growth. Many children will not give any indication that the stimulus is too loud until a loudness discomfort level has been exceeded. Merely increasing the stimulus until the child shows signs of loudness discomfort may result in significant over-stimulation, and there have been many anecdotal cases of children refusing to go in the programming room or wear their speech processors after an experience like this. Clearly, a safer and more reliable method of establishing the upper boundary of the electrical dynamic range is required.

To make the audiologist's job even more challenging, it is essential to perform regular retunes with children. This is because children demonstrate significant program changes over the first two years after switch-on. T-levels have been shown to increase over the first year then stabilize in the second year. C-levels tend to increase over a two-year period (Henkin et al., 2003). Careful behavioural observation of the child is critical when programming changes have been made, and this is essential both during

Susan Hammel
Adrienne Ulrich
Amanda Curtis
Binita Shethna
Bobbie Monroe
Denis Barrell
Joanne Restivo
4778
Kim Maho
47765457
Margaret Chapman
Saul Strieh
Shridhar Kulkarni

the programming session and then afterwards by parents and teachers. However, with younger and younger children receiving implants, it is clear that alternatives to individual behavioural measures on every channel must be sought. Research has addressed the issue of how to achieve acceptable and accurate programs that result in equivalent performance as time-efficiently as possible. Many of these new techniques were developed and validated on adults and are highly applicable to those working with children. These approaches to programming use either modified behavioural techniques or rely on objective measures to program the device and these will be explored next.

## Objective measures in programming

When it is not possible to obtain reliable behavioural responses, the solution often lies in a greater reliance on objective measures (Brown, 2003). As we have seen, this is often the case when programming young deaf children but is also applicable with adults with learning difficulties and even adults with long-term deafness who find loudness judgements challenging. Further details about performing objective measures in cochlear implantation are covered in Chapter 11; however, some of the clinical applications are addressed here.

### Electrically evoked stapedial reflex (ESRT)

The ESRT is also referred to as the electrically evoked auditory reflex (EART). For the purposes of this chapter, the term ESRT will be used throughout. It is a technique by which electrical stimulation is delivered via the implant and used to elicit the stapedial reflex. This can either be observed directly during the implant surgery or measured using a probe in the ear canal using standard immittance equipment. With a wide recording window and the auditory stimulus deactivated, an ipsilateral or contralateral acoustic reflex may be recorded and the threshold determined.

The ESRT may be recorded intra-operatively and post-operatively. The purpose of intra-operative recordings is as a brief assessment of device function as soon as the electrode array has been inserted in the cochlea. It also serves as a quick check of the peripheral pathway and lower brainstem. Typically, the reflex is determined by the visual observation of the stapedial muscle while it is exposed. The effects of general anaesthesia and the use of muscle relaxant will have an effect on ESRT thresholds, and this must be taken into consideration if the ESRT is used subsequently in programming. One study showed that maximum comfortable loudness (MCL) levels were lower than intra-operative ESRTs initially but that they increased to over 70% of the ESRT value after six months. A higher correlation with MCLs was found at the apical portion of the array, which may be due to the proximity of the electrodes to the modiolus (Allum et al., 2002).

Many studies have addressed the use of the ESRT to estimate behavioural comfort levels, particularly in children, and there are conflicting conclusions as to whether the ESRT is a useful predictor of the MCL. One study showed that ESRTs were closer to comfort levels in children than in adults and that, although the ESRT was acceptably close to comfort levels in some patients, they significantly over- or under-estimated C-levels in many patients in the study (Spivak and Chute, 1994). This and other research suggests that the ESRT should be used cautiously in programming but that it is useful to determine a level that should not be exceeded in the programming of challenging cases (Zehnder et al., 1999).

However, other studies have suggested a closer relationship between the ESRT and the MCL (Shallop and Ash, 1995). A high correlation was found between the MCL and ESRT in experienced adult Combi 40 users (Stephan and Welzl-Muller, 2000). Hodges et al. (1997) found that the ESRT was an accurate and quick method of estimating maximum comfort levels and was therefore useful in initial programming. When ESRTs were used to set C-levels, research showed that performance with ESRT-based programs was at least equivalent to that with conventionally programmed programs (Spivak et al., 1994).

As addressed earlier, if a child is over-stimulated he or she may become reluctant to enter the programming room and may even refuse to wear the speech processor. Hence the ESRT may be used as a basis for conditioning behavioural responses and a guideline for setting maximum comfort loudness levels in young children (Hodges et al., 1999). One study showed that when C-levels were set using the ESRT they were consistently lower than C-levels set behaviourally. Moreover, the children using these programs wore them for longer and had fewer episodes of loudness discomfort to environmental sounds (Bresnihan et al., 2001).

Whether ESRTs can be helpful in programming or not, it has been shown that the reflex is absent in approximately 30% of patients regardless of middle ear status. It is suggested that the absence of a reflex may reflect areas of poor neural survival and that the level of maximum tolerable stimulation is reached before the reflex can be elicited (Todd et al., 2003).

## Electrically evoked auditory brainstem response

The EABR is a technique that may also be used intra- and post-operatively. Intra-operative EABR thresholds have been found to be higher than post-operative thresholds (Brown et al., 1994) and may be used to check the correct positioning of the device and also its function (Kileny et al., 1997). Post-operative recordings can also be used to assess electrode failure when behavioural assessment is not possible (Truy et al., 1998).

Again, many studies have looked at how the EABR wave V threshold relates to behavioural program levels in a variety of different cochlear implant systems. Much of the data suggest that the EABR threshold typically lies within the electrical dynamic range and that the thresholds follow the profile of the T-level across the electrode array (Brown et al., 1994). Great inter-subject variability has been noted; indeed, another study found that the EABR threshold exceeded the upper limit of the electrical dynamic range in one subject (Firszt et al., 1999). In order to determine whether the EABR threshold is affected by proximity to the modiolus, the difference in threshold between two Nucleus devices, the CI24M straight array and the precurved modiolar-hugging CI24R, was compared. Interestingly, there was no difference in EABR thresholds with the CI24M or the CI24R even though the precurved CI24R is designed to lie closer to the neural elements (Hay-McCutcheon et al., 2002).

It may be that alternative parameters, such as slope and growth rate (Nikolopoulos et al., 1997) and also morphology and latency (Truy et al., 1998) should be examined in analysis of the EABR response. Despite the existing research demonstrating the value of measuring the EABR, the amount of new research in this area has declined and this may be a result of the introduction of systems capable of measuring the electrically-evoked compound action potential (Brown, 2003).

## Electrically evoked compound action potential

The ECAP is a relatively new tool used to measure the whole nerve compound action potential via the implant itself. This feature is known as Neural Response Telemetry (NRT) in the Nucleus system and Neural Response Imaging (NRI) in the Advanced Bionics system. Both use similar principles and are discussed in greater detail in Chapter 11. Again, these measures may be performed during surgery, typically as the surgeon closes the wound, and also post-operatively. Studies have shown that intra-operative NRT thresholds are higher than those obtained post-operatively (Hughes et al., 2001), and this must be accounted for when using intra-operative results in programming.

Various methods have been described as to how to use the NRT threshold, or T-NRT, to assist in programming the device. Some of these techniques are now incorporated into the programming software.

### Progressive preset MAPs

This technique has been investigated for use in programming young children and is based on the intra-operative T-NRT alone without any behavioural T/C information on individual channels. An offset is used to determine the T- and C-levels where the T-level is fixed at 40 units below the T-NRT. The C-level is set at 30 units below the T-NRT and then progressive MAPs are automatically generated with increasingly wider dynamic ranges. The C-levels are raised in steps of 10 units gradually over time until they are set at the T-NRT itself. Careful observation of the child's responses is required as each MAP is activated and global modifications employed where required (Ramos et al., 2003). However, research into the use of this method with adults at switch-on has suggested that MAPs with C-levels set close to or at the intra-operative T-NRT are likely to significantly exceed behavioural comfort levels across the electrode array. Great caution is recommended in order to ensure that over-stimulation does not occur when using the progressive preset MAP method with children (Craddock et al., 2003b).

### T/C offset

While the T-NRT alone is not strongly correlated with behavioural T/C levels, the T-NRTs usually lie within the electrical dynamic range and typically follow the profile of the MAP. It is possible, therefore, to determine the offset between the T-NRT and the T/C level at a medial channel and then apply this offset to the remaining channels. This way, a MAP can be created that is more highly correlated with the behavioural program levels (Brown et al., 2000; Hughes et al., 2000). However, it has now been suggested that this high correlation may be due to the fact that program levels in monopolar stimulation are fairly flat and that the T/C offset adds little to the program prediction than might be achieved by using a flat MAP (Brown, 2003).

Nonetheless, the T/C offset method has been validated as a means of device fitting via speech perception measures. Speech performance at lower presentation levels (55 dBSPL) with experienced adult users was equivalent with NRT-based MAPs fitted using this technique (Seyle and Brown, 2003). Another multi-centre study showed that speech performance at 70 dB(A) was not significantly different when experienced adult subjects were tested with NRT-based MAPs and behaviourally measured maps. It was found, however, on examination of the group data, that there was a slight over-estimation of basal C-levels when using this technique in the ACE strategy, and this is likely to have resulted from the use of one offset only, which creates a uniform dynamic range across the array (Craddock et al., 2003a).

### The 3-offset method

Further research has shown that using three offsets, one in each section of the electrode array, achieves MAPs that are very close to behavioural program levels and that performance with these MAPs is at least equivalent to that with behavioural programs. This technique, known as the 3-offset method, can also be used to create switch-on programs for adults based on the intra-operative T-NRTs. Moreover, this study has also shown that it is not necessary to measure the T-NRT on every channel, which is another laborious task in itself. Instead, the T-NRT may be measured on five channels and the rest interpolated with no loss of accuracy. The 3-offset method provides a quick and accurate method of creating programs that are acceptable to patients even at switch-on and result in performance that is equivalent to that achieved with behaviourally measured programs (Craddock et al., 2003b).

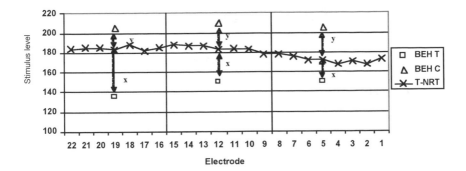

**Figure 12.3** The 3-offset method. The T-NRT is measured on five channels spaced across the array with the remaining values interpolated. Behavioural measures are made on three channels (5, 12 and 19). The offset between the T-NRT and T-level (x) and C-level (y) is determined at these points. The offset is applied to the other channels in each section. This is a typical example of post-operative levels in adults.

This method is clearly applicable for use with young children. Concentration may be given to determining reliable responses on three key channels, one in each section of the array, and then the program can be produced on the basis of the behavioural information combined with the intra-operative ECAP data. The '3-offsets', indicated by 'x' and 'y' in Figure 12.3, take into account the changes in dynamic range across the electrode array and also the fact that the intra-operative T-NRTs are likely to be above behavioural C-level. This inclusion of limited behavioural information reduces the risk of over-stimulation.

*Shift and tilt*

Smoorenburg has also examined the relationship between the T-NRT or ECAP threshold and T/C levels. He concluded that the relationship could be more fully described by analysis of the tilt in the profile in which the ECAP thresholds were highly correlated with behavioural T-levels. In this method, the T-levels are set so the profile is that of the ECAP thresholds. In live mode, the T-levels are globally increased until speech is just detected. These levels are called T-NEW. Next, the C-NEW is determined by shifting all C-levels upward until live speech is perceived as comfortably loud. Hence, there is a constant dynamic range across the electrode array. The profile is then tilted to optimize sound quality. Although the T-NEW levels may be significantly lower than behavioural T-levels due to loudness summation, no deterioration in speech scores was noticed when subjects were fitted with these NRT-based MAPs (Smoorenburg et al., 2002). Adjustment of the shift and tilt is relatively straightforward and has the potential to be used by patients for self-programming in the future (Smoorenburg, 2004).

# New features for quicker programming

It is evident that reducing the amount of time spent programming speech processors is becoming more essential due to the increasing clinical pressures on the audiologist. Many of the features designed to assist in programming the more complex cases may also prove useful in making time spent with routine review appointments as efficient as possible.

## Do T-levels matter?

As we have seen, several studies have suggested that the setting of T-levels has little effect on speech performance (Fu and Shannon, 2000; Smoorenburg, 2002). Some of the newer features in programming software dispense with the need to measure T-levels at all. The Combi 40+ system from Med-El sets all T-levels to a minimum for this reason as their research has also shown that this has little or no significant effect on soundfield thresholds (Boyd, 2000). Similarly the Soundwave software from Advanced Bionics has a feature that automatically sets T-levels to the minimum value or to 20% of the M-level.

## Interpolation

The benefit of monopolar stimulation is that the profile of the T- and C-levels tends to be fairly stable; therefore interpolation is more reliable in monopolar than bipolar stimulation. Also, estimations of program levels are better for those implanted at a younger age but are less reliable for those with severe cochlear damage (Sainz et al., 2003a). Hence, interpolated program levels can be safely used in monopolar mode, and programming systems have features that make it easy to do. Research with the Nucleus device showed that interpolation of MAP levels was possible at all stimulation rates and for widely spaced electrodes and resulted in accurate levels requiring only minor modifications (Plant and Psarros, 2000). The Med-El Combi 40+ system also enables interpolation to be performed on the basis of limited behavioural data (Durst et al., 2003). Again, this has obvious advantages for use with young children when there are no objective data available. Attention may be given to determining reliable behavioural measures on just a few channels spaced across the array and the remaining levels can be safely interpolated.

'Soundwave' from Advanced Bionics employs a 'speech burst' feature where M-levels are set in groups of four using a broadband stimulus. It has been shown that M-levels set using these speech bursts need less adjustments in live mode (Hughes, 2003). Using the automatic T-levels, a 16-channel program can be created very quickly from just four psychophysical measurements.

## Statistical methods

Finally, a new approach to programming is based on the fact that many patients have similar programs and that a patient's program could be generated based on these average levels. Govaerts et al. (2003) describe the 'Automated tuning' technique in which the fitting parameters are determined statistically, based on the patient's case history, epidemiological data and any other objective measures that have been determined. An Automatic Map Generator produces a series of programs and four of these can then be loaded into a speech processor for the patient to try sequentially. Validation of the program is achieved using the Auditory Speech Sound Evaluation, or 'ASSE', test, which gives an indication of whether the patient can differentiate speech sounds (Govaerts et al., 2003).

Statistical analysis in the determination of program levels has been used in other research and, although there are differences between programs created this way and behavioural programs, acceptable programs were achieved in 90% of patients in one study (Sainz et al., 2003b). Another method, known as the Standard Map fitting technique, also uses statistical data with the Med-El device. T-levels are set to a minimum with MCLs based on mean data. On going live, the MCLs are kept low and increased until they are comfortable. Preliminary research has shown little difference in performance between the behavioural, or Custom Map, and the Standard Map (Boyd, 2003).

# Conclusion

Programming cochlear implants can be an extremely straightforward task. Using default parameters, interpolation of levels and new features for the swift and accurate setting of program levels, an audiologist can create an acceptable program for a patient in a relatively short time. This has clear advantages in busy clinics and also opens up new possibilities, such as local service centres, the ability to offer cochlear implants to patients with restricted access to a larger cochlear implant team and even patients being able to program their own speech processors at home. The difficulty is that not everyone can be programmed using these default parameters, or individuals may not achieve their best performance using these programs. As we have seen, conventional behavioural methods are not possible in some situations, and there is now a greater reliance on the use of objective measures in programming and verifying programs. The techniques involved in obtaining accurate objective measures and then applying these to programming can be extremely complex.

It is usually obvious whether a particular patient is going to be challenging to program. If your next switch-on is an 18-month-old congenitally deaf child, it is clear that you are going to need some intra-operative measurements available to assist you in setting program levels. An adult whose surgery was complicated and insertion abnormal is likely to have highly unusual mapping parameters. However, it is not always possible to determine in advance whether a case is going to be easy or challenging, and so audiologists have to be prepared to modify their programming methods to solve unforeseen difficulties. There is no doubt that programming can very rapidly become extremely complex, involving the modification of a vast range of programming parameters. While it has been impossible to address all of these potential challenges in this chapter, the aim has been to demonstrate that the overall responsibility of programming cochlear implants must remain with a highly qualified professional.

# References

Allum JH, Probst R, Greisiger R (2002) Relationship of intraoperative electrically evoked stapedius reflex thresholds to maximum comfortable loudness levels on children with cochlear implants. International Journal of Audiology 41: 93–9.

Baskent D, Shannon R (2003) Speech recognition under conditions of frequency-place compression and expansion. Journal of the Acoustical Society of America 113: 2064–76.

Boyd P (2000) The effects of electrical threshold setting on free-field thresholds and speech discrimination in users of the Med-El Combi 40 system. Paper presented at the 6th International Cochlear Implant Conference, Miami, USA.

Boyd P (2003) Standard map fitting for the young child. Paper presented at the Audiological Management of Cochlear Implantation in Young and Challenging cases, Nottingham, UK.

Bresnihan M, Norman G, Scott F et al. (2001) Measurement of comfort levels by means of electrical stapedius reflex in children. Archives of Otolaryngology: Head and Neck Surgery 127: 963–6.

Brickley G, Boyd P (2000) Considerations in initial tuning of Med-El Combi 40 series cochlear implants. Paper presented at the 5th European Symposium on Paediatric Cochlear Implantation, Antwerp, Belgium.

Brown CJ (2003) Clinical uses of electrically evoked auditory nerve and brainstem responses. Current Opinion in Otolaryngology: Head and Neck Surgery 11: 383–7.

Brown CJ, Abbas PJ, Fryauf-Bertschy H et al. (1994) Intraoperative and postoperative electrically evoked auditory brainstem responses in nucleus cochlear implant users: implications for the fitting process. Ear and Hearing 15: 168–76.

Brown CJ, Hughes ML, Luk B et al. (2000) The relationship between EAP and EABR thresholds and levels used to program the Nucleus 24 speech processor: data from adults. Ear and Hearing 21: 151–63.

Busby PA, Whitford LA, Blamey PJ et al. (1994) Pitch perception for different modes of stimulation using the cochlear multiple-electrode prosthesis. Journal of the Acoustical Society of America 95: 2658–69.

Cochlear Ltd (2001) Input Signal Processing for Optimal Performance. N94452F, 1-8. Cochlear Ltd. White Paper. 1-1-2001.

Craddock LC, Cooper HR, Davies M et al. (2003a) Comparison between NRT-based maps and behaviourally measured maps at different stimulation rates: a multi-centre investigation. Cochlear Implants International 4(4): 161–70.

Craddock LC, Cooper HR, Weigman J et al. (2003b) Using intra-operative NRT thresholds for initial programming in adults: an evaluation of two methods. Paper presented at the 4th International Symposium on Electronic Implants in Otology and Conventional Hearing Aids, Toulouse, France.

Dawson, PW, Skok M, Clark GM (1997) The effect of loudness imbalance between electrodes in cochlear implant users. Ear and Hearing 18: 156–65.

Durst C, Joseph J, Khan S et al. (2003) Estimation of map psychophysics levels from limited behavioural data with the Med-El Combi 40+ cochlear implant system. Paper presented at the Audiological Management of Cochlear Implantation in Young and Challenging Cases, Nottingham, UK.

Firszt JB, Rotz LA, Chambers RD et al. (1999) Electrically evoked potentials recorded in adult and pediatric Clarion implant users. Annals of Otology, Rhinology and Laryngology (suppl. 177): 58–63.

Franck KH, Shah UK, Marsh RR et al. (2002) Effects of Clarion electrode design on mapping levels in children. Annals of Otology, Rhinology and Laryngology 111: 1128–32.

Frijns JH, Klop WM, Bonnet RM et al. (2003) Optimizing the number of electrodes with high-rate stimulation of the Clarion CII cochlear implant. Acta Oto-Laryngologica 123: 138–42.

Fu QJ, Shannon RV (2000) Effects of dynamic range and amplitude mapping on phoneme recognition in Nucleus 22 cochlear implant users. Ear and Hearing 21: 227–35.

Govaerts P, Yperman M, De Ceulaer G et al. (2003) Beyond automated fitting. Paper presented at the Audiological Management of Cochlear Implantation in Young and Challenging Cases, Nottingham, UK.

Hay-McCutcheon MJ, Brown CJ, Clay KS et al. (2002) Comparison of electrically evoked whole-nerve action potential and electrically evoked auditory brainstem response thresholds in Nucleus CI24R cochlear implant recipients. Journal of the American Academy of Audiology 13: 416–27.

Henkin Y, Kaplan-Neeman R, Muchnik C et al. (2003) Changes in time in the psycho electric parameters in children with cochlear implants. International Journal of Audiology 42: 274–8.

Henshall KR, McKay CM (2001) Optimizing electrode and filter selection in cochlear implant speech processor maps. Journal of the American Academy of Audiology 12: 478–89.

Hodges AV, Balkany TJ, Ruth RA et al. (1997) Electrical middle ear muscle reflex: use in cochlear implant programming. Otolaryngology: Head and Neck Surgery 117: 255–61.

Hodges AV, Butts S, Dolan-Ash S et al. (1999) Using electrically evoked auditory reflex thresholds to fit the Clarion cochlear implant. Annals of Otology, Rhinology and Laryngology (suppl. 177): 64–8.

Holden LK, Skinner MW, Holden TA et al. (2002) Effects of stimulation rate with the Nucleus 24 ACE speech coding strategy. Ear and Hearing 23: 463–76.

Hughes ML, Brown CJ, Abbas PJ et al. (2000) Comparison of EAP thresholds with MAP levels in the Nucleus 24 cochlear implant: data from children. Ear and Hearing 21: 164–74.

Hughes ML, Vander Werff KR, Brown CJ et al. (2001) A longitudinal study of electrode impedance, the electrically evoked compound action potential, and behavioural measures in Nucleus 24 cochlear implant users. Ear and Hearing 22: 471–86.

Hughes R (2003) New developments in programming using Hi-Res. Paper presented at the Audiological Management of Cochlear Implantation in Young and Challenging Cases, Nottingham, UK.

James CJ, Blamey PJ, Martin L et al. (2002) Adaptive dynamic range optimization for cochlear implants: a preliminary study. Ear and Hearing 23: 49S–58S.

Kileny PR, Zwolan TA, Boerst A et al. (1997) Electrically evoked auditory potentials: current clinical applications in children with cochlear implants. American Journal of Otology 18: S90–S92.

Lynch C, Craddock L, Crocker S (1999) Developing a child-centred approach for paediatric audiologists: a model in the context of cochlear implant programming. The Ear 1: 10–16.

Mo B, Harris S, Lindback M (2002) Tinnitus in cochlear implant patients – a comparison with other hearing-impaired patients. International Journal of Audiology 41: 527–34.

Moore BCJ (2003) Coding of sounds in the auditory system and its relevance to signal processing and coding in cochlear implants. Otology and Neurotology 24: 243–54.

Muller-Deile J (1997) Which sensitivity should a child use? American Journal of Otology 18: S101–S103.

Nikolopoulos TP, Mason SM, O'Donoghue GM et al. (1997) Electric auditory brain-stem response in pediatric patients with cochlear implants. American Journal of Otology 18: S120–S121.

Parkinson A, Arcaroli J, Staller SJ et al. (2001) The Nucleus 24 Contour Cochlear Implant System: Adult Clinical Trial Results. N94685F, 1-8. Cochlear Ltd. Cochlear White Paper, 1-6-2001.

Plant K, Psarros C (2000) Comparison of a Standard and Interpolation Method of T-and C-level Measurement, Using Both Narrowly Spaced and Widely Spaced Electrodes. Cochlear White Paper N94320F, 1-4. 1-10-2000.

Plant K, Whitford L, Psarros C (2000) Strategy Comparison for Nucleus 24 Recipients with a Limited Number of Available Electrodes. Cochlear White Paper N94317F, 1-4. 2000.

Ramos AM, Maggs J, Cafarelli Dees D et al. (2003) Use of intra-operative NRT data in the initial fitting of very young children: preliminary findings. Paper presented at the Conference on Implantable Prostheses, Asilomar, USA.

Ruckenstein M, Hedgepeth C, Rafter K et al. (2001) Tinnitus suppression in patients with cochlear implants. Otology and Neurotology 22: 200–4.

Sainz M, de la Torre A, Roldan C et al. (2003a) Analysis of programming maps and its application for balancing multichannel cochlear implants. International Journal of Audiology 42: 43–51.

Sainz M, de la Torre A, Roldan C (2003b) Application of statistical analysis of the programming maps for fitting cochlear implants in children. Cochlear Implants International 4: 59–60.

Seyle K, Brown CJ (2003) Speech perception using maps based on Neural Response Telemetry measures. Ear and Hearing 72S–79S.

Shallop JK, Ash KR (1995) Relationships among comfort levels determined by cochlear implant patient's self-programming, audiologist's programming, and electrical stapedius reflex thresholds. Annals of Otology, Rhinology and Laryngology (suppl. 166): 175–6.

Skinner MW, Holden LK, Holden TA et al. (1995) Comparison of procedures for obtaining thresholds and maximum acceptable loudness levels with the nucleus cochlear implant system. Journal of Speech and Hearing Research 38: 677–89.

Skinner MW, Holden LK, Holden TA (1997) Parameter selection to optimize speech recognition with the Nucleus implant. Otolaryngology: Head and Neck Surgery 117: 188–95.

Skinner MW, Holden LK, Holden TA et al. (1999) Comparison of two methods for selecting minimum stimulation levels used in programming the Nucleus 22 cochlear implant. Journal of Speech, Language and Hearing Research 42: 814–28.

Skinner MW, Holden LK, Holden TA et al. (2000) Effect of stimulation rate on cochlear implant recipients' thresholds and maximum acceptable loudness levels. Journal of the American Academy of Audiology 11: 203–13.

Skinner MW, Holden LK, Whitford LA et al. (2002a) Speech recognition with the Nucleus 24 SPEAK, ACE and CIS speech coding strategies in newly implanted adults. Ear and Hearing 23: 207–23.

Skinner MW, Arndt PL, Staller SJ (2002b) Nucleus 24 advanced encoder conversion study: performance versus preference. Ear and Hearing 23: 2S–17S.

Smoorenburg GF, Willeboer C, van Dijk JE (2002) Speech perception in Nucleus CI24M cochlear implant users with processor settings based on electrically-evoked compound action potential thresholds. Audiology and Neuro-Otology 7: 335–47.

Smoorenburg GF, Van Zanten B (2004) Frequency and map changes: the course of fittings over the years. Paper presented at the 5th European Investigators Conference, Vienna, Austria.

Spivak LG, Chute PM (1994) The relationship between electrical acoustic reflex threshold and behavioural comfort levels in children and adult cochlear implant patients. Ear and Hearing 15: 184–92.

Spivak LG, Chute PM, Popp AL et al. (1994) Programming the cochlear implant based on electrical acoustic reflex thresholds: patient performance. Laryngoscope 104: 1225–30.

Stephan K, Welzl-Muller K (2000) Post-operative stapedius reflex tests with simultaneous loudness scaling in patients supplied with cochlear implants. Audiology 39: 13–18.

Stoddart RL, Cooper HR (1995) Electrode complications in 100 adults with multichannel cochlear implants. Journal of Laryngology and Otology (suppl. 24): 18–20.

Summerfield A, Marshall D (1995) Cochlear Implantation in the UK 1990–1994. Report by the MRC Institute of Hearing Research on the Evaluation of the National Cochlear Implant Programme. 1-28 MRC-IHR. London: HMSO.

Sun JC, Skinner MW, Liu SY et al. (1999) Effect of speech processor program modifications on cochlear implant recipients' threshold and maximum acceptable loudness levels. American Journal of Audiology 8: 128–36.

Todd NW, Ajayi E, Hasenstab MS et al. (2003) Childhood otitis media and electrically elicited stapedius reflexes in adult cochlear implantees. Otology and Neurotology 24: 621–4.

Truy E, Gallego S, Chanal JM et al. (1998) Correlation between electrical auditory brainstem response and perceptual thresholds in Digisonic cochlear implant users. Laryngoscope 108: 554–9.

Tyler R, Dunn C, Witt S et al. (2004) Bilateral results in patients with the CII plat-
form. Paper presented at the 5th European Investigators Conference, Vienna,
Austria.

Vickers D, Nunn T, Boyle P (2004) Investigating the effect of rate on electrical
dynamic range. Poster presentation at the British Society of Audiology Short
Papers Meeting on Experimental Studies of Hearing and Deafness, London,
UK.

Wilson BS, Finley CC, Lawson DT et al. (1993) Design and evaluation of a continuous interleaved sampling (CIS) processing strategy for multichannel
cochlear implants. Journal of Rehabilitation Research and Development 30:
110–16.

Zehnder A, Allum JH, Honegger F et al. (1999) The usefulness of intraoperatively registered, electrically evoked stapedius reflex for the programming of
cochlear implants in children. HNO 47: 970–5.

Zeng FG, Grant G, Niparko J et al. (2002) Speech dynamic range and its effect on
cochlear implant performance. Journal of the Acoustical Society of America
111: 377–86.

# CHAPTER 13

# Adult rehabilitation

GEOFF PLANT

## Introduction

There have been many exciting and innovative changes in cochlear implant technology over the past 25 years. These changes, which include the progression from single-channel to multi-channel devices, improved speech processing and coding strategies and bilateral implantation, have resulted in great improvements in speech perception skills which have led in turn to increased client satisfaction.

It is, perhaps, these great improvements which have meant that approaches to aural rehabilitation and speech communication training have not received similar attention over the past 20 or so years. In the early days of cochlear implant research, great emphasis was placed on the need for systematic training, and some excellent programs were developed. Pioneers in this area, such as Norma Norton at the House Clinic in Los Angeles, developed programs that helped adult clients take full advantage of the limited information provided by single-channel devices. The improvements in speech understanding that resulted from this training showed the potential of cochlear implants and encouraged the research and development that has resulted in the greatly improved devices available to deaf adults and children in the early twenty-first century.

It would be hard to find any clinician who would debate the value of, and the need for, a systematic (re)habilitative approach for deaf children with cochlear implants. This usually includes activities aimed at improving the child's speech perception and production skills and often involves preparing the child's parent(s) to provide ongoing training in the home environment. The situation for adults with cochlear implants, however, is considerably more controversial. There are many clinicians who doubt that it is necessary to provide adult clients with anything more than an orientation to the implant, instruction in its use and properly selected speech processor programs or maps, which may need to be modified over time. If a client returns expressing dissatisfaction with her/his implant and the speech information being provided, the response is often to provide a new map, in the hope that this will solve the client's problems. Approaches that emphasize the need for speech communication training (practice in auditory and/or auditory-visual speech perception) and/or counseling are often seen as being unnecessary, especially when the client appears to be having few difficulties adjusting to the auditory signal provided by her/his implant.

This chapter will argue that rehabilitation needs to be seen as an important part of the cochlear implant procedure adopted with adult clients. It will also argue that almost all adult clients, not just those who are experiencing difficulties, would benefit from some systematic rehabilitative intervention following cochlear implantation.

## Goals of rehabilitation

Webster's *Dictionary* defines rehabilitation as, 'to put back in good condition; re-establish on a firm, sound basis'. This definition is in keeping with the aims of aural rehabilitation programs adopted with deafened adults. The effects of an acquired profound hearing loss on speech perception are well recognized. They include a sharp decline in the individual's ability to understand speech via audition only, and their attempts to compensate for this through an increased dependence on or, in some cases, substitution of the visual sense via lipreading, sign, fingerspelling, writing etc. There are also usually changes in the deafened adult's speech production skills, although these vary considerably from person to person. These effects relate directly to communication skills, but as Hogan (2001) has pointed out, 'people do not go deaf in a social vacuum' (ibid., p. 3) and 'irrespective of when the onset of deafness occurs in a person's life, its impact is profoundly social' (ibid., p. 42). These effects can include changes in the dynamics of family life, altered relationships in the workplace and in the community as a whole, and a diminished sense of self (Hogan, 2001).

It is unrealistic to expect that the fitting of a cochlear implant to an individual will solve all of the problems created by her/his deafness. In some cases, testing will show that the implanted adult is able to understand speech with a very high degree of proficiency, attaining a performance level that approximates 'normal' speech understanding. For example, I have recently worked with an adult deafened nine years prior to implantation, who was able to make a complex phone call on the day his implant was activated. Live-voice testing of this subject using the CUNY Sentence Lists (Boothroyd et al., 1985), presented via audition only, yielded a mean score of 99.4% correct. This represents exceptional performance, however-er. As exceptional are the small number of subjects who appear to derive only marginal benefit from their implants. The performance level of the vast majority of implanted adults lies somewhere between these two extremes, but almost all report that their speech understanding post-implant is considerably better than their pre-implant performance.

It is extremely rare to be confronted by an implanted adult who maintains that her/his performance level pre-implant was better than that obtained following implantation. In my clinical experience, I've found that systematic testing almost always reveals a substantial improvement in the post-implant period, and that the subject's dissatisfaction is related to unrealistic expectations. That is, s/he expected to hear normally with the implant, and anything less than this unattainable goal is deemed a failure. Clinicians delight in recounting stories of such clients, who call them on the phone to complain that the implant is providing limited benefit!

One of the major aims of rehabilitation has to be to help the client to obtain optimal performance with her/his implant, and to ensure that this is achieved as quickly as possible. Obviously, this doesn't mean that all subjects will attain or even approach the performance level obtained by exceptional users such as the one cited above. Rather, it means that the subject should be provided with assistance and training that enables her/him to function at her/his optimal level. This is particularly important in the first few months following 'switch on'.

Another primary aim should be to maximize the client's ability to understand speech through listening alone. In cases where auditory-alone speech understanding is not possible, or where performance falls below that required for even, for example, a simple conversation, attention needs to be paid to ensure that the client is provided with opportunities to maximize the use of the auditory signal as a supplement to lipreading.

Attention also needs to be paid to reducing the social effects resulting from the client's deafness. Often the improved speech understanding that follows implantation substantially reduces many of these problems spontaneously. Clients who have avoided social settings, such as dinner parties or business meetings, suddenly find that they are able to take part in such events with little difficulty, and their patterns of communication behavior and expectations are radically changed. Others require extensive counseling before they are prepared to take a step towards resuming such social interactions.

Similarly, some clients may evidence great improvements in their self-perception when their ability to understand speech and to contribute meaningfully to conversations is enhanced by their implant. Others may need to be provided with a large number of experiences and activities that demonstrate their enhanced performance before they start to see themselves in a more positive light. I remember working with one client whose auditory-alone speech understanding was excellent, but when I commented on this to her she evidenced disbelief. Over time, I realized that during her many years of deafness she had regarded her speech perception skills as being poor and this had permeated into her view of her own competence in many other areas. Providing this client with activities that demonstrated her communication competence also had very positive effects on her self-perception.

Other clients may require a more specific rehabilitative approach that targets the psychosocial effects of acquired deafness. The goals of such an approach are to help clients '(1) become aware of the impact of deafness in their lives, (2) while developing new attitudes about themselves and others and (3) while developing a new communicative skills set that enables them to begin living their life in a new and proud fashion' (Hogan, 2001, p. 148).

Another goal of rehabilitation should be to help the client adapt to the signal provided by her/his implant. In cases where the client has had a long-term hearing loss, the implant may provide information that has not been available to her/him for many years. For example, many long-term hearing aid users become adept at using an auditory signal that is devoid of high-frequency speech sounds, using visual cues and their language knowledge to 'fill in the gaps'. An auditory signal that provides access to high-frequency consonants such as [s], [sh] and [ch] may be quite disconcerting, and the client may need specific training that helps her/him re-assimilate this information, which may, at first, act as a distracting 'noise'. One client with a long-term hearing loss described this new high-frequency-rich signal as sounding as if there were someone whispering in the background whenever anyone spoke. Helping this client to initally cope with, and then use, high-frequency speech information was an important goal in her rehabilitation program.

# Approaches to speech communication training

Traditionally, approaches to speech communication training have been divided into two broad categories: analytic and synthetic. This nomenclature dates from the pioneering work of early lipreading teachers, such as Edward Nitchie and Karl Brauckmann, and describes processing strategies which today are usually referred to as bottom-up and top-down, respectively.

Analytic approaches concentrate on training the deafened client to discriminate between minimal units of speech. At the segmental level this might involve discriminating between the voiced and voiceless stops in word pairs such as 'pit/bit', 'pat/bat', 'port/bought' etc., or the high and low vowels [i] and [a] in 'heat/heart', 'key/car', 'cheese/chars' etc. The assumption underlying analytic training is that an improved ability to discriminate between minimal speech contrasts will result in an improved perception of words, phrases, sentences and connected discourse.

The synthetic approach to lipreading instruction was based on the premise that 'the ability to predict meaning, rather than identifying individual speech components, should be the paramount aim in visual training' (Sanders, 1971, p. 280), and many working in auditory training eventually adopted this philosophy. In the synthetic approach, the materials used closely mirror the everyday communication process, and focus on sentence length materials. The person being trained is encouraged to use all of her/his language knowledge to derive meaning. This includes a native speaker's implicit understanding of the phonological, syntactic and collocational (the arrangements of words) rules of her/his language. Thus the person with a hearing loss can use her/his knowledge of these *global cues* to predict, deduce and understand what is being said.

There have been few studies investigating the effectiveness of the two approaches. Those that have been reported show that training using either analytic or synthetic materials can result in enhanced speech perception. For example, Walden et al. (1981) report improved speech perception skills for hearing aid users following intensive analytic training, while Rubinstein and Boothroyd (1987) show improvements in performance following synthetic training. One important study that may have particular relevance for adults with cochlear implants was conducted by Alcantara et al. (1990) in an investigation of an electrotactile aid, the 'Tickle-Talker'. This study strongly supported a combined analytic/synthetic approach, and this result, coupled with clinical observation, has influenced the form of the training materials I have developed over the past decade.

A further influence has been the reality of everyday conversations, which require both top-down and bottom-up processing strategies. There are occasions when contextual information provides no assistance in identification, and the receiver is forced to rely upon the acoustic-phonetic structure of the speech signal. I also feel there is a particular relevance for analytic training to help clients with long-standing hearing losses adapt to the new signal provided by their cochlear implants.

## Analytic approaches

Analytic training provides the client with the opportunity to focus on the acoustic cues that characterize a selected consonant or vowel. In 'AUDI-TRAIN' (Plant, 2001a) there is a series of exercises designed to introduce clients newly fitted with cochlear implants to a range of consonants and vowels. In each case, a short story is used that provides the client with the opportunity to hear the target phoneme in a variety of positions in real words. The clinician reads the story aloud to the client, who is provided with a copy of the text in which each word containing the target is bolded. For example, the first paragraph of the story introducing the voiceless sibilant [s] is shown below.

> I have often wondered whether my **parents displayed** a **sick sense** of humor when they named their children. There were three of us – my two **sisters** and me. Our **surname** was **Sullivan-Smith** and that was bad enough when we were going to **school**. Anyone with a hyphenated name

was regarded with **suspicion** by the other children, who **saw** it as positive proof of **snobbery**.

Plant, 2001a, p. 14

Wherever possible, this is followed by exercises that contrast words differing only in that one contains the target phoneme, while the other does not. Word pairs focusing on [s] in the initial position include 'sought/ought', 'sage/age', 'sin/in' etc., while 'ice/eye', 'pats/pat' and 'ace/A' are examples of final contrasts. Such exercises provide the client with the opportunity to focus on the particular target in a relaxed, non-stressful situation. S/he is asked to follow the story as it is read, not to repeat or answer questions related to the text.

Once two or more targets are introduced, they can be contrasted with each other in simple discrimination exercises. If possible, targets introduced early in training should be those that will create the fewest difficulties for clients. For example, consonants that differ in their voicing characteristics (voiced vs. voiceless) are usually an easy discrimination task, as are some manner of articulation contrasts. Place of articulation contrasts (for example exercises contrasting [p], [t] and/or [k]) are usually quite difficult, and should be avoided at first in analytic training.

Wherever possible, real words are used as the training items. 'Analytika' (Plant, 1994) is a useful source, but there are some circumstances in which the use of nonsense syllables can provide useful information to aid in the development of an individualized training program. For example, the consonants [p, t, k, b, d, g, f, v, h, s, z, sh, ch, j, w, r, l, y, m, n] can be presented for identification in an [aCa] format, and an analysis made of the client's responses to determine her/his areas of strength and weakness. The set of consonants shown has the advantage of using normal orthographic representation, and has been chosen for this reason.

The consonants can be presented for identification in three sensory conditions – auditory only, visual only and auditory-visually – to help determine the effect on overall identification and any changes in the client's response patterns. For example, clients may evidence difficulties in specifying correct place of articulation in the auditory-alone condition but have little difficulty when the materials are presented auditory-visually or visual only. Conversely, the client will almost certainly have great difficulty with voicing and some manners of articulation when the materials are presented visual only. Allowing the client to experience these differences in performance may also serve to indicate the value of the information provided by her/his implant.

Once areas of difficulty have been specified, training can be provided that contrasts these items in meaningful words and/or nonsense syllables. This should indicate whether the client can benefit from training or whether alternatives such as auditory-visual presentation, the use of Clear Speech (Picheny et al., 1985) or the use of appropriate repair strategies need to be considered. It is important that the client be provided with not only an awareness of the contrasts that create difficulties for her/him, but also a realistic means of overcoming these problems in everyday life. It should also be stressed that, although important, analytic training is only one component in an overall program and should occupy no more than 25% of a training session. In my own clinical work, I try to provide analytic training at the beginning of a session, as it can be quite a stressful activity requiring a great deal of concentration on the part of the client.

# Synthetic training

Synthetic training should be the major component of the training program provided to adults with cochlear implants. The materials used for training should replicate normal everyday communication situations, phrases, sentences and connected discourse as closely as possible. Clinicians should also seize opportunities for conversation with the client. Although some clients will complain that conversations are not 'real work', such opportunities to practice the 'give and take' of everyday communication should not be ignored. However, therapists need to be aware that a long-term hearing loss may result in the development of 'compensatory' strategies, such as the use of monologue, which reduce the role of the communication partner to that of affirmation, or very simple, predictable responses. The therapist should therefore ensure that the conversation is truly two-way.

The synthetic materials in 'AUDITRAIN' (Plant, 2001a) provide a wide range of activities that increase in difficulty over time. Initial activities include simple exercises such as looking at numbers, days of the week, dates, playing cards etc., and are designed to provide the client with confidence in her/his ability to follow and understand speech. This is particularly important if the client has a long-term hearing loss and has experienced great difficulty in most communication situations. Building up her/his confidence in her/his ability to understand speech via audition only, or in some cases auditory-visually, is an important step on the way to the successful use of the information provided by the cochlear implant.

The 'Barrier Game' is the referential communication exercise recommended in 'AUDITRAIN'. With this technique, the clinician and the client have an identical set of postcards. At first, the cards can form the basis of a simple conversation, as the clinician asks questions, makes comments etc. regarding them. Later, the clinician can instruct the client to place the cards in a different order. These instructions can involve merely naming each object depicted but, as the client's competence increases, the clinician may describe each item in varying degrees of detail.

'AUDITRAIN' also contains a series of Question and Answer topics. This technique involves providing the client with a list of questions related to a specific topic such as: 'Sweden', 'Finland', 'Kangaroos and Wallabies' and 'Carl Nielsen'. The client asks each question in turn, and the clinician provides the answer. Detailed information that enables the clinician to construct an appropriate response for individual clients is provided in the program. The response may need to be kept relatively simple for some clients, while others will be able to cope with far more complex materials.

Many adults initially find longer sentences extremely difficult, and it is recommended that clinicians use a technique referred to as *expansion* to help the client to understand progressively longer and longer speech sequences. The clinician may provide a relatively short response at first, and then, if the client is able to understand, make it a little longer, and see what effect this has on understanding. For example, if the question was 'Where is Sweden?' the clinician might initially respond, 'Sweden is in the north of Europe.' If the client understands this, the clinician might then present each of the following sentences in turn.

'Sweden is a large country in the north of Europe.'

'Sweden is a large country in the north of Europe. It's part of Scandinavia.'

'Sweden is a large country in the north of Europe. It's part of Scandinavia. The other Scandinavian countries are Denmark, Norway and Finland.'

Each sentence takes the previous one as its core, with the client moving from the familiar to the unfamiliar. One of the advantages of this technique is that the materials can be used with a wide range of clients. The level of complexity can be adjusted to meet the particular needs of an individual client, and as her/his ability to understand speech increases, so too can the difficulty of the response.

'AUDITRAIN' also contains a number of sets of 50 sentences built around specific themes. For example, one set is built around the theme, 'Things people say about reading' and a sample is provided below.

The number of words in the sentences varies considerably, and is provided in parentheses, so that the therapist can observe what effect, if any, this has on the client's ability to repeat each one. If the client has difficulty with longer sentences, they can be broken down into shorter segments for initial presentation, and then presented in their entirety. The use of the expansion technique can also be used to improve the client's ability to cope with progressively longer and longer segments.

Another technique, based on a technique described by Hagerman (1982), involves the use of a set of pictures arranged so that they form a short phrase. An example is provided in Figure 13.1. The client's task is to pick which of the items in each column is presented in each phrase. For example, the clinician might say 'two blue rabbits' or 'five black fish' and the client has to repeat what was said.

This technique was initially developed for use with clients with limited auditory-alone skills, but it can also be used with clients with much more developed skills. When the materials are presented to clients with poorer performance levels, the therapist should take care to use 'Clear Speech', produce the words clearly and leave a short pause between each item. When presented to clients with better auditory skills, however, a far more

| 2 | BLACK | 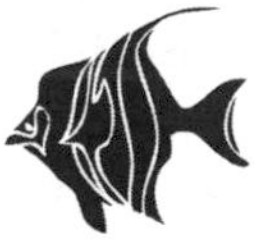 |
| 3 | BLUE | 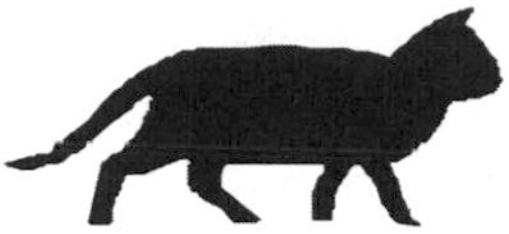 |
| 4 | RED | 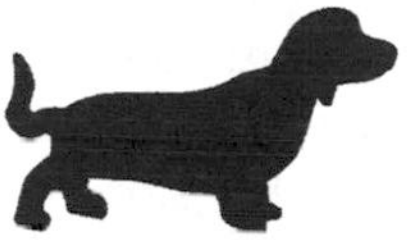 |
| 5 | YELLOW | 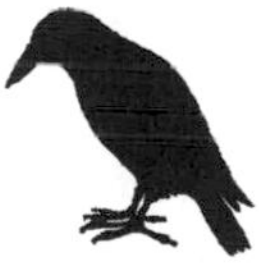 |
| 6 | GREEN | 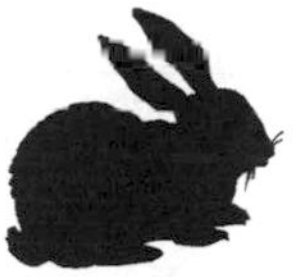 |

**Figure 13.1** Picture Matrix used to generate short phrases for identification.

natural speaking style can be adopted, resulting in blurred word boundaries and far more pronounced co-articulatory effects. This makes the task considerably more difficult, and may serve as a good introduction to the difficulties that occur when speakers use a faster rate.

## Picture-based training materials

Over the past few years, the need for training materials that cater for adults with limited reading skills has become apparent. This creates a series of unique problems for anyone developing aural rehabilitation materials for adults. The materials must be interesting and relevant, and this can be difficult to achieve without the use of the written word. It is also very important that the materials do not appear to be 'talking down' or condescending to the client. Further, the lack of reading skills can be a source of great embarrassment and, as a result, the use of non-test-based materials needs to be introduced carefully. However, as is often the case, I have found that these materials, developed for a very specific group of clients, have applications for many others.

Techniques such as the 'Barrier Game' are suitable for clients with poor reading skills, but there was a need for a far more comprehensive range of materials. 'Syntrain' (Plant, 2002b) represented an attempt to meet this need. The materials, which are all picture-based, include exercises contrasting sets of words with differing syllabic patterns presented in isolation and in progressively more complex phrases and sentences. Other exercises involve spondaic and trisyllabic words, both in isolation and in sentences, and theme-based sets of sentences with pictures providing contextual cues to aid in identification. The materials are designed to allow for varying levels of complexity. For example, at first the client

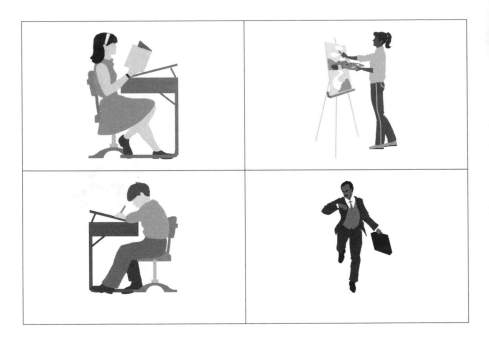

**Figure 13.2** A set of pictures used as stimulus items in 'Syntrain'. Source: Plant (2002b).

may be asked to differentiate between a set of five words presented in a random order. Then s/he can be provided with a clue sentence or set of clue sentences, and be required to identify the object described.

Figure 13.2 shows a set of pictures taken from 'Syntrain'. At first, each of the pictures is introduced and identified as: 'A girl is reading', 'A woman is painting', 'A boy is writing' and 'A man is running'. The four sentences are then presented several times in a random order, and the client is asked to repeat each one. The sentences can then be expanded upon, and the client asked to repeat what was said. For example, the clinician might say, 'A boy is writing', 'A boy is writing a report', 'A boy is writing a report in his book' etc. In this way the original materials can become progressively more and more complex and present real challenges to the client.

# Speech tracking

Speech tracking (De Filippo and Scott, 1978), a procedure 'for training and evaluating the reception of ongoing speech', is one of the most widely used techniques in aural rehabilitation training. In this procedure, the clinician reads from a prepared text, phrase by phrase, for a predetermined time period; I recommend five minutes. The task of the client is to repeat exactly what the speaker said. If the client does not give a verbatim response, the clinician has to apply a strategy to overcome the breakdown. This can involve repeating what was said, the use of clue words or providing a paraphrase of what was originally presented. The clinician goes on to the next segment only when the receiver is able to repeat correctly every word of the original segment.

At the end of the time period, the number of words repeated correctly is counted then divided by the time elapsed to derive the client's tracking rate, expressed in words-per-minute (wpm). For example, if a client repeats 250 words in five minutes, her/his tracking rate would be 50 wpm.

Speech tracking has been criticized as a test instrument because of problems created by such variables as speaker characteristics, receiver characteristics and text complexity. Given these concerns, it is not surprising that Tye-Murray and Tyler (1988) caution against the use of speech tracking for across-subject test designs. They do, however, recognize its value as a training procedure.

I have always found speech tracking a very useful technique to use with most adult clients. It provides practice in the perception of connected materials and, provided care is taken in the selection of the text used, a high interest level can be maintained. I have found fiction written for adolescents and young adults to be the most suitable source of materials for presentation in speech tracking. Such texts are usually entertaining, and their style more closely related to conversational English than books aimed at an adult audience. There have been occasions, however, where more complex materials have been required, and in these cases I have successfully used some of the Sherlock Holmes stories of Sir Arthur Conan Doyle.

Clients' responses to speech tracking have been uniformly positive, and most derive considerable satisfaction from observing a rise in their tracking rate over the course of training. A client once compared his tracking rate to his golf handicap. He noted that the only difference was that he wanted his tracking rate to rise and his golf handicap to go down!

Over the past ten years, I have used the KTH or Kungl Tekniska Högskolan (Royal Institute of Technology) Tracking Procedure (Gnosspelius and Spens, 1992; Spens, 1992), a computer-controlled modification of De Filippo and Scott's original procedure, and have found this a very useful means of presenting training materials to a wide range of clients and recording their results. This approach uses live-voice presentation, but with a pre-determined segment length and the use of only one repair strategy: repetition. If a client fails to correctly identify any word after three presentations, its written form is shown to her/him via either a computer monitor or on paper.

At the end of each tracking session, several different measures are automatically calculated. These include the client's tracking rate, her/his ceiling rate (the time taken to present and respond to a line that is identified correctly after only one presentation), the proportion of blocked words and the number of words that have to be displayed in writing.

Figures 13.3 and 13.4 present tracking rates and ceiling rates for materials presented auditory-visually (Figure 13.3) and auditory only (Figure 13.4) to DJ, an adult cochlear implant user. Note that each datum point represents the mean of five x 5-minute tracking sessions.

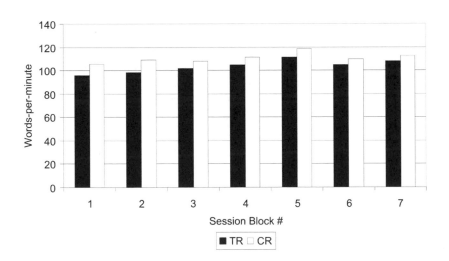

**Figure 13.3** Tracking rates (TR) and ceiling rates (CR) obtained by DJ, an adult cochlear implant subject, for materials presented auditory-visually. Each datum point represents the mean score obtained for five 5-minute tracking sessions.

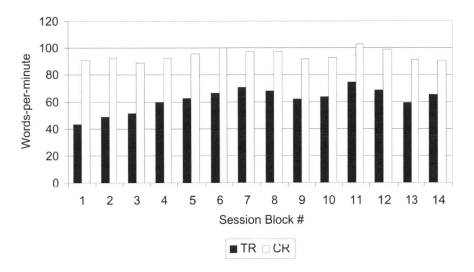

**Figure 13.4** Tracking rates (TR) and ceiling rates (CR) obtained by DJ, an adult cochlear implant subject, for materials presented auditory-only. Each datum point represents the mean score obtained for five 5-minute tracking sessions.

The client's tracking rates for the auditory-visual presentations were very high, and were close to ceiling level performance. It is obvious that the client did not require training in this modality; the sessions shown were used at the beginning of each training period to re-familiarize the subject with the story used and to provide him with a 'break' from the much greater effort required for auditory-only presentations. When the materials were presented auditory-only, his performance was initially around 40 wpm. Following extensive training, his mean tracking rate had risen to around 60–65 wpm. This client greatly enjoyed the challenge of speech tracking, and derived considerable satisfaction from carefully charting his progress from session to session.

There are some clients, however, for whom speech tracking is an unsuitable approach to training. These include anyone with a tracking rate of less than 15–20 wpm. When a client performs at this level, many of the advantages of speech tracking are lost. The benefits of contextual cues to aid in identification can no longer be utilized, and the task starts to resemble the identification of an isolated word or group of words.

'COMMTRAC' (Plant, 1996, 1989) is a modified form of speech tracking developed for use with such cases. In common with conventional speech tracking, the approach uses stories as the stimuli, but it does not require that the client repeat back every word verbatim. A number of stories have been modified for the approach and each is divided into a number of 200-word parts. Each part is then divided into short phrases or sentences for presentation. The therapist presents each line as many times as required (the client can ask for as many repeats as s/he desires) and records the total number of words correctly repeated. The client is then shown the written form, and the therapist moves on to the next line.

This approach provides credit for words correctly repeated, ensures that the client does not become 'bogged-down' by a particularly difficult word or series of words and gives immediate feedback as to the correctness of her/his response. Allowing the client to read each line after it has been presented also provides contextual information and cues which, over time, make the task considerably easier. Even though the approach is aimed at adult clients, the stories used are classic fairy tales, mostly by Hans Christian Andersen. These involve much repetition and relatively simple plot lines, making them very suitable for presentation in this form.

'SpeechTrax' (Plant, 2002a) is the most recent version of this approach. The story used, an adaptation of Andersen's *The Tinderbox*, consists of 53 200-word parts, which also makes it suitable as text for conventional speech tracking.

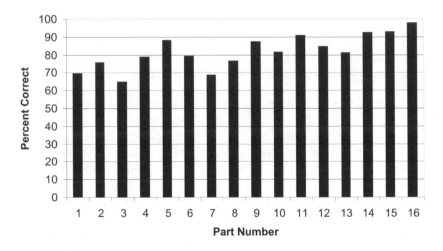

**Figure 13.5** Scores obtained by RR for auditory-only presentations of 'COMMTRAC' materials. Note that alternate lines were presented auditory-only and auditory-visually.

Figure 13.5 presents the scores obtained by RR, a male client in his late fifties who was fitted with a cochlear implant after more than 30 years of deafness following meningitis. This subject found an auditory-only presentation of materials unacceptable, and would become extremely distressed whenever it was attempted. Following extensive counseling, the client agreed to attempt auditory-only training using 'COMMTRAC' materials, but only if each alternate line was presented auditory-visually. The client's score for auditory-only presentations was calculated. Over time, his performance rose from around 70% to better than 90% of words correctly identified. No record was kept of the client's auditory-visual performance, but it was around 100% correct in each session.

As the client's performance improved, so did his confidence in his ability to understand speech via listening alone. Following completion of the 'COMMTRAC' story, training was continued using 'SpeechTrax'. The

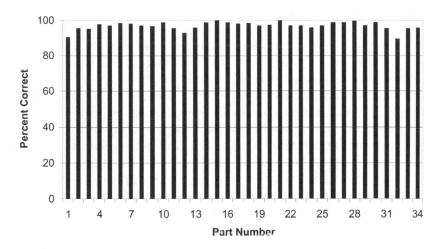

**Figure 13.6** Scores obtained by RR for auditory-only presentations of 'COMMTRAC' materials. Note that all materials after Part 5 were presented auditory-only.

scores obtained are presented in Figure 13.6, and show a consistently high level of performance. It should be noted that following the presentation of Part 5, the client asked that all lines be presented via audition alone. This reflects not only improved performance but also an increased confidence in his ability to understand speech via the implant alone.

Finally, Figure 13.7 presents RR's scores for 35 five-minute auditory-only tracking sessions using the KTH Tracking Procedure. Although RR's tracking rates are quite low, in the range of 25–30 wpm, this performance represents a great improvement over his pre-training performance.

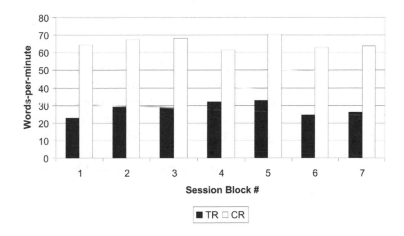

**Figure 13.7** Tracking rates (TR) and ceiling rates (CR) obtained by RR, an adult cochlear implant user, for materials presented auditory-only. Each datum point represents the mean score obtained for five 5-minute tracking sessions.

# Training modalities

Selecting the training modality or modalities – auditory (A), auditory-visual (AV), quiet, noise – used with an individual client is an extremely important part of the aural rehabilitation process. Pre-training testing should provide information on the client's ability to understand speech via listening alone, but the therapist should also be aware that some clients may lack the confidence to attempt the task, and that the test results may not reflect her/his real ability. If a client is reluctant to attempt auditory-only training, the use of closed-set (the client is given a list of alternatives and is asked to indicate which has been presented as the stimulus) analytic materials can reduce the task's complexity and provide cues as to her/his skills. The approach adopted with RR above (alternating A, AV presentations) can also encourage the client to attempt auditory-only tasks secure in the knowledge that half of the materials will be presented in the other, much easier, modality. Over time, more complex open-set synthetic materials can be introduced as the client's performance indicates that her/his skills and confidence are improving.

In auditory-visual training, the aim is to provide the client with exercises that enhance her/his use of the implant as an aid to lipreading and vice versa. If this proves to be excessively easy for a client, the therapist should consider the use of background noise to increase task complexity. It is not necessary to specify the exact signal-to-noise ratio used, or to be overly concerned with the type of noise used. Multi-talker babble has the advantage of replicating, in part, the situations most people with hearing loss report as causing great difficulties, but other noise sources such as machinery, street sounds and music can also be used. More important is for the clinician to ensure that the noise is set at a level that creates some difficulty for the client, but not so great that s/he has to strain to pick up even a few words. The aim is to increase the level of difficulty slightly, not make the task too stressful.

When and if the client is able to understand speech via listening alone to a degree that allows at least some simple conversation, consideration should be given to attempting telephone training. The use of the telephone is an extremely important part of everyday communication, and many clients need to be provided with experiences that allow them to approach this potentially daunting task with confidence. Telephone training using materials with which the client is comfortable and assured of success can provide the confidence needed to attempt telephone use in everyday life.

# Personnel

I am often asked what sort of training therapists need to have before attempting to provide aural rehabilitation training to adults with cochlear implants. This question usually refers to the clinician's academic qualifications, that is should the therapist be an audiologist, speech pathologist, hearing therapist, teacher of the deaf etc? This is difficult to answer, as none of the groups mentioned have necessarily had specific preparation in this area during their training. My response is usually to indicate that a good theoretical and practical knowledge of speech perception (auditory, visual and auditory-visual) by people with hearing loss, combined with practical experience in providing speech communication training to a range of clients with hearing loss, is an invaluable preparation for this work.

Just as important, however, is an awareness of the problems created by hearing loss in the familial, social and vocational lives of people with profound hearing loss. Although there are some therapists who have a profound hearing loss themselves, most will gain this knowledge through observation of and interactions with deafened people. Adults vary greatly in how they react, however, and therapists need to interact with a large number of clients to see the many 'solutions', some positive and some negative, that individuals develop to cope with the acquisition of profound deafness. For example, some clients develop 'positive' strategies such as informing their communication partners about their hearing loss, asking for repeats and providing a précis of what they think has been said. Others 'cope' with hearing loss by the use of 'negative' strategies such as engaging in lengthy monologues that reduce the role of the communication 'partner' to that of a passive recipient. This presupposes a 'willingness to listen' on the part of the therapist, and an acceptance that there are many valid responses to acquired deafness. The skills and knowledge outlined above are probably far more important than any specific academic qualification, and should be primary factors in selecting personnel to work with both newly implanted adults and also with those who experience long-term difficulties in deriving optimal benefit from their implant.

This knowledge and experience implies that clinicians should have spent considerable time working with a wide range of adults with varying degrees of hearing loss prior to providing aural rehabilitation training to adults with cochlear implants. An additional problem is that in-service courses in communication training and other appropriate techniques may be difficult to obtain in some situations. Attending training courses or workshops is one possible solution, and the benefit of serving an internship with an experienced therapist should also be considered. In the long term, it may be necessary for academic institutions to provide short courses aimed at clinicians who wish to specialize in this area of cochlear implant rehabilitation.

## Facilities and resources

Wherever possible, training should be provided in an area that reflects real-life situations, rather than in 'pristine' acoustic conditions. For example, I prefer to work in a quiet office, as this is more typical of everyday listening situations, rather than a sound-treated test booth. The latter has a number of 'advantages' such as reduced background noise and little reverberation, but these are not realistic for most people. The presence of some competing noise – people talking in the next office, the telephone ringing, people walking down the hall – provides clients with experiences that mirror everyday life and can help prepare them for listening in difficult situations.

Some consideration should be given to ensuring that the room has good lighting, so that the client can take full advantage of visual cues. If the room has a window, the therapist should sit facing it with the light shining on her/his face. Therapists should also check for any possible sources of glare, and reduce them if at all possible. I usually sit facing the client, with a small table between us on which written or pictorial materials can be placed. Although I do not make a conscious effort to measure the talker-to-receiver distance, it is usually around 1 metre, which is fairly representative of normal everyday communication.

If materials are presented via listening only, the therapist needs to ensure that the client is not able to see her/his lips. The client can be asked to look down or to close her/his eyes, but usually I recommend the use of an acoustic screen to cover the clinician's face. This consists of an embroidery frame with two sheets of black loudspeaker cloth stretched across it. This effectively removes any possibility of the client seeing the lips but does not degrade the acoustic signal. Sheets of cardboard or the hand may serve to obscure the lips but they also reduce high-frequency speech cues and should not be used.

Access to a personal computer (PC) can be invaluable for record keeping and for the presentation of some training materials. As more computer-based training materials become available, this will become progressively more important. One factor which has held back the implementation of some computer-based materials has been the need to have programs that use speakers with the same dialect as the clients attending a particular clinic. I feel that this is a relatively minor concern, especially when it is considered that we are exposed to many different dialects on a daily basis, via the popular media. Clinicians who wish to use the KTH Tracking Procedure will also need to have access to a PC for presentation of the text for the speaker and to record and analyze the client's responses.

There are currently a number of training resources available on video and CD-ROM for clinic- and home-based training. Access to audiotape, VCR and DVD equipment will become increasingly important as more test and training materials become available in these formats. One exciting prospect of these innovations will be the chance for clients to have access to self-training materials. Although such materials should not be seen as a substitute for a well-trained therapist, they certainly provide a very useful supplement and will allow clients to work at their own rate between training sessions and in situations where they do not have access to a trained clinician.

Clinicians also need to have access to a wide range of training materials to meet the needs of their client group. Each of the cochlear implant manufacturers provides a range of materials for clinical use, and these can be supplemented by other resources such as Hogan's (2001) 'Hearing Rehabilitation for Deafened Adults' and Wayner and Abrahamson's (1998) 'Learning to Hear Again with a Cochlear Implant'.

# Evaluation of performance

Over the past 100 years, almost all aural rehabilitation programs provided to adults with acquired hearing loss have suffered from one major deficit – a lack of any systematic evaluation of the outcomes of training. Unfortunately, this trend, which started with lipreading instruction in the early twentieth century, has been continued by many cochlear implant teams. Programs are provided, but there are few attempts to assess whether they result in improvements in a client's ability to understand speech and her/his social and vocational situation. It is perhaps this lack of systematic evaluation that has resulted in many clinicians feeling that aural rehabilitation is the 'soft' component of hearing health care. Consequently, they doubt its value.

There are many reasons why it is necessary to assess an individual client's performance before, during and after training. The most obvious is to determine whether the training has led to improvements in her/his ability to understand speech, whether it is via audition only or auditory-visually. Systematic evaluation can also highlight areas of concern for individual clients and help determine (a) whether further training is warranted and (b) the direction it should take. For example, many clients report that they have great difficulty with longer sentences. The use of a test such as the CUNY Sentence Lists (Boothroyd et al., 1985), which contains sentences of varying lengths, may verify whether this is a problem, and indicate future training directions.

The materials used for this evaluation should vary from client to client, and be of an appropriate level of difficulty so as to avoid possible floor and ceiling effects. The level of difficulty may also need to be varied depending upon the presentation mode. For example, some clients may be able to cope with complex materials when they are presented auditory-visually, but may require materials at a considerably lower level when they are presented via audition only, or in the presence of competing noise. In my clinical work I prefer in most cases to start with simpler materials and introduce more complex measures if the client's performance warrants it. The test battery I use includes both word and sentence materials and can involve both closed-set and open-set materials. The test materials used include a selection of the following measures:

## Word tests

1. Closed sets of words that vary in their syllabic number and/or type. For example, a test list can contrast sets of monosyllables, spondees (two-syllable words with equal stress on both syllables – football, rainbow etc.), trochees (two-syllable words with primary stress on the first syllable and weak stress on the second – table, rabbit ctc.) and trisyllables (three-syllable words with varying stress patterns – typewriter, paperback etc.). The client is provided with a list of alternatives and has to indicate which was presented as the stimulus. The client can be scored for the number of words correctly identified, as well as for the number of words correctly categorized by their syllabic structure.
2. Closed sets of spondaic words.
3. Closed sets of words that contrast selected consonants or vowels in meaningful words. The newly revised 'Analytika' (Plant, 1994) contains over 600 lists that can be used for this type of testing.
4. Open-set lists of monosyllabic words. There are numerous lists to choose from, and the tests I use currently include the Dahl CVC Word Lists (Plant, 2001b), which consist of words drawn from the 500 most frequently occurring words in spoken American English (Dahl, 1979), and High Frequency Word Lists (Plant, 2001b), which present words consisting of only voiceless consonants and vowels and diphthongs with high second formant frequencies. Clients are scored for the number of words correctly identified and also for the recognition of initial consonants, vowels and final consonants.

## Sentence tests

1. Closed sets of sentences. The client is shown a list of sentences and has to select which one is presented as the stimulus.
2. The HELEN Test (Plant et al., 1982). This test consists of lists of 20 simple questions that require a one-word answer.
3. The BKB Sentences (Bench and Bamford, 1979). Although originally designed for use with hard-of-hearing children, these lists are also suitable for evaluating some adult clients.
4. The Dahl 500 Sentence Lists (Plant, 2001b). These lists of sentences consist only of words from the 500 most frequently occurring words of spoken American English (Dahl, 1979).
5. The CUNY Sentence Lists. Each list contains 12 sentences, ranging in length from 3 to 14 words.

## Speech tracking

Speech tracking is another measure that can be used to evaluate a client's performance over time. It is important to remember, however, that the same speaker should be used for pre- and post-training testing, as speaker characteristics can potentially influence a client's tracking rate (Tye-Murray and Tyler, 1988).

### Self-assessment

Another potentially useful means of evaluating a client's performance is to have her/him rate her/his performance in a variety of situations pre- and post-training. There are a number of scales, originally developed for assessing benefit from hearing aids, which could be adapted for use with adults with cochlear implants. These include the Cox and Alexander's (1995) Abbreviated Profile of Hearing Aid Benefit (APHAB), which assesses aided and unaided performance, and the considerably longer Hearing Performance Inventory (Giolas et al., 1979).

Another potential approach is that adopted in the Dillon et al. (1997) Client Oriented Scale of Improvement (COSI). In this measure, the clinician and client specify important situations in which the client 'would like to hear more clearly' at the initial interview (Dillon, 2001, p. 361). At the completion of the rehabilitation process, the client is asked '(a) how much more clearly they now hear in that situation, and (b) how well they hear in that situation' (Dillon, 2001, p. 361). This approach has the advantage of assessing the listening situations that the client rates as being of importance and may provide useful insights into the client's performance in everyday life.

## Conclusion

Although cochlear implants have provided great benefit for many adults with acquired losses, there still exists a need for aural rehabilitation training to ensure that implanted adults derive optimal benefit from their devices. The type of training adopted should be determined by the client's specific needs and concerns, and should take account of her/his familial, social and vocational situation. There is also a need for the systematic evaluation of the programs and procedures adopted to ensure that they are meeting the specific needs of individual clients. Over time, such evaluations should result in the provision of more appropriate programs and materials for use with adults with cochlear implants.

## References

Alcantara JI, Cowan RSC, Blamey PJ et al. (1990) A comparison of two training strategies for speech recognition with an electrotactile speech processor. Journal of Speech and Hearing Research 33: 195–204.

Bench J, Bamford J (eds) (1979) Speech-Hearing Tests and the Spoken Language of Hearing-Impaired Children. London: Academic Press.

Boothroyd A, Hanin L, Hnath T (1985) A sentence test of speech perception: reliability, set equivalence and short-term learning. Internal Report No. RC 110, City University of New York Speech and Hearing Sciences Research Center.

Cox R, Alexander G (1995) The abbreviated profile of hearing aid benefit. Ear and Hearing 16: 176–86.

Dahl H (1979) Word Frequencies of Spoken American English. Essex, CT: Verbatim.

Dillon H (2001) Hearing Aids. Sydney: Boomerang Press.

Dillon H, James A, Ginis J (1997) Client Oriented Scale of Improvement (COSI) and its relationship to several other measures of benefit and satisfaction provided by hearing aids. Journal of the American Academy of Audiology 8: 27–43.

De Filippo CL, Scott BL (1978) A method for training and evaluating the reception of ongoing speech. Journal of the Acoustical Society of America 63: 1186–92.

Giolas T, Owens E, Lamb S et al. (1979) Hearing Performance Inventory. Journal of Speech and Hearing Disorders 44: 169–95.

Gnosspelius J, Spens K-E (1992) A computer-based speech tracking procedure. STL-QPSR (The Speech Transmission Laboratory – Quarterly Progress and Status Report), Royal Institute of Technology (KTH), Stockholm, Sweden, 1/1992, 131–7.

Hagerman B (1982) Sentences for testing speech intelligibility in noise. Scandinavian Audiology 11: 79–87.

Hogan A (2001) Hearing Rehabilitation for Deafened Adults: A Psychosocial Approach. London: Whurr.

Picheny MA, Durlach NI, Braida LD (1985) Speaking clearly for the hard of hearing. I: intelligibility differences between clear and conversational speech. Journal of Speech and Hearing Research 28: 96–103.

Plant G (1989) COMMTRAC: Modified Connected Discourse Tracking Exercises for Hearing Impaired Adults. Chatswood, NSW: National Acoustic Laboratories.

Plant G (1994) Analytika: Analytic Testing and Training Lists (revised 2004). Somerville, MA: The Hearing Rehabilitation Foundation.

Plant G (1996) COMMTRAC: Speech Tracking Exercises for Hearing Impaired Adults (revised edn). Somerville, MA: The Hearing Rehabilitation Foundation.

Plant G (2001a) AUDITRAIN: An Auditory and Auditory-Visual Training Program. Innsbruck: Med-El.

Plant G (2001b) Speech Stuff: Speech Testing and Training Resources for Teenagers and Young Adults. Somerville, MA: The Hearing Rehabilitation Foundation.

Plant G (2002a) SpeechTrax. Innsbruck: Med-El.

Plant G (2002b) Syntrain: Synthetic Training Exercises for People with Hearing Loss. Innsbruck: Med-El.

Plant G, Phillips D, Tsembis J (1982) An auditory-visual speech test for the elderly hearing-impaired. Australian Journal of Audiology 4: 62–8.

Rubinstein A, Boothroyd A (1987) Effects of two approaches to auditory training on speech recognition by hearing-impaired adults. Journal of Speech and Hearing Research 30: 153–60.

Sanders D (1971) Aural Rehabilitation. Englewood Cliffs, NJ: Prentice-Hall.

Spens K-E (1992) Numerical aspects of the speech tracking procedure. STL-QPSR (The Speech Transmission Laboratory – Quarterly Progress and Status Report), Royal Institute of Technology (KTH), Stockholm, Sweden, 1/1992, 115–30.

Tye-Murray N, Tyler R (1988) A critique of continuous discourse tracking as a test procedure. Journal of Speech and Hearing Disorders 53: 226–31.

Walden BE, Erdman SA, Montgomery AA et al. (1981) Some effects of training on speech recognition by hearing-impaired adults. Journal of Speech and Hearing Disorders 24: 207–16.

Wayner DS, Abrahamson JE (1998) Learning to Hear Again with a Cochlear Implant. Austin, TX: Hear Again.

CHAPTER 14
# Paediatric habilitation

ELIZABETH TYSZKIEWICZ AND JACQUELINE STOKES

## Introduction

Implant centres and education services allocate extensive resources to supporting the child and family both before and after the fitting of an implant system. This support occurs in a range of environments, involves a variety of approaches and is delivered throughout childhood. This implies a consensus regarding the need for services above and beyond the simple fitting of the implant equipment or hearing aids. In this chapter, rather than attempt to describe the array of services around the UK, we explore the reasons underlying the need for habilitation and attempt to identify characteristics of good practice.

## Why intervene?

As can be seen from the wealth of information contained in other chapters in this volume, cochlear implants are an impressive technology, which can give a person who is profoundly deaf access to all the sounds of speech. Why, then, do we continue to talk about 'habilitation'? Habilitation may be defined as 'the process by which professionals support a child and family in adapting to hearing loss, getting used to a hearing device and developing the child's language and communication skills' (Edwards and Tyszkiewicz, 1999). Is it not sufficient simply to ensure that the technology is optimally fitted, early in the child's life, and treat our young implant users exactly as we treat their peers with normal hearing? It appears intuitively correct to say that, once the sensory input (hearing) has been restored, the human brain, with its powers of adaptation and information processing, will do the rest.

Observation and evidence, on the other hand, show that this is not the case. The young implant user's experience is 'abnormal' in a number of significant ways, and habilitation seeks to redress this through an enhanced version of normal experience. Factors to be taken into account are:

1. Implants are routinely monaural in the UK, for a number of reasons, and the child will therefore have either a monaural listening experience or a significantly less comprehensive signal from a hearing aid in the non-implant ear.
2. An implant system cannot be worn for a full 24 hours, so the child's total 'listening time' in a day is significantly reduced compared to his hearing peers. The device must be removed when sleeping, bathing, swimming etc.
3. The child does not benefit from the efficiency that normally hearing ears provide when listening in noise, or at a distance, which means reduced opportunities for incidental learning through overhearing.
4. A paediatric cochlear implant user is usually making a late start in the acquisition of auditory processing, or returning to auditory learning after a significant trauma (such as in the case of deafness caused by meningitis). Learning begins after a period of sensory deprivation, in which the brain has had limited opportunities to establish processing for auditory input. As Carol Flexer says:

> Auditory stimulation is necessary for the development of critical auditory brain centres.
>
> Flexer, 1999

Young children are highly reliant on a strong interactive framework in the early stages of language learning. The social interactionist theory of language acquisition assumes that learning is:

> A product of the child's early social interactions with the important people in his life [...] the child communicates and interacts socially with other people before he is able to produce language forms [...] the child's attempts to communicate and socialize prompt his parents and other caregivers to provide the language appropriate for these exchanges.
>
> Hulit and Howard, 1997

The young implant user is likely to have received less benefit from this early stimulation as a result of poor access to sound. Many of the child behaviours that provoke adult communicative input are triggered by the child's auditory responses to voice or to sound in his environment. An infant with profound hearing impairment does not, for example, turn to the sound of someone entering the room or of a dog barking, each of which would cause the adult carer to provide verbal input and interaction. The child starts his listening life with a lower level of competence in the basics of communicative interaction, such as the taking of verbal turns or joint attention to an object of interest. Habilitative programmes can only be effective if they address this need, as an integral part of the child's early auditory development.

Children also become implant users at a range of ages and stages. Habilit-ation programmes must be highly individualized, and of excellent quality, in order to allow each child to fulfil the excellent potential represented by an optimally fitted implant system. The other elements in the equation are the child as eager learner and the support of his family. With the expanding referral criteria for implants, a young implant user may be an infant, a child or a teenager. Each of these paediatric patients starts out with a highly indi-vidual history of hearing loss and previous auditory development.

Although cochlear implants are recognized as an increasingly sophisti-cated and effective aid to sound perception, all studies of user outcome show a wide spread of results in speech perception, spoken language development, educational achievement and user satisfaction. The implant fits into a complex habilitative framework, in which a range of variables affects the results of intervention. Some correlations are well documented, such as duration of deafness (Waltzman and Cohen, 1998; Kirk et al., 2002) or communicative environment (Osberger et al., 2000). Other variables cannot be measured as reliably, but have a bearing on any child's learning: level of ability and motivation, presence of other sensory or cognitive dif-ficulties, family and social environment etc.

Children who have severe to profound hearing impairment are some-what more at risk, as a group, of additional difficulties that affect learning (Condon, 1991). The goal of post-implant intervention is to establish the optimal programme for the individual, and constantly review expecta-tions to ensure that each implant user's full auditory potential is achieved.

**Good practice**

The cochlear implant technology described elsewhere in this book has impressive potential to provide access to sound, and therefore to spoken communication, and participation in mainstream society. We acknowl-edge that intervention, or 'habilitation', is required to optimize this benefit for the wide range of users in the paediatric population. The next area for discussion is, therefore: what are the elements of good practice?

# Mastery of the technology

Unlike adult users with previous hearing experience, young children starting out with their cochlear implant systems have no point of com-parison to enable them to judge the quality of the signal they are receiving. They are totally dependent on the adults around them to main-tain, troubleshoot and monitor their equipment.

More than that, it is vital for the adults to know what the child can be expected to hear using the device. They may not know immediately from the child's responses what he does hear, but must have a strong and confident understanding of the potential of a correctly fitted and mapped cochlear implant device: the child should be able to hear quiet speech sounds across the frequency range. If the appropriate electrical stimulation is present, these responses will emerge shortly after activation of the device. It becomes possible to teach the child appropriate reactions to auditory signals in his environment (e.g. when someone knocks, we need to turn and look at the door) and to set up tasks which confirm that sound detection is occurring (e.g. a conditioned response to a speech stimulus). Really effective habilitation involves training the adults around the child to be knowledgeable about what to expect. They become skilled observers of emerging auditory behaviours, and promoters of auditory learning. Habilitationists need to do more than assert that the child is progressing in his auditory skills. They must also ensure that carers are independent assessors of their child's responses, aware of auditory behaviours such as stilling (stopping body and eye movement briefly in response to a stimulus), turning, imitating sound or understanding through audition without additional cues.

Most cochlear implant equipment is relatively robust and stable, but glitches in electronic devices can occur anywhere and at any time. This has considerable implications for the technical and clinical 'after sales' support provided by cochlear implant centres. The vigilant monitoring of equipment function and a constant effort to optimize its performance are the foundations of all habilitation. Such monitoring implies a range of activities, from daily checking of the child's reception of sound (see emerging auditory behaviours, above) to the provision of excellent, rapid spares and repairs services and, of course, a high standard of programming and clinical care. Time spent using less-than-optimal equipment is wasted learning time and will have a negative impact on the outcome for the child. People throughout his environment need to have the confidence and knowledge to support his use of the technology. This creates the need for a network of good communication, involving families, clinical centres, implant manufacturers, education and therapy services, community audiology clinics, health visitors, nursery nurses and others. There is an encouraging variety of creative solutions in the UK to address the problems presented by round-the-clock maintenance, such as websites with question-and-answer services, back-up packs provided at a small cost for families on holiday or training for school staff in troubleshooting.

Like all technology, implants are developing and changing very fast. Information has to be constantly updated and disseminated, and further training provided. A child who grows up with optimally functioning equipment will be best able to make independent judgements of sound quality, and to take responsibility for his own use of technology.

# A foundation in normal developmental processes

If a child requires such planned, intensive input, is it not better to place him in a specialized setting to be taught by experts? This is a reasonable assumption to make, given the tremendous task faced by a new implant user. However, it must be challenged because we know that in many cases an implant provides real potential for the child to be educated alongside his hearing peers.

> Listening is not a mechanical decoding skill. It is a complex and problematic aspect of communication and thinking [...] Listening is thinking; as we listen we make all kinds of judgements and choices.
>
> Haynes, 2002

In fact, the greatest challenge is to ensure that the habilitation programme has its roots deeply embedded in our knowledge of the role played by audition in typical, normally hearing development. The child has undergone a period of sensory deprivation and the purpose of habilitation following cochlear implantation is to trigger the developmental processes arrested by the hearing loss. The first step is to capture the child's auditory attention and enable him to make the link between the sound and its meaning. For example, the child understands that a knock on the door means someone is there.

The habilitation programme then aims to move the child rapidly through the language learning process of the child with intact hearing. This implies a proactive habilitative approach where the adults purposefully attempt to teach the child what to listen for. Otherwise, the cochlear implant merely increases the quantity and volume of sound the child hears, and learning is likely to remain random and unfocused. Carol Flexer makes a distinction between the development of specific listening skills through learning and practice that leads to proficiency, and the learning acquired through general experience. She compares the listening skills of a trained ornithologist, who can differentiate the calls of many birds, to the rest of us, who, while able to hear the bird song, can identify very few.

> The goal in teaching listening skills to children who have hearing problems is to make them as proficient listeners as possible.
>
> Flexer, 1999

Post-implant rehabilitation programmes in the UK frequently follow a prescribed hierarchy of 'listening' exercises. These involve, for example, contrasts between musical instruments, forced-choice discrimination between long and short speech sounds or the type of exercise in which a child moves the train in response to 'choo choo' or the car in response to 'beep' (Archbold and Tait, 2003). These tasks do not fit readily into a framework based on normal development. The goal of habilitation, rather, is to develop the language learning process by providing highly enhanced auditory input within a strong communicative framework. A simple rule of thumb to evaluate the helpfulness of a proposed activity is to ask whether a hearing child of the same age or stage would benefit from doing it in order to learn to communicate. It is also a concern that many auditory training activities imply a very low expectation of both the implant and the child's ability to use it. Expecting a child to throw a bean bag at a picture of a triangle when he hears it struck, or at a picture of a drum in response to the drum-beat, has no musical or speech discrimination value. Sometimes, such material is used even in cases where parents already report the child responding correctly to the phone and the doorbell at home.

Historically, exercises with low functional value such as these have been recommended for many young implant users. They are derived from adult auditory training, where the tasks are designed to help the deafened adult associate the new sound sensation from the implant with his already well-established language knowledge (Tye-Murray, 1997). When adapted for use with children, they become further reduced and devoid of linguistic content because the child has limited linguistic knowledge. This leads to exercises such as long versus short discrimination, which many children and parents find frustrating and meaningless. A habilitation approach based on this model has a tenuous link to our model for children's auditory development based on normal processes of spoken language acquisition. If we agree that effective intervention enhances 'normal' processes, rather than replacing them, this type of exercise is unlikely to be included, since it has no equivalent in the experience of a typically developing child. Those children who have had a successful outcome from this type of habilitation are likely to be accessing intensive auditory and spoken language stimulation in their homes and schools in any case. A revised view of the priorities in paediatric habilitation may offer those children who are less successful the opportunity to fulfil more of their potential as implant users.

Implicit in a proactive habilitation approach is the recognition that effort is a positive aspect of learning (Vygotsky, 1978). In the presence of a disability it is sometimes hard to see a child's struggle in this positive light. The tendency is to help the child meet his needs without effort because we judge the challenge to be too great for him. For example, the adult might give the child with hearing impairment a sign or a lipreading cue to help him understand what is said. In doing so, the adult saves the child from having to expend effort to make use of his new-found auditory sense to solve the communication problem. This eliminates the need to learn to make meaningful use of audition, and a habilitative opportunity is wasted.

There are potentially helpful parallels with other developmental processes facilitated by parents, such as a child learning to crawl. The adult puts the child on the floor because he needs to learn to crawl and he will not learn this skill in his baby seat. The parent believes that he will learn to crawl, that he will need plenty of opportunities and that he does not need to be protected from having to try. The parent recognizes his motivation to crawl, sees his effort and knows that his drive to get about will enable him to achieve it. Through habilitation, this same learning process is nurtured in the beginning listener. The child's expenditure of effort is the outward evidence of his desire to communicate, and his reward is 'solving the problem'. This effort to learn goes on throughout all aspects of normal development in children and continues into adulthood. Further reading of Vygotsky and other theorists shows that this does not, of course, mean that the child with a new implant device is to be 'thrown in at the deep end' and left to puzzle out alone the meaning of the environmental sounds and speech he hears.

> Children, even quite young ones, will not let themselves be passively led. They will actively invent and discover, using what we tell them as a starting point. But we must try not to hinder them by putting them down at starting points from which the road is unnecessarily long and hard.
>
> Donaldson, 1983

As Donaldson points out, the second key aspect associated with the benefit of allowing learners to expend effort is ensuring the size of the challenge is not too great. Goals must lie within the area of the child's capability and understanding, with the help of the more knowledgeable adults. A child will not crawl before he can sit, and the beginning auditory learner also needs adult carers who have a sound working knowledge of the successive stages he needs to reach in order to achieve competence in the use of his device for communication.

Take the example of James who is aged three, with one year's implant use. He can hold his own in a conversation about a familiar topic in a one-to-one setting with a friendly adult.

What skills has James yet to acquire, and how do they fit into the developmental sequence? This information, which will indicate what needs to be worked on next, is examined with reference to the typical three-year-old, bearing in mind James' hearing age is one year. The professionals who deliver habilitation to him and to his family identify his next goals and work to structure and support his learning. This requires the gathering of detailed information in at least the following areas: the length of utterance James understands and uses, his repair skills, his ability to communicate with other children, the type and complexity of questions he uses and understands and how he manages in noise. When the information is available, learning goals are set and then broken down into manageable steps. Adults who understand the underlying structure support the child in achieving them.

For example, when sharing a story such as 'The Three Little Pigs', James may understand the plot line but is unable to express how events are linked to each other. A number of specific sentence structures are targeted, with the adult providing the first part of the utterance and allowing the child to complete it: 'The pig is scared because ...' 'The wolf blows down the house so that ...' This tactic is discussed and rehearsed with the child's parents, and opportunities for further practice in the home environment are identified. The technique is explained, and its links to auditory recall, verbal reasoning and expressive language are clarified. Once this skill is acquired, the next step will be for the child to generate the whole utterance himself. Carers need to know that this is 'where they are headed', so that specific goals always fit into a framework, which is made explicit to them.

As this example illustrates, the cochlear implant is intricately involved in a complex developmental process of language acquisition. Rather than creating a need for separate, specific 'listening exercises', it is a tool to enable spoken language development to occur within the strong social context seen in normal language acquisition.

## Authoritative and accurate baseline assessment

If it is acknowledged that habilitation is closely attuned to the cognitive, social and communicative development of each child, it follows that there cannot be a 'cookbook' containing a set of procedures suited to all new implant users, nor indeed the same starting point.

Estabrooks, 1998

Baseline measures need to be easily obtained and intelligible to all those who have a stake in the child's programme. They are the first pointer to the child's individual goals.

Which assessments, then, provide the guidelines for planning effective post-implant habilitation programmes for a population of young cochlear implant users who are diverse in their age, ability, development, social environment and pre-implant experience? The logical choice, given the assumptions we are working under, is norm-referenced assessments of spoken language development. In the UK, we are fortunate in having access to a choice of assessments of communicative development, with norms obtained from large numbers of English-speaking children (e.g. MacArthur Communicative Development Inventories, Pre-School Language Scale, Pre-School CELF (Wiig et al., 1992)). Some US material is available in British versions, and there is some interesting material from this side of the Atlantic, particularly at more advanced levels of language use (e.g. Assessment of Comprehension and Expression, 6–11 (Adams et al., 2001)). Communicative competence, which provides the framework within which the language is used, is assessed with reference to typical development through structured observation and the recording of age-appropriate communicative behaviours (e.g. Pragmatics Profile) and of play development, which is a strong indicator of cognitive and communicative level. Margaret Donaldson expresses this link as follows:

A child's ability to learn language is indeed something at which we may wonder. But his language-learning skills are not isolated from the rest of his mental growth. There is no reason to suppose that he is born with an 'acquisition device' which enables him to structure and make sense of the language he hears while failing to structure and make sense of the other features in his environment. On the contrary it now looks as though he first makes sense of situations (and perhaps especially those involving human intention) and then uses *this* kind of understanding to help him make sense of what is said to him.

Donaldson, 1983

This reminds us, yet again, that assessments and/or interventions that are embedded in a normal developmental framework are of most use both in evaluating progress and in setting goals.

Young implant users are routinely assessed as to their auditory detection levels, speech perception, speech production, language, cognition including play, social communication skills and educational attainment. To be of benefit to post-implant habilitation, relevant assessments need to be administered in a way that is effective and time-efficient. In addition, children who are implant users undergo assessment in many different settings, with the potential for duplication and poor dissemination of results, which then cannot usefully be incorporated into the child's programme.

There is a range of reasons for collecting information through assessment: to inform planning for the child, to diagnose a particular difficulty (e.g. oro-motor assessment when speech production presents difficulties), to measure progress and to collect research data. A child can spend a high proportion of his contact hours with specialist professionals being assessed, without a coherent plan of action necessarily emerging from the process.

The test battery administered to young implant users is often an amalgamation of assessments selected by the different professionals in the implant team. As a result, a standard report may represent many hours undergone by the child and family yielding a relatively small amount of information that is relevant to the habilitation programme. If data is being collected for research purposes, it is of course an ethical requirement that this is kept separate from clinically relevant assessments, and that the child and family's informed consent is obtained.

The topic here, however, is assessment directly relevant to habilitation, measuring what the implant is enabling the child to do, and what the next steps are. Clinicians use assessment to establish a baseline for intervention and the planning of habilitation. Service users (children and their families) and support professionals will benefit most from assessment if they know what the testing is for, and what information it contains to point to the next stage of development and aid in setting targets (Dyson, 1987). Children are most likely to be compliant, and to give accurate responses, if assessment is planned, purposeful and time-efficient.

In establishing a habilitation baseline, the following areas are assessed: audition, play and cognition, and communicative competence. The three-year-old child who has sharp auditory responses, immature symbolic play and few single words will have a very different habilitation plan from a child who has poor auditory responses but more age-appropriate play and communicative competence. Every child has a characteristic profile, which may change at different assessment points. The goal of habilitation is to bring each area within normal limits if the child has that potential, and this shapes his individual programme.

An effective assessment battery usually includes both norm- and criterion-referenced material and attempts wherever possible to use tests suitable for the chronological age bracket the child falls into. In addition, well-documented, structured observation by parents and professionals is a vital complement to formal evaluation.

A framework for the initial evaluation of a two-year-old beginning implant user might typically comprise:

*Auditory awareness*
Parental report and structured co-observation in deliberately contrived situations

*Speech perception*
Ling test of auditory perception and production (Ling, 2002)

*Linguistic knowledge*
MacArthur CDI (Fenson et al., 1993)
Pre-School Language Scale (PLS) (Zimmerman et al., 1997)

*Social communication skills*
Pragmatics profile (Dewart and Summers, 1995)

*Play/cognition*
Symbolic Play Test (Lowe and Costello, 1988)

These measures provide a baseline that directly informs habilitation planning. They need to be repeated at six-monthly intervals and the plan adjusted accordingly.

Since habilitation workers are in regular contact with young implant users, assessment results may be accumulated over a number of sessions until a complete picture emerges.

To be really effective, the plan and the progress reports must be disseminated to relevant adults across all the environments in which the child finds himself, starting with his parents. An enormous amount of energy, expertise and hard work can go into producing abundant paperwork about the young implant user as a result of over-assessment and somewhat unfocused assessment batteries. This hard work could be of immense benefit were it to be redirected into targeted assessment, followed by goal setting and implementation.

It cannot be stressed sufficiently that, while the formal information described above is extremely important in habilitation planning, it is always supplemented by informal observations of the child's functioning in a range of settings. The protocol for presenting items in a norm-referenced test is restrictive. Formal language assessments like the Pre-School Language Scale (Zimmerman et al., 1997) require set formulations, without repetitions, and may not allow the child to display his full ability. Observation and reporting, when they are accurate and well structured, are valuable elements within the assessment battery.

Reported information and observation must, however, refer to a clear framework to avoid inaccuracy and lack of relevant information. This is evident in such statements as:

'He is starting to know the difference between speech and non-speech stimuli such as music.'

'He gave some lovely responses to a variety of presentations across the speech frequency range.'

Cochlear implant centre report, 2003

In order for the above to be usable observations, supporting evidence needs to be recorded. Valid observation looks for repeatable behaviours and is consistent between observers. It is different from general impressions or opinions, and is a reliable tool for planning.

## The child's family

For typically developing children, parents and other closely involved carers are the principal source of language stimulation in the early years. All speakers develop their initial communication skills within the family and this is generally recognized as both appropriate and effective, with very little outside intervention being necessary. In the case of a hearing impairment the situation alters somewhat and other adults will become involved. It is vitally important that the child's parents remain firmly at the centre of both decisions and processes.

Many parents faced with the daunting prospect of trying to 'close the gap' between a young implant user's chronological age and communication ability feel an understandable desire to place their children in the hands of 'experts'. There is increasing evidence that children who are hearing aid or implant users from a young age, and are well supported, can access mainstream education (Archbold et al., 2002). However, the reality seems very different when a child's communication ability is mismatched with the demands of the educational environment. It may seem safer and even more effective to place the child in a specialized environment where there is established expertise in the support of young children who are 'deaf'. Parents and extended families are increasingly recognized as the primary source of learning for the developing child, regardless of disability. Habilitation support must do more than merely acknowledge the importance of the parent/carer. It should enable and inspire that person to experience both the effort and the satisfaction of being the main agent of their child's progress.

Intervention that helps parents enjoy their infants and that strengthens parental sensitivity, responsiveness, and skill creates a parent–child system in which the parent experiences success and the infant progresses to his maximum potential.

Bromwich, 1978

The prevailing philosophy in the UK favours what may be described as generalized support rather than direct intervention. It encourages parenting behaviours that are as close as possible to what would occur in the absence of a disability. Thus parents are advised to behave and talk 'naturally' to their child with hearing impairment. If we accept that there is a 'natural' way to talk to a three-year-old, for example, we can then examine some of the features of that conversation. These are as follows: there is satisfying communication occurring for both participants, there is a shared topic known to both participants, each participant adds new information and, if there is a breakdown in communication, both will have a means of clarifying the situation. When there is a mismatch between a child's chronological age and his level of communicative competence, as is frequently the case with a young implant user, many of these features are missing in the child's contribution to the conversation. The parent talking 'normally' realizes that the conversation is not progressing and feels dissatisfied. Parents know that talking to a three-year-old with a hearing impairment and delayed communicative competence is not 'natural' and requires much more conscious effort on their part. The experience of parenting a young implant user is necessarily different from that which the parent may have had with the child's hearing siblings. The need for intervention could not be illustrated more clearly than by this comment from a mother of two children, one of whom has a profound hearing impairment:

Watching my second (normally hearing) two-year-old son learn to speak, I have living proof every day that the naturalness in communicating with a hearing child is purely the result of his hearing, not of myself 'being natural'. They just trigger the responses in the mother. And I find myself triggered thus all day long by my youngest and I listen with amazement that he freely repeats every new word he hears.

Parent, personal communication 2002

Many new implant users have previously well-established communication strategies using non-verbal means. A child who comes to implant use with good lipreading skills could improve measurably and become an excellent lipreader without using anything like the full potential of the implant. It is sometimes argued that relying on lipreading and not developing the child's listening potential does not matter, as long as the child is learning to talk. On the other hand, lipreading does not enable the child to speak on the phone, listen to music, hear his mother comforting him from another room or know what the teacher in the hall is saying. For many paediatric users, the implant does have the potential to enable these and other goals to be achieved.

Inevitably, there are some patients for whom the implant cannot work to its full potential. This may be attributable to physiological factors (poor neural survival or ossified cochlea) or factors related to learning (auditory processing or language difficulties) which limit benefit. Starting out in a well-structured auditory programme that has clearly defined goals gives such users the best chance of having their specific needs identified. Adaptations can then be made to the habilitation based on documented evidence, including the use of sign language, and input from other specialist professionals such as occupational therapists. As Robbins (2000) puts it, 'The child will move along a continuum to become as auditory as is possible for him or her.'

In addition, a number of young implant users' families make an informed choice to educate them in an environment that includes both speech and sign language. Research indicates clearly that strong spoken language input results in the most favourable spoken language outcomes (Osberger et al., 2000), but some families and educators accept this limitation as a necessary consequence of wishing to incorporate sign into their communication.

In the early stages of implant use, the child needs to discover that sound has meaning and provides valuable, useful information. The challenge for the parent is to make the new meaningless sensory input over-ride the already well-established processing on other modalities. It is an understandable, but mistaken, assumption that fitting a device as sophisticated as a cochlear implant while a child is very young will bring auditory development back in line with the norm. The two-year-old hearing child has a highly tuned auditory system that has been in use since birth and has already stored a rich database. The two-year-old new implant user has a very different starting position, with little of this knowledge in place. At a point between these two are those children who change over from being effective hearing aid users to using an implant, whose rate of learning often demonstrates the benefits of their previous listening experience. They have many of the auditory processing abilities they need already in place and because of this can more easily take on board the new information provided by the implant. The better established the child's auditory processing system is, the easier it is for him to receive and interpret new information.

For every child, the starting point needs to be established using appropriate assessment, and this information needs to be shared with the parents. Once parents have a good understanding of what to work towards, the habilitation programme needs to provide them with the means to do so, through specific practical guidance and access to the theoretical information that underpins it.

For example, a beginning listener aged ten months shows enjoyment and interest in perceiving through audition the sound 'aaaaaah' associated with a toy aeroplane. After many models from therapist and parents, and plenty of silent pauses, the child takes the aeroplane and imitates action and sound. Although fun and satisfying in the short term, this episode in isolation will be of no lasting benefit to the child and family unless it is underpinned by the background information. Intuitively, 'aaaah' is not the sound associated with planes for English-speaking children, but it is chosen deliberately for its audibility (high intensity, mid-frequency), duration (longer presentations give the beginning listener the time needed to process a sound) and ease of production (the child need only vocalize with open mouth to imitate the sound accurately). The association of a sound with a particular object is the precursor to labelling objects with their names, and the opportunity to imitate establishes auditory feedback (imitating what you have heard). This background information, together with the successful episode involving the child, is distilled for the parents into a set of 'take-home messages' which incorporate all this information:

- My child needs simple, meaningful, easy-to-hear sounds which catch his auditory attention.
- My child needs time to think and process.
- My child hears and can imitate speech sounds and therefore, in due course, words.
- My child can learn to 'label' an object with the appropriate word, and sound–object associations such as 'aaaah' for aeroplane are the first step towards this goal.

These messages and their underlying principles enable the child's parents and other carers to present information to him in a way that maximizes the learning potential of their everyday activities. The habilitation programme steadily builds up the parents' background knowledge and provides them with ideas and examples for putting it into practice in their individual situations and with their particular child. Clearly, within this model of practice, there cannot be a hierarchy of goals and achievements that are applicable to every young implant user. Skilled and knowledgeable professionals are required to co-work closely with families, devising programmes suited to their individual needs and making knowledge accessible to those closest to the child.

A model of support in which parents, who are the most important adults in the child's life, and professionals, who are knowledgeable about the disability, work closely towards shared goals is very appealing in theory. It is often challenging to achieve in practice.

In a laudable effort to be flexible and accommodating, input from professionals can become so non-directive that it leaves the family confused as to what the programme and targets actually are. On the other hand, as discussed in the preceding paragraph, there is unlikely to be much benefit from a set of specific auditory exercises without the relevant individualized coaching and support.

When the parent–professional partnership for post-implant habilitation is working well, there is joint planning, continual re-evaluation of progress, active problem solving and shared high expectations. Unsurprisingly, parents report a range of quality in services around the UK (Bamford et al., 2000; Robinshaw, 2001). Professionals are often aware of a mismatch between their agenda and the family's, and are uncertain as to how to resolve this conflict in the best interests of the child. There is a strong movement within support service provision towards the establishment of transparent, accountable practice in the field (ESPP project, Department for Education and Skills, 2004), with service users and providers consulting together to produce policies and materials.

## Conclusion

In due course, the very young implant user grows up and needs to have access to information and take responsibility for his use of the equipment. The purpose of the habilitation programme is, after all, to allow him to become a fully independent member of society. A twelve-year-old may need to attend a workshop where he can learn about the fitting, functioning and reasons for the implant he had fitted as a toddler. A seven-year-old may develop an interest in using the telephone and require training and support to achieve this with his family. A student setting off to college may benefit from information about listening tactics and assistive devices to ensure he gains maximum benefit from his new learning environment. In all cases, the device is the means to an end, and habilitation maps out the route. A generation of children is growing up who demonstrate what can be achieved with excellent technology, in conjunction with a family and educational environment, which provide a solid framework for auditory learning.

## References

Adams C, Coke R, Crutchley A et al. (2001) Assessment of comprehension and expression 6–11. Windsor: NFER Nelson.

Archbold S, Nikolopoulos T, Lutman M et al. (2002) The educational settings of profoundly deaf children with cochlear implants compared with age-matched peers with hearing aids: implications for management. International Journal of Audiology 41(3): 157–61.

Archbold S, Tait M (2003) Facilitating progress after implantation. In: Cochlear Implants for Young Children, 2nd edn. London: Whurr.

Bamford J, Davis A, Hind S et al. (2000) Evidence on Very Early Service Delivery: What Parents Want and Don't Always Get. Chicago: Phonak AG.

Bromwich R (1978) Working with Parents and Infants, an Interactional Approach. Austin, TX: Pro-Ed.

Condon M-C (1991) Unique challenges, children with multiple handicaps. In JA Feigin, PG Stelmachowicz (eds), Pediatric Amplification, Omaha: Boys Town National Research Hospital.

Department for Education and Skills (2004) Developing Early Intervention and Support for Deaf Children and their Families (UK: www.espp.org.uk). London: DfES Publications.

Dewart H, Summers S (1995) Pragmatics Profile of Early Communication Skills. Windsor: NFER Nelson.

Donaldson M (1983) Children's Minds. London: Flamingo/Open University Press.

Dyson S (1987) Reasons for assessment: rhetoric and reality in the assessment of children with disabilities. In: T Booth, W Swann (eds), Including Pupils with Disabilities. Milton Keynes: Open University Press.

Edwards J, Tyszkiewicz E (1999) Cochlear implants. In J Stokes (ed.), Hearing Impaired Infants: Support in the First Eighteen Months. London: Whurr.

Estabrooks W (ed.) (1998) Cochlear Implants for Kids. Washington: AG Bell.

Fenson L, Dale PS, Reznick JS et al. (1993) The MacArthur Communicative Development Inventories. San Diego: Singular.

Flexer C (1999) Facilitating Hearing and Listening in Young Children. London: Singular.

Haynes J (2002) Children as Philosophers. London: Routledge Falmer.

Hulit LM, Howard MR (1997) Born to Talk: An Introduction to Speech and Language Development. Boston: Allyn and Bacon.

Kirk K, Miyamoto R, Lento C et al. (2002) Effects of age at implantation in young children. Annals of Otology, Rhinology and Laryngology 111: 102–8.

Ling D (2002) Speech and the Hearing Impaired Child: Theory and Practice, 2nd edn. Washington: AG Bell.

Lowe M, Costello A (1988) Symbolic Play Test, 2nd edn. Windsor: NFER Nelson.

Osberger MJ, Zimmerman-Phillips S, Fisher L (2000) Relationship between communication mode and implant performance in paediatric Clarion patients. In S Waltzman, N Cohen (eds), Cochlear Implants. New York: Thieme Medical.

Robbins AM (2000) Recommendations to implant teams. Loud and Clear 4(2). Valencia, CA: Advanced Bionics Corporation.

Robinshaw HM (2001) Service provision for pre-school children: parents' perspectives. Early Child Development and Care. 168: 63–93.

Tye-Murray N (1997) Communication training for older teenagers and adults: listening, speechreading and using conversation. Washington: AG Bell.

Vygotsky LS (1978) Mind in Society. Cambridge, MA: Harvard University Press.

Waltzman S, Cohen N (1998) Cochlear implantation in children younger than 2 years old. American Journal of Otology 19: 158–62.

Wiig EH, Secord W, Semel E (1992) CELF Preschool, Clinical Evaluation of Language Fundamentals – Preschool. London: The Psychological Corporation.

Zimmerman IL, Steiner VG, Pond EP, adapted for UK by J Boucher, V Lewis (1997), Pre-School Language Scale – 3 (UK). London: The Psychological Corporation.

# CHAPTER 15

# Soundfield hearing for patients with cochlear implants and hearing aids

RICHARD S. TYLER, CAMILLE C. DUNN, SHELLEY A. WITT, WILLIAM NOBLE, BRUCE J. GANTZ, JAY T. RUBINSTEIN, AARON J. PARKINSON AND STEVE C. BRANIN

## Introduction

There are several important issues that need to be discussed in order to fully understand and question the potential advantages associated with bilateral cochlear implants. Our approach in this chapter is to propose what we believe are the key questions involved in considering bilateral cochlear implantation.

## What are the likely mechanisms of binaural interactions?

Binaural hearing depends on the ability to process temporal, level and spectral information available at both ears. Both psychoacoustical and physiological models have evolved over the years (e.g. Yost, 1974; Zurek, 1993; Hartmann and Constan, 2002). Excellent reviews of the broader perspectives of spatial hearing, including the cocktail party effect, are also available (Cherry, 1953; Cherry and Sayers, 1959; Yost and Gourevitch, 1987; Yost and Guzman, 1996; Blauert, 1997; Gilkey and Anderson, 1997; Dubno et al., 2002; Plomp, 2002; Litovsky et al., 2004). In this chapter, we will discuss a few of the likely mechanisms associated with binaural hearing with cochlear implants and hearing aids.

### 1. Ignoring one of two ears

One advantage of binaural hearing is having the opportunity to choose which ear to attend to. To accomplish this, the brain receives input from both ears, locks onto the side with the better signal-to-noise ratio and inhibits the input from the side with the poorer ratio. This task is accomplished by a brain mechanism that attends to one ear while in the background monitoring the less clear side in case the optimal ear changes.

## 2. Listening when the information is the same at each ear

In some situations, the sound at both ears is exactly the same. For example, this might happen when listening to a talker who is directly in front of you either in a quiet environment or with background noise emanating from the same location as the talker. This could also happen when the talker and/or noise is directly behind the listener. In all of these situations, a 'front-back' confusion can occur. Spectral and level cues for predictable sources, and particularly visual cues, often help resolve this front-back confusion.

When information is the same at both ears, there is a binaural advantage often referred to as binaural summation. This occurs due to a brain mechanism that combines or sums the information from each ear to provide an overall increase in loudness of the signal. For example, the loudness of a soft sound would be greater when listening with two ears compared to one. Binaural summation typically refers to either an improvement in threshold (typically on the order of 3 dB for normal listeners) or a similar increase in loudness. Another way to think about the advantage of listening when the information is the same at each ear is that there are two versions of the same signal. Even though the information may be redundant, having redundant information can be useful in less-than-optimal listening situations.

To understand the mechanisms that might be responsible for these advantages, it is important to consider that, even when listening in quiet, there is inherent uncorrelated noise present in the auditory system on both sides. The mechanisms by which the same information from both sides is combined might involve:

- a better representation of the stimulus because it is coded twice;
- ongoing sampling of the stimulus on each side to take advantage of short term changes in signal-to-noise differences

## 3. Combining different information from each ear

In many realistic listening situations, the target (usually speech) or background noise is closer to one ear than the other. We have already discussed above how the brain might attend to information coming from one ear and not the other. But can the brain combine different information from both ears to improve performance? The answer is 'yes'. This is accomplished by neural interactions when either the noise or the signal is similar in both ears. It results in improved understanding over monaural listening.

Markides (1977) credits Koenig (1950) for coining the term 'squelching' to describe the boosting of the effective signal-to-noise ratio under binaural listening conditions. Masking level difference experiments, performed under earphones, highlight some of these squelch effects (e.g. Hirsch, 1948; Hall et al., 1984).

We have described the combination of different information between ears as a result of acoustic differences. However, results from different signal processing and/or different patterns of hair cell/neural survival across the two ears may also exist. When this happens, the brain must integrate the different information from each ear to provide a complete signal. Hearing aid algorithms were proposed decades ago in an attempt to divide the spectrum between ears (e.g. Franklin, 1981; Tyler, 1986a). Another example requiring such integration would be an individual with a low-frequency hearing loss in one ear and a high-frequency hearing loss in the other ear.

# What are the potential benefits of having two implants?

Bilateral cochlear implantation offers a number of potential advantages. In the following four tables we group these potential advantages into four categories: localization, speech perception, sound quality and a miscellaneous category.

### 1. Localization

Bilateral cochlear implants have the potential of improving localization, particularly in the horizontal plane. In contrast, vertical plane localization, which is dependent upon pinna-related cues, has not been strongly documented as a potential advantage of binaural hearing (e.g. Byrne and Noble, 1998) (see Table 15.1).

**Table 15.1** Benefits of horizontal plane localization

| Benefit | Description |
|---------|-------------|
| Sense of motion | Improvement in following a moving sound source |
| Talker location | Identification of a talker during a group conversation |
| Safety | Improvement in spatial awareness of one's acoustic environment |
| Auditory scene analysis | Segregation of different sound sources in the environment |
| Locating sound sources out of sight | Improvement in the ability to locate sounds behind you or in poor light conditions |

## 2. Speech perception

Binaural listening has shown improvements in speech understanding in quiet and in noise for normal-hearing individuals and bilateral hearing aid users (Koenig, 1950; Carhart et al., 1967; Day et al., 1988; Kaplan and Pickett, 1981; Zurek, 1993; Dillon, 2001). This same potential exists for bilateral cochlear implant recipients. It is assumed that low-level sounds should be more audible because of binaural summation. Although the gain control for a unilateral implant recipient can be adjusted to amplify quieter sounds, a binaural cochlear implant recipient has the potential to make use of a wider range of amplification due to a possible binaural summation effect. Studies suggest that loudness discomfort levels are not necessarily reduced by acoustic binaural hearing (Dillon, 2001); however, this deserves further study (see Table 15.2).

**Table 15.2** Benefits to speech perception

| Benefit | Description |
| --- | --- |
| Ignoring one of two ears | Attending to the ear directed away from a competing noise source |
| Listening when information is the same at each ear | Improvement in the sensitivity of softer sounds (e.g. consonant recognition), whispered speech or speech at a distance |
| Combining different information from each ear | Improvement of speech perception due to squelching of noise |

## 3. Qualitative advantages

There are also many potential qualitative advantages of binaural hearing (Table 15.3), including a more natural, balanced sound and an improved 'ease of listening' (Byrne, 1980; Balfour and Hawkins, 1992). Since most adult cochlear implant recipients are postlingually deafened, binaural

**Table 15.3** Benefits to sound quality

| Benefit | Description |
| --- | --- |
| Externalization | Perceiving sound as originating from its source, not from inside the head |
| Three-dimensional sound perception | Perceiving sounds within the relative location or distance that they occur, resulting in a more naturally sounding environment |
| Balanced sound | Perceiving sound that is equal across the two ears |
| Clearer | Sound appears sharper |
| Fuller | Sound is richer and complete |
| Ease of listening | Less effort is required to listen |

implantation provides an opportunity to return hearing status to something closer to what they were accustomed to, possibly resulting in a better quality of life.

### 4. Miscellaneous advantages

If hearing can be improved with two cochlear implants compared to one, this could lead to an increase in secondary benefits, such as better speech production or improved language development in children (Tyler et al., 1986). Table 15.4 identifies some of these additional potential advantages. One advantage of having two cochlear implants is the increased signal processing options. For example, with two cochlear implants you can selectively choose the most effective channels across ears or send different signals to each ear to try to maximize performance. These types of unique programming algorithms are not available when programming a single device. Stimulating both ears might also reduce auditory deprivation. When fitting binaural hearing-impaired patients with one hearing aid, further hearing loss can continue at a greater rate in the unaided ear (Silman et al., 1984; Neuman, 1996).

**Table 15.4** Potential miscellaneous benefits of bilateral cochlear implants

| Benefits | Description |
| --- | --- |
| More signal processing alternatives | More combined channels are available |
| | Signal processing strategies can be designed to complement ears |
| Prevention of neural atrophy | Stimulation can retard degeneration |
| Always having one working device if one fails | If one device breaks down, the other working device will prevent the user from not hearing any sound |

# Binaural hearing in the real world

Listening to sound in the everyday world requires the monitoring of multiple auditory streams of information (Noble, 1983; Bregman, 1990; Gatehouse and Noble, 2004). In any given period of time, from a few seconds to longer, one audible signal (or sometimes two) will be present in the foreground of a listener's experience (i.e. the item given primary attention). This signal could be a person speaking, music playing, an animal calling or an object, person or machine involved in some activity. In all cases, the signal or signals may be stationary or mobile. Within the same time period, the listener also monitors a range of other sounds. At any time, the sounds that are not in the foreground could become more significant (i.e. growing louder, growing softer, changing direction or changing in content) and could require more of the listener's attention.

Simultaneous and overlapping auditory streams will almost always have spatial distinctness because they occur in different places and/or over different pathways of movement. Informational masking, however, can occur due to acoustic properties or common content of one signal relative to another. In order to monitor auditory streams effectively and to be able to distinguish one sound from another, listeners must be able to spatially segregate, localize and track sound. Spatial segregation is especially important in the release from informational masking (Kidd et al., 1993). However, localization or being able to identify the particular whereabouts of a sound also plays a role. Because signals can change, for example the sound of a vehicle from behind turning a corner will necessitate the listener's head to turn to track this 'opposite' direction, tracking is an important component of auditory monitoring.

Effective auditory monitoring in the everyday world requires distributing attention across all of the types of auditory streams previously mentioned. In some cases visual and other sensory inputs may do all or part of the work. However, for situations where visual input is not available, the auditory system plays a crucial role in maintaining the effectiveness of the connection to the real world.

The capacity for effective auditory monitoring depends on a functioning binaural system. The ability to segregate, localize and track audible signals is due to interaural differences and their transformations. For example, identifying the location of a stationary object requires the use of interaural differences in time, level and frequency spectra. In contrast, identifying the location of a moving object requires a combination of rate of change of time, level and frequency spectra together with change in overall signal level.

Gatehouse and Noble (2004) examined the relationship between disability and handicap by administering the Speech, Spatial and Qualities of Hearing Scale (SSQ) to a sample of hearing clinic clients (n = 153). The disability dimension of the SSQ covers all elements of hearing for speech (i.e. one-on-one and group conversations, speech in stationary noise and reverberant conditions and with background competing speech, with and without full visual contact with other speakers, in contexts of rapid switching of speakers and in contexts of trying to follow simultaneous speech streams), spatial hearing (i.e. direction, distance, movement, indoors and outside) and quality of sound (i.e. segregation, recognizability, naturalness and listening effort). Handicap was defined as social restriction and emotional distress due to hearing impairment.

Results indicated that non-traditional areas of speech perception that require divided and rapidly switching attention were more strongly linked with the experience of the handicap rather than the traditional speech perception domains such as one-to-one or group conversation, or conversation in noisy backgrounds. Furthermore, it was these non-traditional speech-hearing contexts that were also related to spatial hearing functions, especially the detection of the direction of movement. In addition, dynamic spatial hearing functions were more closely linked to handicap experience than to other more stationary features of spatial hearing. Segregation, identification and listening effort were more strongly linked with the experience of handicap. These outcomes are consistent with the conceptual analysis given earlier of how hearing is actually used in the real world.

Interestingly, asymmetry of hearing loss appeared to play a prominent role in the disability–handicap link. An additional analysis with a sub-sample of 50 listeners who had one better ear and one worse ear was completed. Spatial hearing function, as expected, was found to be more of a disability in the asymmetry group and was especially strong as a driver of handicap experience.

Taken altogether, these results confirm the real-world conceptual analysis that hearing under conditions that are demanding and require a shifting of attention, abilities that rely on effective spatial hearing, underpins a sense of good connection with one's surroundings. It follows that unilateral cochlear implants may not serve the most critical domains of auditory connection with the real world.

## What are the risks of getting two implants?

There are risks which are present with monaural implantation but are more serious with bilateral implantation. These include potential damage from electrode insertion and electrical stimulation. There may be unknown long-term effects.

Implantation can reduce residual acoustic hearing, and the consequences of this are also greater with binaural implantation. This applies to signal processing that includes acoustic and electrical hearing in the same or both ears. In addition, the insertion of electrodes into the cochlea and the consequent destruction of cochlear tissue in both ears may limit the individual from taking advantage of future implant designs and/or molecular and genetic treatments.

Many of the surgical risks involved in receiving two implants are similar to or only slightly greater than when receiving one implant (Gantz et al., 2002). These risks, including infection and the use of an anesthetic, are relatively small. The potential loss of blood with bilateral surgery is an additional issue to consider, particularly in young children. Another concern is a disruption of bilateral vestibular input.

## Who should get two implants?

Traditionally, guidelines for implantation have depended on how much benefit is obtained from hearing aids, and how much benefit might be expected from a cochlear implant. However, we have argued (Tyler and Witt, 2003) that for both monaural and binaural implantation it is critical to determine the contribution from each ear individually, as well as binaurally. Speech perception tests should be conducted with the patient using hearing aids testing the left, right and binaural conditions. The results from each individual ear can be compared to determine the best monaural condition and, perhaps most important, the best monaural condition can be compared to the binaural condition to determine if there is a binaural advantage.

Documenting preoperative hearing aid benefit is necessary when considering cochlear implant candidacy for children and adults. However, hearing aid benefits, particularly those that contribute to speech and language development in infants and very young children, are often challenging to document until children are older (Barker and Tomblin, 2004). Delays in determining cochlear implant candidacy may have a negative effect on language acquisition (Tomblin et al., in press).

Staggered bilateral implantation may partially alleviate this problem but is much more costly and may potentially miss a window of binaural plasticity.

Table 15.5 lists the principles involved in considering binaural implantation. We refer to poor, medium and high speech perception scores, realizing that this is arbitrary. The actual values will depend on the test and will change as overall implant performance improves.

**Table 15.5** Principles involved when considering bilateral implants

| Aided binaural test results | Binaural implant decision |
| --- | --- |
| If binaural scores are high, and both ears are contributing: | Do not implant |
| If binaural scores are high, one ear not contributing: | Implant poorer ear to improve spatial hearing |
| If binaural scores are medium, both ears are contributing equally: | Implant binaurally<br>Do not implant (conservative approach) |
| If binaural scores are medium with one ear contributing more than the other and the best monaural is equal to the binaural score (no binaural benefit): | Implant poorer ear to improve spatial hearing<br>Implant better ear to improve speech in quiet<br>Implant binaurally to improve spatial hearing and speech in quiet |
| If binaural scores are medium with one ear contributing more than the other and the best monaural is less than the binaural score (is binaural benefit): | Do not implant to preserve current performance levels<br>Implant poorer ear to improve binaural benefit and to preserve better ear<br>Implant better ear to improve speech in quiet |

**Table 15.5** continued

| Aided binaural test results | Binaural implant decision |
| --- | --- |
| | Implant binaurally to improve speech in quiet and spatial hearing |
| If binaural scores are medium with one ear not contributing and best monaural is equal to the binaural score (no binaural benefit): | Implant poorer ear to improve spatial hearing and speech in quiet<br>Implant binaurally to improve speech in quiet and spatial hearing |
| If binaural scores are poor with one ear contributing more than the other: | Implant binaurally |
| If binaural scores are poor, ears contributing equally: | Implant binaurally |

# How should two implants be fit?

To facilitate binaural performance for individuals with two implants, the devices must be fit appropriately. Bilateral cochlear implants are typically fit similarly to bilateral hearing aids, where each aid is fit separately, then both are turned on and in a sound field with a talker directly in front, one or the other or both is/are adjusted until the overall loudness is appropriate and the sound is balanced between the two sides. With cochlear implants, the initial fitting involves maximizing the dynamic range on each electrode. Then, the overall level is adjusted for one device with only that device turned on. Subsequently, both devices are turned on and the overall gain for one of the devices is either increased or decreased until the loudness produced by the two devices is similar. Owing to binaural summation effects, a comfortable listening volume for the bilateral fitting typically requires less gain than for the unilateral fitting. This might increase the dynamic range and allow the maximum output level to be increased.

We also believe the fitting procedure for amplifying speech to audible and comfortable levels recommended by Tyler (1986a; see also Tyler, 1991) can be easily adopted to bilateral cochlear implant fittings. The intent is to adjust a device so that noise bands in different frequency regions are all judged to be comfortably loud. The 1/3-octave bands are presented at the average level of conversational speech in each frequency region. For example, a 500 Hz narrow band noise is presented at 60 dB HL. The right implant (left implant off) is adjusted so that the noise is perceived as being at the most comfortable listening level (MCL). Then the same adjustment is made with the left implant. Next, both implants are turned on, and any further adjustments are made so that the noise is perceived at the MCL in both ears. Sound at this frequency should then be perceived as centered. The procedure is then repeated with a 4000 Hz 43 dB SPL noise band. This is the average level of conversational speech in this frequency region. The procedure is then repeated for a low-level sound just above threshold, and then with a high-level sound just below the uncomfortable loudness level. Additional frequency bands can be added if necessary. In some patents, readjustments of the 500 and then 4000 Hz band may be helpful to account for inter-band loudness interactions. Additional frequency bands can also be used. The procedure ensures that speech is perceived at a comfortable level throughout the frequency range and is balanced throughout the frequency range over the levels tested. Under computer control, the strategy is fast and efficient.

# How should the benefits of two implants be measured?

Studies involving bilateral cochlear implantation have primarily focused on three areas of potential benefit: localization, speech perception in noise and subjective advantages. Tests should be determined by the particular experimental question. For example, different tests could be used for determining selection criteria, fitting effectiveness, to monitor progress or to determine if two devices are better than one.

### 1. Localization

Horizontal localization ability is typically measured using an array of speakers. Initially, bands of noise were used as stimuli for experiments. Our early experience was that patients with one cochlear implant could localize above chance. This ability was attributed to the repeated presentations of the same broadband stimuli, a situation that does not occur in real life. Some of our patients learned that noise on the opposite side of their implant had a higher-pitch quality due to the head shadow effect and thus were able to score above chance even when the stimulus level was roved. We consider this an artifact, and therefore now use everyday sounds as stimuli (Kramer, 1998).

### 2. Speech perception in noise

The ability to understand speech in noise is influenced by spatial separation. Various speaker configurations can be used, but a common one is with the speech in front and the noise located at 90° to the left or right. This configuration results in the best representation of the speech at both ears and the maximum difference between the noise at both ears.

## Subjective advantages

The Speech, Spatial and Qualities of Hearing Scale (SSQ) (Gatehouse and Noble, 2004) discussed earlier in this chapter and the Iowa Spatial Hearing Questionnaire (ISHQ) (see Appendix 15.A) are two subjective measures than can be administered to assess binaural function. Both questionnaires attempt to evaluate the ability to understand speech in a variety of spatial situations, as well as directionality of sound stimuli. The SSQ scale ranges from 0 (not at all) to 10 (perfectly), while the ISHQ scale ranges from 1 (very difficult) to 100 (very easy). The higher the score on the questionnaires, the better the patient perceives they are able to use spatial cues to localize sounds and understand speech in noise.

# How well do patients with bilateral cochlear implants hear?

Several groups have now reported the benefits obtained from two cochlear implants (e.g. van Hoesel et al., 1991, 1993, 2002; van Hoesel and Clark, 1999; Schön et al., 2002; Gantz et al., 2002; Tyler et al., 2002a; Müller et al., 2002; Wilson et al., 2003). In general, most bilateral implantees benefit from the ability to attend to the side with the better signal-to-noise ratio, and from improved horizontal plane localization. Benefits from binaural summation and squelch are present in only some patients.

## 1. Localization

Patients with bilateral cochlear implants generally show improved horizontal localization over time. Figure 15.1 shows the averaged responses for an eight-speaker everyday sounds test. The horizontal axis represents each speaker, while the vertical axis represents the patient's response. Perfect localization would be graphed showing a diagonal line. Average total root mean square (RMS) error is shown in degrees at the top of each graph. RMS-average error takes into account variability and standard error in patient responses. The smaller the RMS-average error, the better the localization ability.

Figure 15.1 shows the improvement in localization abilities for one patient from pre-implantation with bilateral hearing aids (top panel) to post-implantation (bottom panel) with bilateral cochlear implants. Also shown are the results for each implant separately. Bilateral pre-implantation results with two hearing aids show a RMS-average error of 37° with the patient perceiving the sound as originating from the center, regardless of the location of the loudspeaker from which the sound originated. The results from bilateral implants show an improvement in localization with the RMS-average error being reduced to 15°, with responses more closely following the eight-speaker array. Data for individual ears show that this patient cannot localize with only one cochlear implant. In this subject, sound is always perceived as coming from the side with the unilateral cochlear implant worn monaurally.

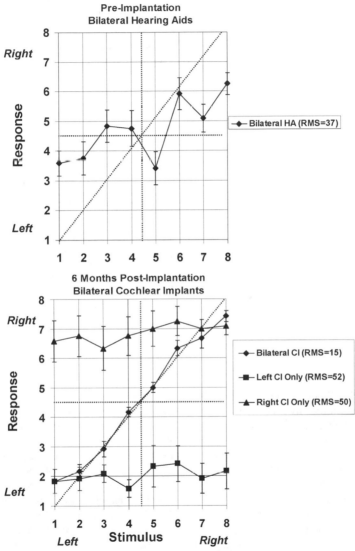

**Figure 15.1** Averaged responses for an eight-loudspeaker everyday sounds localization test. The horizontal axis of each graph represents the presentation loudspeaker, while the vertical axis represents the patient's response. Average total root mean square (RMS) error is shown in degrees in the legend of each graph. In the top panel, localization abilities are shown for one patient with pre-implant bilateral hearing aids. The RMS error is 37° with most responses toward the patient's 0° azimuth. In the bottom panel, localization abilities are shown for the same patient, now with bilateral cochlear implants. When wearing one implant, the patient localizes to the side of the implant.

## 2. Speech perception

Figure 15.2 shows average performance from 23 patients on the City University of New York CUNY Sentences (Boothroyd et al., 1985) in noise. Each of the four panels contains the same data, but is highlighted in different ways. The darkened bars focus on particular benefits. By displaying the entire data set the contribution of each ear is evident in each condition. The signal-to-noise ratio (S/N) was adjusted individually from a +5 S/N to a +10 S/N to minimize ceiling or floor effects.

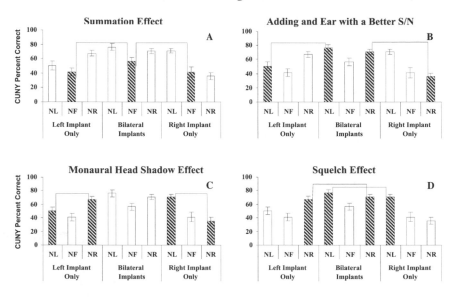

**Figure 15.2** Speech perception abilities are shown for 23 patients with bilateral cochlear implants. In each panel, the vertical axis represents the percentage correct for CUNY Sentences. The horizontal axis represents scores for the left and right implants only and with bilateral implants. In all conditions, error bars indicate significance for the sentences played at the patient's 0°-azimuth with noise emanating at the patient's 0°-azimuth (NF) or 90° to the left (NL) or right (NR) of the patient's 0°-azimuth. The S/N varied among the 23 bilateral patients from a +5 S/N to a +10 S/N to minimize the chance of a ceiling or floor effect. In Panel A, the darkened bars compare the left and right cochlear implants with NF to the bilateral implants with NF. Average results suggest a significant improvement in speech perception in the bilateral condition: a summation effect. In Panel B, the darkened bars compare the left implant with NL to the bilateral implant with the NL and the right implant with NR to the bilateral implant with the NR. Both comparisons show significant improvements in average sentence recognition in the bilateral condition when adding an ear with a better S/N. In Panel C, darkened bars compare the magnitude of head shadow effect when comparing the left implant with NL to the left implant with NR and right implant with NR to the right implant NL. Both comparisons show a significant improvement in average sentence recognition: a head shadow effect. In Panel D, darkened bars compare the left implant with NR to the bilateral implant NR and the right implant NL to the bilateral implant NL. Both comparisons show no significant improvement in average sentence recognition when adding an ear with a poorer S/N.

# Summation

Some bilateral cochlear implant listeners benefit when there is redundant information in both devices. This benefit is due to a 'summation' effect. The darkened bars in Figure 15.2a show results from the noise front (NF) condition with their left and right implants and bilaterally. Sentence recognition is significantly better with two devices worn than with either device alone. When comparing individual scores, however, only 8 out of the 23 listeners had a significant summation advantage.

# Adding an ear with a better signal-to-noise ratio

Figure 15.2b shows the average benefit of adding an ear with a better sig-nal-to-noise ratio, related to the head shadow effect. The darkened bars compare two different listening configurations: (1) the left implant only with the noise facing left (NL) condition to the bilateral condition with the noise facing left and (2) the right implant only condition with the noise facing right (NR) to the bilateral condition with the noise facing right. For both listening configurations a bilateral improvement is found. Individual data for the total 23 bilateral patients show that 13 benefited from what is likely to be mediated by a head shadow effect. This analysis is conserva-tive because it is using the best monaural condition as the baseline.

In this panel it is also possible to examine the contributions of each ear separately. For example, there is no difference between the use of the right implant when noise was on the left compared to the bilateral implant condition with the noise left. This suggests the brain is ignoring the ear with the poorer signal-to-noise ratio, while paying attention to the ear with the better signal-to-noise ratio.

# Monaural head shadow effect

The head shadow effect is due to the head and shoulders acting as a phys-ical barrier between the signal and the noise and so listeners have the capability to turn their head so that one ear has a better signal-to-noise ratio. Although patients with only one cochlear implant have the ability to benefit from this cue, having two cochlear implants guarantees that there is always an ear with a better signal-to-noise ratio.

The darkened bars in Figure 15.2c shows the magnitude of the head shadow effect with each unilateral device by comparing the difference in unilateral performance when noise is facing the unilateral device versus when the noise is on the opposite side. Average data show a magnitude of head shadow effect of 26% for the left implant and 35% for the right implant.

# Adding an ear with a poorer signal-to-noise ratio

The darkened bars in Figure 15.2d compare the average benefit of adding an ear with a poorer S/N, referred to as binaural squelch, in two different listening configurations: (1) the left implant with the noise facing right to the bilateral condition with the noise facing right and (2) the right implant with the noise facing left to the bilateral condition with the noise facing left. On average, no binaural squelch effect was found for the group in either listening configuration.

Although average data did not show an effect, individual data for 12 out of 23 listeners did show a binaural squelch effect for one ear. Thus, almost half of the individuals in this sample were able to take advantage of the binaural squelch effect in one condition.

# Spatial quality

Figure 15.3 shows an example of a bilateral cochlear implant patient who has completed the Speech, Spatial and Qualities of Hearing Scale (SSQ) and the Iowa Spatial Hearing Questionnaire (ISHQ) pre-operatively and

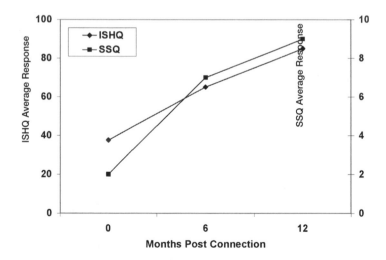

**Figure 15.3** Shown is the subjective ability to understand speech and directionality of sound in a variety of spatial situations with the Speech, Spatial and Qualities of Hearing Scale (SSQ) (Noble and Gatehouse, 2004) and the Iowa Spatial Hearing Questionnaire (ISHQ). The higher the score on the questionnaires, the better the patient perceives they are able to use spatial cues to localize sounds and understand speech. The SSQ scale ranges from 0 (not at all) to 10 (perfectly), while the ISHQ scale ranges from 1 (very difficult) to 100 (very easy). Subjective ratings from a bilateral cochlear implant patient who has completed the SSQ and ISHQ pre-operatively and at 6 and 12 months post-implantation indicate that aspects of spatial hearing have improved with time post-implantation.

at six and 12 months post-implantation. Results indicate that with time this patient reports spatial hearing has improved dramatically, and that realization of these benefits in real life may take at least 12 months of binaural implant use. These finding are typical among bilateral implant recipients at the University of Iowa.

## Will a single cochlear implant work with a hearing aid in the other ear?

Some, but not all, patients with a cochlear implant and a hearing aid on contralateral ears receive binaural advantages (Chmiel et al., 1995; Armstrong, et al., 1997; Simon-McCandless and Shelton, 2000; Ching et al., 2001a, 2001b, 2004; Tyler et al., 2002b; Hamzavi et al., 2004). It is thought that the amount of residual hearing in the aided ear, as well as the way the cochlear implant and hearing aid are fit, could account for some of the variation in the binaural advantages among these listeners.

Listeners with one hearing aid and one cochlear implant have at least two major disadvantages. First, the signal presented to each ear is quite different. Secondly, there may be important time delays introduced by different signal processing between the hearing aid and cochlear implant. In Figure 15.4 sentence recognition results are shown for three subjects with

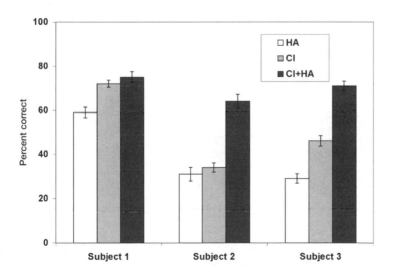

**Figure 15.4** Sentence recognition scores with noise facing the cochlear implant are shown for three patients wearing a hearing aid and a cochlear implant on contralateral ears. Standard error bars are shown to indicate significance. Subject one shows no bilateral advantage. Subject two shows the hearing aid and cochlear implant scores contributing equally to the bilateral advantage. Subject three shows a bilateral advantage. In this case, the hearing aid contributes to the binaural score even though it is performing much more poorly than the cochlear implant.

a cochlear implant and hearing aid on the contralateral ear. These three subjects were chosen to represent different outcomes. For all subjects, the sentences were presented from the front with the noise facing the subject's better ear, which happened to be the subject's cochlear implant side. Subject 1 shows no bilateral benefit. The individual hearing aid score is above chance (50%); however, the cochlear implant is the dominant ear with no difference shown between the bilateral score and the implant only score. Subject 2 shows a large bilateral benefit. The individual cochlear implant and hearing aid scores are relatively even and a large bilateral advantage is observed. Subject 3 also shows a bilateral advantage, but with the cochlear implant likely to be providing more information.

## Will a combined cochlear implant/hearing aid in one ear work with a hearing aid in the other ear?

Gantz and Turner (2003), Turner et al. (2004) and Von Ilberg et al. (1999) propose stimulating low-frequency regions with a hearing aid and high-frequency regions with a short-electrode implant (see also Wilson et al., 2003) within the same ear. Many of these patients will use a hearing aid on the unimplanted side. Performance of one patient in each of these listening conditions is shown in Figure 15.5. Results are shown with

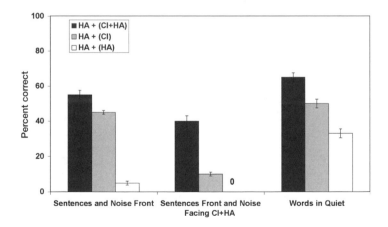

**Figure 15.5** Speech perception results are shown with sentences and noise facing front, sentences from the front with the noise facing the implanted ear, and with words in quiet for one patient with a combined cochlear implant and a hearing aid on one ear with a hearing aid on the contralateral ear. Standard error bars are shown to indicate significance. Results are shown in three conditions: (1) hearing aid on contralateral ear and combined cochlear implant and hearing aid [HA + (CI+HA)], (2) hearing aid and cochlear implant on contralateral ears [HA + (CI)] and (3) bilateral hearing aids [HA + (HA)]. Speech perception in noise and in quiet is best when the patient is wearing the combination cochlear implant and hearing aid with the hearing aid on the contralateral ear.

sentences and noise facing front, sentences from the front with the noise facing the implanted ear and with words in quiet. Speech perception in noise and in quiet is best when the patient is wearing the combination short electrode and hearing aid unilaterally with another hearing aid in the contralateral ear. Information across ears can be combined.

## Can a directional microphone serve the same purpose as two cochlear implants?

Virtually all microphones on hearing aids and cochlear implants are directional. That is, they are more sensitive to sounds from the front than they are from the sides or from the back. Microphones and circuits can be designed to be very directional (e.g. Ricketts, 2000), in the extreme case where any sound from the back or from the side is not perceived. This could be desirable, because usually speech is from the front and noise is from somewhere else or the listener can physically turn to create such an environment. This has an obvious potential advantage for speech perception in noise, and this advantage can occur with only one device.

The difficulty with directional microphones is that there are frequently sounds that originate from the back or side that are important. Normally, with binaural hearing the listener hears sounds from all directions and attends to the most important or salient one. This is critical if a new talker arrives from the side, or if a dangerous object approaches from behind. Highly directional microphones reduce the chance of this new information being heard. Therefore, directional microphones (even bilateral directional microphones) are not a substitute for binaural hearing and could actually impair binaural hearing.

## Can two microphones and one implant work as well as two implants?

It is reasonable to consider a more cost-effective alternative to bilateral cochlear implants that involve the use of bilateral microphones with the output being delivered to a unilateral cochlear implant (Tyler et al., 1992; Pedley, 1998). This concept has been used for many years in patients using a BICROS hearing aid system (Bilateral Contralateral Routing Of Signals) (Skinner, 1988; Dillon, 2001). Such patients typically have a 'dead' ear on one side and usable hearing on the other. A microphone is placed over each ear, and the output from each microphone is simply added and routed (wireless systems are now available) to the hearing side.

There are possible advantages to such a system, but also disadvantages. One way to think about this is to consider the monaural implant patient as the baseline. What are the relative advantages of giving this person a second microphone on the other side, or a second implant?

First, consider speech and noise from the front. A second microphone simply adds the same signal to the first. There is no difference in the signal-to-noise ratio and no expected difference in performance. A second implant activates a second neural channel and allows for the possibility of binaural summation.

Second, consider the speech from the front and noise on the side of the monaural implant. Adding a second microphone could improve performance moderately, because the lesser noise from the second microphone would be added to the greater noise originating from the implant microphone (the second microphone has less noise because it is shadowed by the head). Adding a second implant also picks up the signal from the side with the better signal-to-noise ratio. The second implant should result in better performance than the second microphone because the bilateral implant patient could be able to ignore the sound from the implant on the noise side. The patient with the second microphone does not have this option.

Third, consider the speech from the front and noise on the opposite side of the monaural implant. Adding a second microphone should make performance worse because the greater noise from the second microphone would be added to the stimulus originating from the implant microphone. Adding a second implant also picks up the signal from the side with the worse signal-to-noise ratio. However, the second implant should result in better performance than the second microphone because the bilateral implant patient could ignore the sound from the implant on the noise side. The patient with the second microphone does not have this option.

A fourth consideration is localization. Localization, theoretically, should be impossible with two microphones stimulating one implant. Localization is possible and common with two implants.

From the above arguments it appears that adding a second microphone will not provide the same benefits as adding a second implant. However, there are some situations where adding a second microphone may improve performance over a monaural implant. When the second microphone has a better signal-to-noise ratio, the performance should be better with two microphones. However, it seems that this would be offset by the equally probable event that the second microphone will have a poorer signal-to-noise ratio. There are perhaps at least two exceptions to this scenario. First, having two microphones might make it easier for the person to position themselves in a listening situation with a favorable signal-to-noise ratio. Secondly, in quiet situations without any noise, having a second microphone will increase the chance that a microphone will be close to the signal, avoiding the head shadow and facilitating the reception of quiet speech. One may argue that the limited benefits provided by a second microphone do not warrant further development and use in light of the possibility of much greater binaural benefits provided by bilateral cochlear implants.

# What signal processing might facilitate two cochlear implants?

Bilateral cochlear implants provide a unique opportunity to provide complementary information across ears. Typically, cochlear implants provide a series of electrical pulses to the auditory nerve, although analog waveforms are also used (Abbas, 1993). The pulses delivered are determined by the characteristics of the sound stimulus and the processing parameters of the device. Simply giving someone a second similar implant results in two processors functioning independently. There is no opportunity to control the relative timing among pulses between the two devices. All present commercial devices, and all the data referred to above, are of this type.

The areas in which signal processing for two devices might further be explored can be divided into two large categories: those requiring coordinated, or synchronized, processing, such as using one processor for two ears, and those that do not require coordinated processing. The former can be further divided into two categories: those that still attempt to provide true binaural hearing in the absence of synchronized processing and those that use the two ears as independent avenues or 'channels' to the central auditory system.

## 1. Uncoordinated independent processing

We have found that some patients benefit from dividing information across the two ears and letting the brain integrate the partial information from each ear to make sense of the whole signal. For example, some bilateral patients receive a significant binaural advantage in noise when frequency information is filtered across the two ears creating an interleaved binaural strategy. Specifically, in one ear frequency information from only the even filters is made audible, while frequency information from only the odd filters is made audible in the other ear. The two ears act as independent avenues or 'channels' of information that the brain has to integrate together to create a whole signal. Figure 15.6 shows the range of improvement found for two patients when comparing scores obtained while wearing their standard strategy versus this unique bilateral interleaved strategy.

## 2. Uncoordinated binaural processing

With unsynchronized processors, there is the potential for the interaural phase differences between pulses to vastly exceed the maximal interaural time differences (ITD) that are normally used by the binaural system for sound localization and binaural masking level differences (BMLD) ($\sim$700 $\mu$S). The ITD of any temporal fine structure represented in the stimulus-evoked auditory nerve spike train will be randomized due to the unpredictable nature of the unsynchronized processor outputs. Under such circumstances, binaural cues to localization will be limited to those provid-

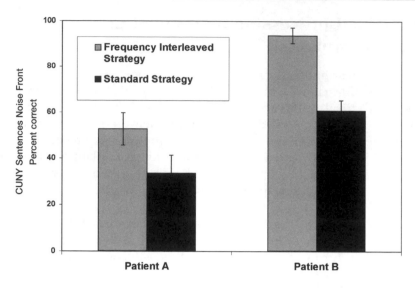

**Figure 15.6** Speech perception results are shown with sentences and noise facing front for two bilateral cochlear implant patients. The light bars represent scores when bilateral interleaved strategies are used and the dark bars represent scores when all channels are used on each implant (standard strategy). Standard error bars are shown to indicate significance. Results show significant benefits of wearing the bilateral interleaved implant programs over the programs with all channels.

ed by interaural intensity differences (IID) and ITD of envelope information. Likewise, any possibility of a BMLD or binaural squelch will depend on the ITD of envelope information. For broadband stimuli rich in frequencies below 1500 Hz, such as speech, the ITD of temporal fine structure dominates the binaural perception of laterality (Henning and Ashton, 1981; Bernstein and Trahiotis, 1985; Wightman and Kistler, 1992). Nevertheless, it has been demonstrated that envelope-based ITD cues for frequencies above 1500 Hz can provide some lateralization even if these cues are dominated by those based on fine structure (Bernstein and Trahiotis, 1985). Recent physiological studies demonstrate neurons in the inferior colliculus of cats, which are primarily sensitive to envelope-based ITDs, even at low frequencies (Joris, 2003). Thus while coordinated processing is necessary to represent fine-structure-based ITDs, the dominant binaural cue for speech, envelope-based ITDs and IIDs may still both be available to users of unsynchronized bilateral cochlear implants. The fact that squelch effects are observed in some bilateral users (see above in this chapter) suggests, but does not prove, that such ITD cues can be used effectively, particularly since current processing strategies do not appear to adequately represent fine-structure information (Rubinstein and Hong, 2003).

## 3. Coordinated processing

Coordinated processing can be thought of as the output of two microphones, each located on one side of the head, delivered to a single processor. This single processor could in turn be programmed to coordinate or synchronize the electrical pulses sent to each cochlear implant. When a sound is presented directly in front of a bilateral cochlear implant patient, the sound will reach each microphone at the same time. A single processor could then deliver electrical pulses to each implant at exactly the same time. Recall that with uncoordinated or independent processors there is no control over the precise timing of pulses between the two implants.

When a sound source is off to the left side, sound would naturally reach the left microphone first before it reached the right microphone. With a single processor, the processor could be set to deliver pulses to the left implant slightly before delivering pulses to the right implant. Presumably, the brain could then easily detect that the sound is on the left side.

This is a rather simplistic strategy, as in real life there are a series of pairs of pulses, with objects moving in the horizontal and vertical planes, changing their levels and distance. The trailing pulse of one pair might also be matched by the brain with a leading pulse from the following pair. Nevertheless, such fine control of pulses between devices will be necessary to convey highly sophisticated and valuable characteristics of normal spatial hearing.

Van Hoesel and Tyler (2003) report on one attempt to use coordinated processors, which they refer to as 'peak derived timing'. The pulses were coordinated by determining the positive peak of the input waveform in each filter band arriving at each microphone. No benefits were observed in four subjects compared to the clinical uncoordinated devices. Wilson et al. (2003) studied one subject and found similar results. Additional, clever algorithms need be to be devised and tested. The 'right' approach could have enormous benefits (see also Lawson et al., 1998).

## Are two implants cost-effective?

With the growing interest in the potential benefits of bilateral implantation, there has been concern regarding the increased costs. Our summary above suggests that there are important potential advantages of two implants, but is the benefit sufficient?

First, here are some general principles that perhaps we could all agree on:

- Two implants almost always result in better hearing than one implant.
- If a choice has to be made between providing one person with two implants and two people with one implant, then it is almost always better to provide two people with one implant.
- Two implants are more expensive.
- Two implants provide greater risks.

The additional costs of binaural implants include:

- a longer and more involved surgery;
- the cost of a second implant device;
- greater fitting time;
- additional maintenance;
- more frequent battery charging and/or replacement.

We suggest that it is too soon to answer this question. One of the biggest obstacles is that a value must be placed on monaural and on binaural hearing. This will undoubtedly require arbitrary subjective judgments about the quality of life, the meaning of life and happiness. Hasty statements may hinder a serious understanding of the relevant issues. Individual needs and listening circumstances will undoubtedly play an important role in evaluating benefit. For example, a deaf–blind person could benefit substantially from being able to localize and, one could argue, should always be considered for two implants.

## What needs to happen to improve binaural cochlear implant performance?

Synchronized processing (van Hoesel and Tyler, 2003) has the potential to allow for two extremely promising avenues of binaural implant signal processing. One approach involves pitch or place matching of bilateral electrodes (e.g. Long et al., 2003; Wilson et al., 2003). In the normal auditory system and in some implant recipients, this has been shown to dramatically improve ITD sensitivity. It has not yet been demonstrated to improve binaural benefit in implant patients, but the necessary studies have not been performed. Another approach, possibly complementary with the first, is to attempt better fine-structure representation with each implant's signal processor. As suggested by Smith et al. (2002), such strategies would not only improve music perception and sound quality transferred by a single cochlear implant but also improve the ITD representation of bilateral cochlear implants since such cues are dominated by fine structure. The feasibility of improving fine-structure representation using a novel signal processing strategy has been demonstrated for unilateral implants (Hong and Rubinstein, 2003; Hong et al., 2003; Rubinstein and Hong, 2003), and preliminary speech perception measures demonstrate improvement in background noise in some subjects using such strategies. It remains to be seen whether using such an approach bilaterally, with or without pitch matching of electrodes or with a contralateral hearing aid, can improve ITD cues and restore true binaural hearing. Nevertheless, the future of this particular area of cochlear implant technology appears extremely bright. Many of the cost-benefit analyses discussed earlier in this chapter would be substantially affected by the restoration of squelch effects to bilateral cochlear implant recipients.

# Conclusions

There are numerous potential benefits from spatial hearing, not the least of which involves improved hearing in noise, localization and a perception of experiencing a true sound environment. There are also risks for trying to provide spatial hearing through bilateral cochlear implants. Nonetheless, preliminary data indicate that real advantages can be obtained from two implants that cannot be obtained with two microphones and one implant, one cochlear implant and one hearing aid on opposite ears or with directional microphones. There are also many opportunities to improve bilateral signal processing, including contributions in fitting algorithms that consider two devices. Recent efforts to streamline fitting by reducing time or optimizing for the 'average' patient needs to be considered with great caution. Future advances in bilateral cochlear implants will improve benefits to hearing-impaired people wearing binaural cochlear implants, binaural hearing aids and a variety of combinations of binaural hearing aids and cochlear implants. This is both exciting and necessary in our attempt to restore hearing as closely as possible to normal.

## Acknowledgements

Supported in part by research grant 2-P50-DC00242 from the National Institutes on Deafness and Other Communication Disorders, National Institutes of Health, grant RR00059 from the General Clinical Research Centers Program, Division of Research Resources, National Institutes of Health, the Lions Clubs International Foundation and the Iowa Lions Foundation. We would also like to thank Beth Macpherson for her helpful editing comments.

# References

Abbas PJ (1993) Electrophysiology. In RS Tyler (ed.), Cochlear Implants: Audiological Foundations. San Diego: Singular Publishing.

Armstrong M, Pegg P, James C et al. (1997) Speech perception in noise with implant and hearing aid. American Journal of Otology 18: S140–S141.

Balfour PB, Hawkins DB (1992) A comparison of sound quality judgments for monaural and binaural hearing aid processed stimuli. Ear and Hearing 13(5): 331–9.

Barker BA, Tomblin JB (2004) Comparing bimodal perception skills in infant hearing-aid and cochlear-implant users. Archives of Otolaryngology: Head and Neck Surgery 130(5): 582–6.

Bernstein LR, Trahiotis C (1985) Lateralization of low-frequency, complex waveforms: the use of envelope-based temporal disparities. Journal of the Acoustical Society of America 77(5): 1868–1880.

Blauert J (1997) Spatial Hearing: The Psychophysics of Human Sound Localization. Cambridge, MA: MIT Press.

Boothroyd A, Hanin L, Hnath T (1985) A Sentence Test of Speech Perception: Reliability, Set Equivalence, and Short-term Learning. New York: Speech and Hearing Sciences Research Center, City University of New York.

Bregman AS (1990) Auditory Scene Analysis: The Perceptual Organization of Sound. Cambridge, MA: MIT Press.

Byrne D (1980) Binaural hearing aid fitting: research findings and clinical application. In ER Libby (ed.), Binaural Hearing and Amplification. Chicago: Zenetron.

Byrne D, Noble W (1998) Optimizing sound localization with hearing aids. Trends in Amplification 3(2): 51–73.

Carhart R, Tillman TW, Johnson KF (1967) Release of masking for speech through interaural time delay. Journal of the Acoustical Society of America 42: 124–38.

Cherry EC (1953) Some experiments on the recognition of speech, with one and two ears. Journal of the Acoustical Society of America 25: 975.

Cherry EC, Sayers B (1959) On the mechanism of binaural fusion. Journal of the Acoustical Society of America 31: 535.

Ching TY, Psarros C, Hill M (2001a) Hearing aid benefit for children who switched from the SPEAK to the ACE strategy in their contralateral Nucleus 24 cochlear implant system. Australian and New Zealand Journal of Audiology 22: 123–32.

Ching TY, Psarros C, Hill M et al. (2001b) Should children who use cochlear implants wear hearing aids in the opposite ear? Ear and Hearing 22(5): 365–80.

Ching TY, Incerti P, Hill M (2004) Binaural benefits for adults who use hearing aids and cochlear implants in opposite ears. Ear and Hearing 25: 9.

Chmiel RA, Clark J, Jerger J et al. (1995) Speech perception and production in children wearing a cochlear implant in one ear and a hearing aid in the opposite ear. Annals of Otology, Rhinology and Laryngology (suppl. 166): 314–16.

Day G, Browning G, Gatehouse S (1988) Benefit from binaural hearing aids in individuals with a severe hearing impairment. British Journal of Audiology 22(4): 273–7.

Dillon H (2001) Hearing Aids. New York: Thieme.

Dubno JR, Ahlstrom JB, Horwitz AR (2002) Spectral contributions to the benefit from spatial separation of speech and noise. Journal of Speech, Language and Hearing Research 45: 1297–1310.

Franklin B (1981) Split-band amplification: a HI/LO hearing aid fitting. Ear and Hearing 2: 230–3.

Gantz BJ, Turner CW (2003) Combining acoustic and electrical hearing. Laryngoscope 113: 1726–30.

Gantz BJ, Tyler RS, Rubinstein JT et al. (2002) Binaural cochlear implants placed during the same operation. Otology and Neurotology 23: 169–80.

Gatehouse S, Noble W (2004) The Speech, Spatial and Qualities of Hearing Scale (SSQ). International Journal of Audiology 43(2): 85–99.

Gilkey RH, Anderson TR (1997) Binaural and spatial hearing in real and virtual environments. Mahwah, NJ: Lawrence Erlbaum.

Hall JW, Tyler RS, Fernandes MA (1984) Factors influencing the masking level difference in cochlear hearing-impaired and normal-hearing listeners. Journal of Speech and Hearing Research 27: 145–54.

Hamzavi J, Pok SM, Gstoettner W et al. (2004) Speech perception with a cochlear implant used in conjunction with a hearing aid in the opposite ear. International Journal of Audiology 43: 61–5.

Hartmann WM, Constan ZA (2002) Interaural level differences and the level-meter model. Journal of the Acoustical Society of America 112(3): 1037–45.

Henning GB, Ashton J (1981) The effect of carrier and modulation frequency on lateralization based on interaural phase and interaural group delay. Hearing Research 4: 185–94.

Hirsch IJ (1948) Influence of interaural phase on interaural summation and inhibition. Journal of the Acoustical Society of America 20: 536–44.

Hong RS, Rubinstein JT (2003) High-rate conditioning pulse trains in cochlear implants: dynamic range measures with sinusoidal stimuli. Journal of the Acoustical Society of America 114(6): 3327–42.

Hong RS, Rubinstein JT, Wehner D et al. (2003) Dynamic range enhancement for cochlear implants. Otology and Neurotology 24: 590–5.

Joris PX (2003) Interaural time sensitivity dominated by cochlea-induced envelope patterns. Journal of Neuroscience 23(15): 6345–50.

Kaplan H, Pickett J (1981) Effects of sensorinerual hearing loss on loudness discomfort level and most comfortable level judgements. Journal of Speech and Hearing Disorders 21: 680–1.

Kidd G, Mason CR, Deliwala PS et al. (1993) Reducing informational masking by sound segregation. Journal of the Acoustical Society of America 95(6): 3475–80.

Koenig W (1950) Subjective effects in binaural hearing. Journal of the Acoustical Society of America 33: 537–8.

Kramer SE (1998) Assessment of hearing Disability and Handicap. Unpublished dissertation, p43.

Lawson DT, Wilson BS, Zerbi M et al. (1998) Bilateral cochlear implants controlled by a single speech processor. American Journal of Otology 19: 758–61.

Litovsky RY, Parkinson A, Arcaroli J et al. (2004) Bilateral cochlear implants in adults and children. Archives of Otolaryngology: Head and Neck Surgery 130(5): 648–55.

Long CJ, Eddington DK, Colburn HS et al. (2003) Binaural sensitivity as a function of interaural electrode position with a bilateral cochlear implant user. Journal of the Acoustical Society of America 114(3): 1565–74.

Markides A (1977) Binaural Hearing Aids. London: Academic Press.

Müller J, Schön F, Helms J (2002) Speech understanding in quiet and noise in bilateral users of the Med-El Combi 40/40+ cochlear implant system. Ear and Hearing 23(3): 198–206.

Neuman AC (1996) Late-onset auditory deprivation: a review of past research and an assessment of future research needs. Ear and Hearing 17(suppl. 3): 3S–13S.

Noble W (1983) Hearing, hearing impairment and the audible world: a theoretical essay. Audiology 22: 325–38.

Noble W, Gatehouse S (2004) Interaural asymmetry of hearing loss, Speech, Spatial and Qualities of Hearing Scale (SSQ) disabilities, and handicap. International Journal of Audiology.

Pedley K (1998) Comparison of conventional and dual microphone cochlear implant headsets – a case study. Australian Journal of Audiology 20(1): 17–20.

Plomp R (2002) The Intelligent Ear: On the Nature of Sound Perception. Mahwah, NJ: Lawrence Erlbaum.

Preece JP, Tyler RS, Bergen C (in preparation) A test of localization of environmental sounds.

Ricketts T (2000) Directivity quantification in hearing aids: fitting and measurement effects. Ear and Hearing 21(1): 45–58.

Rubinstein JT, Hong RS (2003) Signal coding in cochlear implants: exploiting stochastic effects of electrical stimulation. Annals of Otology, Rhinology and
Laryngology 112 (suppl. 191): 14–19.

Schön F, Müller J, Helms J (2002) Speech reception thresholds obtained in a symmetrical four-loudspeaker arrangement from bilateral users of Med-El cochlear
implants. Otology and Neurology 23(5): 710–14.

Silman S, Gelfand SA, Silverman CA (1984) Late-onset auditory deprivation:
effects of monaural versus binaural hearing aids. Journal of the Acoustical
Society of America 76(5): 1357–62.

Simon-McCandless M, Shelton C (2000) Cochlear implants and hearing instruments: do they mix? Hearing Review (Nov): 38–48.

Skinner MW (1988) Hearing Aid Evaluation. Remediation of Communication
Disorders Series. Englewood Cliffs, NJ: Prentice-Hall.

Smith ZM, Delgutte B, Oxenham AJ (2002) Chimaeric sounds reveal dichotomies
in auditory perception. Nature 416: 87–90.

Summerfield AQ, Barton GR, McAnallen C et al. (2003) Self-reported outcomes
from bilateral cochlear implantation: auditory performance, quality of life, and
tinnitus. Paper presented at the British Society of Audiology Meeting on
Experimental Papers on Hearing and Deafness, Nottingham, England.

Tomblin JB, Barker BA, Spencer LJ et al. (in press) The effect of age at cochlear
implant stimulation on expressive language growth in infants and toddlers.
Journal of Speech, Language and Hearing Research.

Turner CW, Gantz BJ, Vidal C et al. (2004) Speech recognition in noise for
cochlear implant listeners: benefits of residual acoustic hearing. Journal of the
Acoustical Society of America 115(4): 1729–35.

Tyler RS (1986) Adjusting a hearing aid to amplify speech to the MCL. The
Hearing Journal, August: 24–7.

Tyler RS (1991) What can we learn about hearing aids from cochlear implants. Ear
and Hearing 12(suppl. 6): 177S–186S.

Tyler RS, Berliner K, Demorest M et al. (1986) Clinical objectives and research-design
issues for cochlear implants in children. Seminars in Hearing 7(4): 433–40.

Tyler RS, Opie JM, Fryauf-Bertschy H et al. (1992) Future directions for cochlear
implants. Journal of Speech-Language Pathology and Audiology 16(2): 151–64.

Tyler RS, Gantz BJ, Rubinstein JT et al. (2002a) Three-month results with bilateral cochlear implants. Ear and Hearing 23(suppl. 1): 80S–89S.

Tyler RS, Parkinson A, Wilson B et al. (2002b) Patients utilizing a hearing aid and
a cochlear implant: speech perception and localization. Ear and Hearing 23(2):
98–105.

Tyler RS, Witt S (2003) Cochlear implants in adults: candidacy. In R Kent (ed.),
The MIT Encyclopedia of Communication Disorders. Philadelphia: PM Gordon
Associates, pp. 440–4.

van Hoesel RJM, Clark GM (1999) Speech results with a bilateral multichannel
cochlear implant subject for spatially separated signal and noise. Australian
Journal of Audiology 21(1): 23–8.

van Hoesel RJM, Tong YC, Hollow RD et al. (1991) Preliminary studies on a bilateral cochlear implant user. Journal of the Acoustical Society of America (suppl.
88): 193.

van Hoesel RJM, Tong YC, Hollow RD et al. (1993) Psychophysical and speech perception studies: a case report on a binaural cochlear implant subject. Journal
of the Acoustical Society of America 9: 3178–89.

van Hoesel RJM, Ramsden R, O'Driscoll M (2002) Sound-direction identification, interaural time-delay discrimination, and speech intelligibility advantages in noise for a bilateral cochlear implant user. Ear and Hearing 23(2): 137–49.

van Hoesel RJM, Tyler RS (2003) Speech perception, localization, and lateralization with bilateral cochlear implants. Journal of the Acoustical Society of America 113(3): 1617–30.

von Ilberg C, Keifer J, Tillein J et al. (1999) Electro-acoustic stimulation of the auditory system. Annals of Otology, Rhinology and Laryngology 61: 334–40.

Wightman FL, Kistler DJ (1992) The dominant role of low-frequency interaural time differences in sound localization.Journal of the Acoustical Society of America 91(3): 1648–61.

Wilson BS, Lawson DT, Müller JM et al. (2003) Cochlear implants: some likely next steps. Annual Review of Biomedical Engineering 5: 207–49.

Yost WA (1974) Discriminations of interaural phase differences. Journal of the Acoustical Society of America 55(6): 1299–1303.

Yost WA, Gourevitch G (1987) Directional Hearing. New York: Springer-Verlag.

Yost WA, Guzman SJ (1996) Auditory processing of sound sources: is there an echo in here? American Psychological Society 125–31.

Zurek PM (1993) Binaural advantages and directional effects in speech intelligibility. In GA Studebaker, I Hochberg (eds), Acoustical Factors Affecting Hearing Aid Performance. Boston: Allyn and Bacon, pp. 255–76.

# Appendix 15.A

Iowa Spatial Hearing Questionnaire

NAME_____HOSP. #_____
DATE_____TEST SESSION # _____

Please respond to each question with a number from 1-100. Number 1 means the situation would be very difficult. Number 100 means the situation would be very easy.

1....Very Difficult 100....Very Easy

| 1. | A man talking to you is standing in front of you. It is a very quiet room. How well can you understand him? | |
| 2. | A woman talking to you is standing in front of you. It is a very quiet room. How well can you understand her? | |
| 3. | A child talking to you is standing in front of you. It is a very quiet room. How well can you understand the child? | |
| 4. | You are listening to music that is comfortably loud coming from in front of you. It is a very quiet room. How easy or difficult is it to hear the music clearly? | |
| 5. | A man talking to you is standing in front of you. There is a loud fan directly behind him. How well can you understand him? | |
| 6. | A woman talking to you is standing in front of you. There is a loud fan directly behind her. How well can you understand her? | |
| 7. | A child talking to you is standing in front of you. There is a loud fan directly behind them. How well can you understand the child? | |
| 8. | You are listening to comfortably loud music coming from in front of you. There is also a loud fan in front of you. How easy or difficult is it to hear the music clearly? | |
| 9. | A man talking to you is standing in front of you. There is a loud fan off to one side. How well can you understand him? | |
| 10. | A woman talking to you is standing in front of you. There is a loud fan off to one side. How well can you understand her? | |
| 11. | A child talking to you is standing in front of you. There is a loud fan off to one side. How well can you understand the child? | |
| 12. | You are listening to comfortably loud music coming from in front of you. There is also a loud fan off to one side. How easy or difficult is it to hear the music clearly? | |
| 13. | How well are you able to determine the location of a man's voice when you cannot see him? | |
| 14. | How well are you able to determine the location of a woman's voice when you cannot see her? | |
| 15. | How well are you able to determine the location of a child's voice when you cannot see the child? | |
| 16. | How well are you able to determine the location of a music source, say a radio, when you cannot see it? | |
| 17. | How well are you able to determine the location of a man's voice when he is behind you? | |
| 18. | How well are you able to determine the location of a woman's voice when she is behind you? | |
| 19. | How well are you able to determine the location of a child's voice when the child is behind you? | |
| 20. | How well are you able to determine the location of a music source, say a | |

# CHAPTER 16

# The future of cochlear implants

JENNIFER L. SMULLEN, ADRIEN A. ESHRAGHI
AND THOMAS J. BALKANY

## Introduction

As we look to the future of cochlear implants, let us remember how far we have come. Two French physicians, Andre Djourno and Charles Eyries (1957), first stimulated the cochlear nerve electrically during surgery under local anesthesia. Electrical stimulation by an electrode directly on the auditory nerve produced an auditory sensation. The concept of using direct electrical stimulation of the auditory nerve to mimic the transduction function of the cochlea initiated the eventual development of the cochlear implant.

Further work led to the production of a speech processor, which could drive an electrode implanted in the cochlea. By 1982, a single-channel cochlear implant, the House 3M, was available commercially (Figure 16.1). Ten years later, a multichannel device was developed at the University of Melbourne and marketed by Cochlear Ltd (Niparko and Wilson, 2000).

Currently, multichannel electrodes and highly advanced processors make recognition of conversational speech a reality for most cochlear implant recipients. There are presently over 60,000 worldwide cochlear implant recipients. Despite the significant advances of the past 15 years, cochlear implants can still improve, particularly in the areas of music appreciation and speech recognition in noise.

Research continues in many areas of cochlear implantation. In the future, perhaps cochlear implants will provide normal (or better) hearing, replace hearing aids for most indications, prevent further hearing loss and restore hearing through neural regeneration. In the near future, aims are for devices that provide better speech comprehension, easier insertions, expanded usage and retained residual hearing.

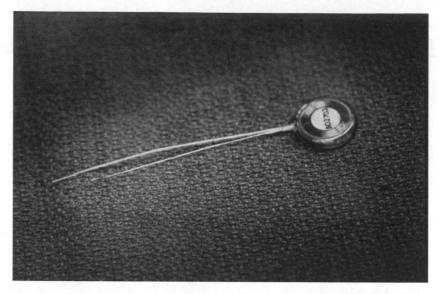

**Figure 16.1** The House 3M single-channel cochlear implant

# Engineering

In the United States there are three FDA-approved devices (Table 16.1).

**Table 16.1** FDA-approved cochlear implant devices.

| Company | Device |
| --- | --- |
| Advanced Bionics Corporation | Clarion |
| Cochlear Limited | Nucleus 24 |
| Medical Electronics Corporation | Med-El |

Patients with the help of their audiologist and surgeon choose the device that best suits their individual needs. Physicians and scientists all over the world are working to improve the current state of the art.

### Electrodes

One area of continued research is electrode design. Great strides have been made from the first single-channel electrode, which provided sound awareness to the current devices (Table 16.2), which optimally can restore near normal hearing.

However, there is still room for further improvement. The ideal number of channels in an implanted electrode is not yet known. In theory, the more specific the stimulation of spiral ganglion cells along the spiral lamina,

**Table 16.2** FDA-approved electrode arrays

| Device | Number of electrodes | Electrode arrays |
| --- | --- | --- |
| Clarion | 16 | Enhanced bipolar<br>HiFocus<br>HiFocus II |
| Nucleus | 22 | 24K<br>24 Double Array<br>Contour |
| Med-El | 12 paired | Combi 40+<br>Combi 40+ Compressed Array<br>Combi 40+ Split Array |

the more similar the firing is to natural hearing and the higher the quantity of information delivered to the brain for processing. However, this theory has its limitations. With current electrode design and positioning, the power needed to produce a stimulus in a few spiral ganglion cells transmits to the surrounding region as well, thus limiting the number of unique electrode sites along the length of the Organ of Corti. New low-power electrodes constructed with thin-film techniques of up to 100 channels could be capable of very localized patterns of stimulation (Parker et al., 1999). The frequency-specific information delivered with such electrodes could lead to improvements in speech and music perception.

Another way to reduce the stimulation thresholds and fine-tune the stimulation pattern is to position the electrode closer to the auditory nerve (Briggs et al., 2001). Already scala tympani insertion places the array closer to the basilar membrane than scala vestibuli insertion. Newer electrodes, such as the Contour, further direct the array toward the spiral ganglion (Balkany et al., 1999). Perimodiolar positioning not only demonstrates decreased stimulation thresholds, but theoretically may allow for more localized neural stimulation to improve speech perception.

The insertion of perimodiolar electrodes, as with all electrodes, carries a risk of intracochlear injury. Fractures of the osseus spiral lamina, spiral ligament tears, organ of Corti disruption and loss of spiral ganglion cells can occur with electrode placement (Balkany et al., 2002; Eshraghi et al., 2003). Electrodes that are narrower, more flexible and with a softer tip may lessen the risk of trauma to the inner ear structures by reducing insertion forces. The preservation of the cochlear anatomy may allow for future use of hybrid devices, newer electrodes or even neural regeneration. Many cochlear implant patients are children with a projected lifespan of decades, and in another 50 years who knows what developments are possible?

New shorter electrodes are under investigation for use in high-frequency sensorineural hearing loss (SNHL). By taking advantage of the tonotopic

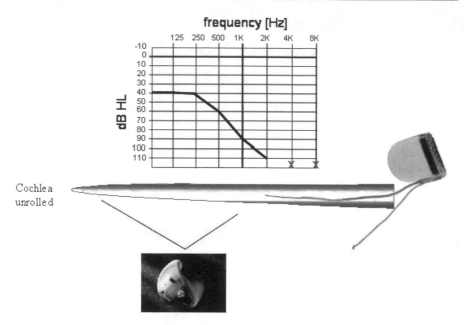

**Figure 16.2** Electro-Acoustic Stimulation. A sample audiogram for an electro-acoustic stimulation candidate. The basal turn of the cochlea is stimulated by the cochlear implant for high frequency representation, and the apical turn is acoustically stimulated by the hearing aid in the lower frequencies.

arrangement of the cochlea, a short electrode stimulates only the basal turn high-frequency areas of the cochlea, thus leaving the more apical segment with residual hair cell function undisturbed for reception of the lower frequencies (Figure 16.2). This allows for electrical replacement of only that portion of the spectrum with the hearing loss. Residual hearing is preserved for bimodal stimulation or to take advantage of future advances.

As technology improves rapidly in the cochlear implant field, many patients are left with older devices and seek modernization. In other instances, it may become necessary to replace the internal device and electrode for device failure, extrusion or wound infection. Currently, the replacement of the internal device requires the complete removal and replacement of the electrode as well as the internal receiver component with the resultant risk of intracochlear trauma from electrode removal and reinsertion. New cochlear implants may be modular, giving the ability to change one or more parts of the implant without incurring the risk and cost of a completely new device.

## Processors

Advances in silicone chip technology have permitted the miniaturization of cellular phones, laptop computers and numerous biomedical devices, including cochlear implants. The external microphone, processor and transmitter of the cochlear implant device were first available only as a bulky body-worn box. Now external devices are as small as five by six centimeters, and some are completely ear-level. More programming strategies are held within the processors, and smaller, faster devices that require less power are under investigation.

## Fully implantable cochlear implant

As rechargeable batteries improve and external devices become smaller and faster, the possibility of a fully implantable cochlear implant comes within reach. Perhaps soon a cochlear implant can be placed within the mastoid cavity leaving no external device or visible implant. This has many benefits for cosmetic, social and compliance issues, especially in children (Maniglia et al., 2001). The totally implantable device would eliminate the need for transcutaneous radiofrequency transmission of the electric signal. The implant would be more cosmetic and more protected within the mastoid cavity. The absence of an external device eliminates the need for manual dexterity in the very young or very old, and would improve compliance. The device could be used 24 hours a day with no need to remove for sleeping or bathing.

One of the challenges of implantable devices is the need for transdermal charging of lithium-ion batteries, or periodic replacement of implanted batteries such as is done with cardiac pacemakers. Lowering the power requirements of the device as previously mentioned prolongs the charge of the batteries and will be essential to make a fully implantable device.

Sound reception is yet another unique problem of the implanted device. Subdermal microphones have reduced sensitivity compared to their external counterparts; so several devices for detection of sound have been proposed and tested. The bioelectric middle ear microphone (BMEM) makes use of the pinna, external auditory canal, tympanic membrane and ossicles for amplification (Goode, 1995; Maniglia et al., 2001). The ossicular movement is then detected and transduced into an electronic signal delivered to the processor. Vibration detection strategies have included a middle ear infrared light with a tympanic membrane reflector (Ko et al., 1995), a magnet on an ossicle over an electromagnetic coil and a piezo-electric cantilever to convert a bending motion into a signal (Yanagihara et al., 1995).

## Hybrids

Another area of research is the use of bimodal speech processing. While the cochlear implant provides electrical stimulation, a hearing aid offers acoustic stimulation in the ipsilateral or contralateral ear. As early as 1993, binaural stimulation with a cochlear implant speech processor and a speech-processing hearing aid for the unimplanted ear was found to be superior to a cochlear implant alone (Dooley et al., 1993). As the results of cochlear implantation improve, people with more residual hearing are becoming

candidates. These patients may have some benefit from traditional amplification. Short electrode arrays for high-frequency hearing loss and improved
surgical techniques preserve residual hearing in the implanted ear (Gantz
and Turner, 2003). Hybrid devices are designed to take advantage of bimodal
input. If the same processor encodes input for both devices, frequency
ranges could be assigned and coordinated for better speech perception and
hearing in noise. Combined electric and acoustic stimulation (EAS) has been
successful in small groups of study patients (Baumgartner et al., 2003). The
brain is able to understand the combination of stimuli and patients report
more natural speech and environmental sounds.

## Objective programming

Programming the cochlear implant device requires three steps. First, perception of auditory stimuli is confirmed. Then the lowest current level of
perception is established for each electrode. Next, the maximum current
level the patient can accept for each electrode is determined. The best
sound perception is achieved when the electric stimulation is consistent
across all electrodes and dynamic range is maximized. Achieving this balance is hard because it relies on the patient's subjective perception of
sound. Particularly in children, this last step can be difficult, creating a
need for an integrated tool to determine the maximum loudness level.
The maximum loudness level corresponds well to the electrically elicited
middle ear reflex (EMR). Using the principle of the stapedial reflex, an
integrated EMR detector could reduce subjective error and assist in the
programming of children (Allum et al., 2002).

A currently integrated tool is Neural Response Telemetry (NRT). NRT
measures whole nerve action potentials. Integrating NRT reverse telemetry eliminates the need for external electrodes as well as the need for a
cooperative child (Gordon et al., 2002). The measurement and clinical
application of this technique are addressed in other chapters.

Electrical Auditory Brainstem Response (EABR), can be performed
intraoperatively or postoperatively (Kubo et al., 2001). The effects of electrical stimulation via an electrode on the promontory or in the round
window can be measured with EABR. This can assist in the prediction of
the usefulness of the cochlear implant. Knowing how well a cochlear
implant could work in a given patient can be used for counseling regarding realistic expectations and to expand candidacy for those in whom the
EABR indicates high likelihood of success despite not otherwise being a
candidate. EABR can also assure that even very young children are receiving benefit from their cochlear implants (Kubo et al., 2001).

## MRI compatibility

Cochlear implant device compatibility with MRI varies (Pappas and Cure,
2002). The Nucleus 24 has a surgically removable magnet, which renders

the device safe for up to a 1.5 Tesla magnet according to the package insert. The Med-El device can be used without alteration in a 1.0 Tesla magnet (Youssefzadeh et al., 1998) and the Clarion device has little risk with a 0.3 Tesla magnet (Weber et al., 1998). Despite all of these advances, we have yet to achieve full MRI compatibility.

New biocompatible materials and fully implantable devices may soon make cochlear implants MRI safe. Currently, the titanium, ceramic and silicone components of the cochlear implant are MRI compatible, and the totally implantable device would eliminate the need for an internal magnet and electromagnetic induction.

## Auditory brainstem implants

The auditory brainstem implant (ABI) is similar to a cochlear implant (Toh and Luxford, 2002) but is reserved for those patients without a functionally intact eighth cranial nerve excluding them from cochlear implant candidacy (Table 16.3).

**Table 16.3** ABI selection criteria

| |
| --- |
| Neurofibromatosis type 2 |
| Age > 12 |
| Requiring surgery (first or second side) |
| Proficiency in the English language |
| Reasonable expectations |

Like a cochlear implant, there is an internal and an external component. The internal device has a 21-channel electrode array, which is placed in proximity to the dorsal and ventral cochlear nuclei in the brainstem, usually at the time of vestibular schwannoma surgery for neurofibromatosis type 2 (NF-2). The electrode is connected to an internal receiver-stimulator. The external component has a microphone, speech processor and a transcutaneous transmitter coil. One important difference is that there is no magnet within the internal device, thus allowing NF-2 patients to undergo their surveillance MRI scanning. In place of a magnet, a retainer disk secures the external transmitter coil. In the United States, the FDA approved the Nucleus multichannel ABI device in the year 2000. Medical Electronics Corporation has a similar device in use in Europe.

Most patients receiving ABI have NF-2, although the criteria are expanding. Colletti et al. (2002) implanted three children with cochlear aplasia and cochlear nerve hypoplasia. After 12 months, one child gained good environmental sound awareness, good speech detection and some speech recognition. The second child had good environmental sound awareness and some speech detection after eight months, while the third child had good environmental sound awareness after only one month.

In a multicenter European study, 11 patients who received ABI were evaluated (Nevison et al., 2002). All 11 continued to be daily users of the implant with high patient satisfaction. They reported ABI improved receiving and differentiating environmental sounds, enhanced speech perception and enhanced lipreading. The House group reports ABI results similar to the early single-channel cochlear implant experience with 85% able to receive auditory sensation (Otto et al., 2002). At 3–6 months, 93% of 55 patients implanted had improved sentence understanding when combined with lipreading cues, although open-set speech recognition is not usually possible.

# Molecular biology

Perhaps some of the most original and promising innovations in cochlear implantation are in the field of molecular biology. Cochlear implants rely on functioning auditory neurons, so it is important to preserve functioning neurons for successful cochlear implantation. The more understanding of the auditory system on a cellular and subcellular level, the more chance there is to manipulate the natural history of hearing loss as we work toward the goals of neural preservation and ultimately neural regeneration. The intracochlear electrode array may serve as the delivery device for new auditory pharmacotherapy.

### Neural preservation

Trauma-induced oxidative stress to the auditory system is known to cause a loss of hair cells and neurons through necrosis and apoptosis (Scarpidis et al., 2003). While immediate necrosis may be difficult to prevent, the delayed nature of apoptosis gives a window to manipulate the intercellular pathways and signaling cascades to prevent further cell death.

One such apoptotic pathway known to affect the auditory system is the mitogen activated protein kinase (MAPK)/ c-Jun N-terminal Kinase (JNK) signal cascade (Scarpidis et al., 2003). An anti-apoptotic molecule termed JNK inhibitory peptide one (JNKI-1) has been shown to nearly stop apoptosis *in vitro*. In addition, when JNKI-1 is delivered to the scala tympani in an animal model, it can wholly prevent gentamicin-induced ototoxicity and sound trauma initiated hearing loss.

Caspase molecules are also known to induce both the intrinsic and extrinsic cell death pathways within the auditory system (Van De Water et al., 2004). Caspase inhibitors are a target of investigation as a means to prevent electrode insertion induced apoptosis in the cochlea. The potential for injection into the cochlea at the time of cochlear implantation or reimplatation make apoptotic pathway inhibitors an ideal intervention to preserve residual hearing during periods of known oxidative stress.

Steroids have an evolving role in cochlear implantation. Steroids have been found to be safe for use in the cochlea (Shirwany et al., 1998). A single application of triamcinoloneacetonide at the time of electrode insertion can reduce the impedances of the electrode arrays long term. The steroid acts to reduce inflammation and scar formation from insertion trauma (De Ceulaer et al., 2003).

Several other protective substances have been found in animal models including antioxidants, ion chelators, glutamate receptor antagonists, nitric oxide synthase inhibitors and blood flow promoting agents (Duan et al., 2002). Perhaps a combination of these therapeutic agents applied through an intracochlear delivery system will prevent hearing loss in susceptible populations.

Experimental cochlear implant devices currently contain drug delivery systems allowing continuous delivery to the auditory system. Otherwise administration of medications to the cochlea is limited to the systemic route or by middle ear instillation with subsequent round window absorption. Systemic delivery requires higher doses than local administration, and whole body absorption, organ targeting and systemic toxicity limit concentrations. Middle ear injection of drugs, such as gentamicin or steroids, eliminates systemic affects but relies on round window membrane absorption from the middle ear. The round window has variable permeability (Chelikh et al., 2003) giving unpredictable intracochlear concentrations of the therapeutic agent. A device inserted directly into the cochlea with the electrode array could deliver exact drug dosages and regulate concentrations within the perilymph for precise delivery without systemic effects or uncertain absorption.

## Neural regeneration

Cochlear implant success relies on functioning neurons. The restoration of neuroauditory pathways requires neuron regeneration, hair cell regeneration and accurate targeting of neurons to hair cells. Loss of hair cells and spiral ganglion neurons has previously been considered irreversible. However, several *in vitro* and *in vivo* studies are aimed at regenerating neurons not only to improve cochlear implantation but also to preserve and restore natural hearing.

The role of neurotrophins in the auditory system is under investigation. In animal models, neurotrophins can induce dendrite regrowth in a manner which is augmented by electrical stimulation (Kanzaki et al., 2002). A cochlear implant with a drug delivery system would be ideal for the application of neuroregulatory molecules and electric stimulation to the auditory system.

The cochlea may also be suitable for gene therapy. The cochlea is a contained space with relatively easy access making it an ideal target of gene therapy. Numerous studies have focused on gene delivery systems to the inner ear. Luebke et al. (2001) demonstrated that an adenovirus vector could successfully transfect the cochlea without damage. Sekiya et al.

(2000) showed that transfection of the GNDF (glial cell line derived neu-rotrophic factor) gene in the cochlea was protective against gentamicin ototoxicity in an animal model. The introduction of genes into the audi-tory system provides an exciting new way to preserve or restore hearing. A cochlear implant device may serve as the delivery system to the cochlea.

Hair cells and spiral ganglion nerve cell replacement has been the tar-get of stem cell research. The therapeutic value of embryonic stem cells is under investigation in many disorders from multiple myeloma to spinal cord trauma (Catley and Anderson, 2004). Recently, neural stem cells were successfully implanted into the cochlea of transgenic mice (Tateya et al., 2003). The stem cells survived and differentiated into glial cells and hair cells. Potentially, a patient's own stem cells or donor cells delivered through a cochlear implant could be used to regenerate hair cells and auditory neurons. As the understanding of neuron targeting improves, perhaps the restoration of the neuroauditory system through gene thera-py and stem cell research will become a reality.

### Expanding candidacy

Current criteria for cochlear implant candidacy include physiologic age over 12 months with at least a severe bilateral sensorineural hearing loss, an inability to discriminate a significant portion of speech using appro-priate hearing aids and the ability to receive general anesthesia. As cochlear implant technology and the capability to preserve residual hear-ing improve, these criteria may expand to one day include patients with only a moderate sensorineural hearing loss. As objective measures of hearing and surgical techniques improve; perhaps children may no longer have to wait until their first birthday to receive the benefit of a cochlear implant. In the ovine model, Antonelli et al. (2002) demonstrate that in utero cochlear implantation not only is possible but also is able to correct changes in deafness related to central auditory system metabolic activity. With easier insertions and smaller devices, perhaps cochlear implantation may be accomplished under local anesthesia to further include those patients who are not candidates for general anesthesia.

# Beyond hearing

In the future, many innovations could be combined with cochlear implant technology to make the cochlear implant a multi-tasking device. Each patient's implant could be personalized by merely adding a small, silicone chip for each additional function desired.

The cochlear implant works by turning speech into digital information, and speech recognition programs to interpret this digital information already exist. With the addition of a speech recognition program, the patient's spoken commands could be used to control the cochlear implant or any other installed device. Using the cochlear implant technology, the device could respond electrically, which would be perceived by the patient as speech. The cochlear implant would 'talk back'. Only the patient would hear the responses because they would be delivered through the cochlear implant. Voice-activated databases of all kinds could be easily and confidentially accessed. The cochlear implant could replace hand-held computers and time pieces, and even remember voices of people other than the wearer for future identification.

Since the cochlear implant is held within the body, it is in a unique position to monitor physiologic functions. Records of heart rate, blood pressure, electrocardiogram and temperature could be monitored and recorded using the cochlear implant device. In diabetics, a blood sugar monitor with a report heard through the cochlear implant could help with glucose management, and a drug delivery system in the cochlear implant could deliver insulin without the need for painful injections.

Since the cochlear implant can receive the patient's voice and can deliver electrically encoded speech to the auditory nerve, it would only require a transmitter to make the cochlear implant function as a cellular telephone with digital quality sound. In fact, the cochlear implant cellular telephone would be simpler than a standard phone because digital information would not need to be transduced into sound waves. This implanted cellular phone could be voice-operated or could be programmed to access emergency services if the physiology monitors detected any abnormalities.

A popular science fiction movie depicts a future filled with talking robots. One of these robots is used to interpret languages from alien species. Even today we have language interpreting computer programs. By adding a language chip to the cochlear implant, the patient could choose to hear speech in any language. Imagine traveling around the world and listening effortlessly in any country! The cochlear implant could eliminate the need for that robot interpreter. The addition of a global positioning satellite system to the cochlear implant would ensure the patient would never get lost on that worldwide trip.

Cochlear implants have come far from that first experiment in 1957, but in the future, the sky is the limit.

# References

Allum JH, Greisiger R, Probst R (2002) Relationship of intraoperative electrically evoked stapedius reflex thresholds to maximum comfortable loudness levels of children with cochlear implants. International Journal of Audiology 41(2): 93–9.

Antonelli PJ, Gerhardt KJ, Abrams RM et al. (2002) Fetal central auditory system metabolic response to cochlear implant stimulation. Archives of Otolaryngology: Head and Neck Surgery 127(3): 131–7.

Balkany TJ, Cohen NL, Gantz BJ (1999) Surgical technique for the Clarion Cochlear Implant. Annals of Otology, Rhinology and Laryngology 108(suppl. 177): 27–31.

Balkany TJ, Eshraghi AA, Yang N (2002) Modiolar proximity of three perimodiolar cochlear implant electrodes. Acta Otolaryngolica 122(4): 363–9.

Baumgartner WD, Jappel A, Grobschmidt K et al. (2003) Clinical, surgical and histopathologic results from Vienna electroacoustic surgeries (EAS) and temporal bone experiments. Abstracts of the Hearing Preservation Workshop II. Frankfurt, Germany, 17–18 Oct.

Briggs RJS, Tykocinski M, Saunders E et al. (2001) Surgical implications of perimodiolar cochlear implant electrode design: avoiding intracochlear damage and scala vestibuli insertion. Cochlear Implants International 2(2): 135–49.

Catley L, Anderson K (2004) Strategies to improve the outcome of stem cell transplantation in multiple myeloma. Hematology Journal 5(1): 9–23.

Chelikh L, Teixeira M, Martin C et al. (2003) High variability of perilymphatic entry of neutral molecules through the round window. Acta Otolaryngolica 123(2): 199–202.

Colletti V, Fiorino F, Carner M et al. (2002) Auditory brainstem implantation: the University of Verona experience. Archives of Otolaryngology: Head and Neck Surgery 127(1): 84–96.

De Ceulaer G, Johnson S, Yperman M et al. (2003) Long-term evaluation of the effect of intracochlear steroid deposition on electrode impedance in cochlear implant patients. Otology and Neurotology 24(5):769–74.

Djourno A, Eyries C (1957) Prothese auditive par excitation electrique à distance du nerf senroiel à l'aide d'un bobinage inclus à demeure. La Presse Medicale 35: 14–17.

Dooley GJ, Blamey PJ, Seligman PM et al. (1993) Combined electrical and acoustical stimulation using a bimodal prosthesis. Archives of Otolaryngology: Head and Neck Surgery 119(1): 55–60.

Duan ML, Ulfendahl M, Laurell G et al. (2002) Protection and treatment of sensorineural hearing disorders caused by exogenous factors: experimental findings and potential clinical application. Hearing Research 169(1–2): 169–78.

Eshraghi AA, Yang NW, Balkany TJ (2003) Comparative study of cochlear damage with three perimodiolar electrode designs. Laryngoscope 113(3): 415–19.

Gantz BJ, Turner CW (2003) Combining acoustic and electrical hearing. Laryngoscope 113(10): 1726–30.

Goode RL (1995) Current status and future of implantable electromagnetic hearing aids. Otolaryngology Clinics of North America 28(1): 141–6.

Gordon KA, Ebinger KA, Gilden JE et al. (2002) Neural response telemetry in 12- to 24-month-old children. Annals of Otology, Rhinology and Laryngology (suppl. 189): 42–8.

Kanzaki S, Stover T, Kawamoto K et al. (2002) Glial cell line-derived neurotrophic factor and chronic electrical stimulation prevent VIII cranial nerve degeneration following denervation. Journal of Comparative Neurology 454(3): 350–60.

Ko WH, Zhu W, Maniglia AJ (1995) Engineering principles of mechanical stimulation of the middle ear. Otolaryngology Clinics of North America 28(1): 29–41.

Kubo T, Yamamoto K, Iwaki T et al. (2001) Significance of auditory evoked responses (EABR and P300) in cochlear implant subjects. Acta Otolaryngolica 121(2): 257–61.

Luebke AE, Steiger JD, Hodges BL et al. (2001) A modified adenovirus can transfect cochlear hair cells in vivo without compromising cochlear function. Gene Therapy 8(10): 789–94.

Maniglia AJ, Murray G, Arnold JE et al. (2001) Implantable electronic otologic devices: state of the art. Otolaryngology Clinics of North America 34(2): 1–9.

Nevison B, Laszig R, Sollmann WP et al. (2002) Results from a European clinical investigation of the Nucleus multichannel auditory brainstem implant. Ear and Hearing 23(3): 170–83.

Niparko JK, Wilson BS (2000) History of cochlear implants. In JK Niparko, KI Kirk, NK Mellon et al. (eds), Cochlear Implants: Principles and Practices. Philadelphia, Lippincott, Williams and Wilkins, pp. 103–7.

Otto SR, Brackmann DE, Hitselberger WE et al. (2002) Multichannel auditory brainstem implant: update on performance in 61 patients. Journal of Neurosurgery 96(6): 1063–71.

Pappas DG Jr, Cure JK (2002) Diagnostic imaging. Otolaryngology Clinics of North America 35(2): 239–53.

Parker JR et al. (1999) Testing of thin-film electrode arrays for cochlear implants of the future. In B Lithgow, I Cosic (eds), Biomedical Research in the Third Millennium. Proceedings of the Inaugural Conference of the Victorian Chapter of the IEEE Engineering in Medicine and Biology Society, pp. 41–5.

Scarpidis U, Madnani D, Shoemaker C et al. (2003) Arrest of apoptosis in auditory neurons: implications for sensorineural preservation in cochlear implantation. Otology and Neurotology 24(3): 409–17.

Sekiya T, Shimamura N, Hatayama T et al. (2000) Cerebellopontine angle cisternal infusion of NGF, BDNF and NT-3: effects on cochlear neurons disconnected from central target, cochlear nucleus: an in vivo quantitative study. Acta Otolaryngolica 120(4): 473–9.

Shirwany NA, Seidman MD, Tang W (1998) Effect of transtympanic injection of steroids on cochlear blood flow, auditory sensitivity, and histology in the guinea pig. American Journal of Otology 19(2): 230–5.

Tateya I, Nakagawa T, Iguchi F et al. (2003) Fate of neural stem cells grafted into injured inner ears of mice. Neuroreport 14(13): 1677–81.

Toh EH, Luxford WM (2002) Cochlear and brainstem implantation. Otolaryngology Clinics of North America 35(2): 325–42.

Van De Water TR, Lallemend F, Eshraghi AA et al. (in press) Caspases, the enemy within, their role in oxidative stress-induced apoptosis of inner ear sensory cells. Otology and Neurotology. 25(4): 627–32.

Weber BP, Goldring JE, Santogrossi T et al. (1998) Magnetic resonance imaging compatibility testing of the Clarion 1.2 cochlear implant. American Journal of Otology 19(5): 584–90.

Yanagihara N, Gyo K, Hinohira Y (1995) Partially implantable hearing aid using piezoelectric ceramic ossicular vibrator. Otolaryngology Clinics of North America 28(1): 85–97.

Youssefzadeh S, Baumgartner W, Dorffner R et al. (1998) MR compatibility of Med-El cochlear implants: clinical testing at 1.0 T. Journal of Computer Assisted Tomography 22(3): 346–50.

# CHAPTER 17
# A patient's perspective

## JEAN BRIGGS

My name is Jean and I have been a cochlear implantee for nearly six years now. I had hearing problems for a number of years and had a stapedectomy in 1976, which worked well for a while. I then went deaf in my other ear through a blood clot and bleeding, which also damaged my balance down one side. I had to retire from work, as I could not cope. I started to wear a hearing aid in my operated ear and I did so for a number of years. Then eight years ago, after a fall hitting the back of my head, I suddenly became profoundly deaf overnight. I was very scared at the time and I cried, wondering how I would cope.

I had read about cochlear implants in a magazine and I went to see a specialist at our local hospital. After some tests he said he would put me forward for a possible cochlear implant as it was the only thing that would help me to hear – but I had to wait for the next financial year. While I was waiting for an appointment, I felt I had to get out and get on with life and not sit at home and feel sorry for myself. I joined a lipreading class to help me get by. That was a great lifesaver, seeing other people struggling to hear, giving great support to each other. It was a great eye-opener. You don't know what is going on around you until you get involved. I made good friends there. It was very hard being deaf in a hearing world as I knew no deaf people. All my friends and family could hear. Even though I had good support, deafness really knocks your confidence.

However, in May 1997 my appointment arrived. I went to the Queen Elizabeth Hospital in Birmingham to see Mr Ivor Donaldson. He made me feel at ease straight away and we then talked about my problem in great depth. The therapists and students who were sitting in with him asked many questions, which I was able to answer. I then went to Selly Oak Hospital to have more tests, and five months later Mr Donaldson gave me the good news I had been waiting for. I was told I could have the implant. I was over the moon – I wanted it desperately. I had been deaf for just 21 months and, although I coped, I hated it. I was very lucky to get it so soon.

On 6 January 1998 I had my operation. All went well; I just had some facial ache for a couple of days. But the biggest shock was when my bandage came off – half my hair had been shaved off. I didn't expect that, but it was a small price to pay for what was to come (and they do things differently now). Members of the implant team came to see me, which I thought was nice. I was in hospital for six days, with good nursing. I then went home to wait for the big day.

One month later I went for the switch-on. What a wonderful day that was, very emotional, nervous yet excited, wondering how it would be. I met Huw Cooper and he tuned me in and switched on. The first words I heard were Huw saying, 'How are you, Jean?' The words were really clear, which I wasn't expecting. I thought that I would have to learn speech. But it wasn't like that; it was marvellous – to come out of the silence was incredible. I stayed in Birmingham for the next five days, going back each day to see Huw. I had more programming changes and tests to see how I was going on with the programme. I continued to go back for therapy and tests regularly for about nine months. It was all very helpful and each time it got better. To help with my tinnitus I had relaxation classes for a while, which I did with my eyes closed, listening to the therapist. One time I was doing the exercises and I heard my new boots squeak! I just yelled, 'I have heard my boots!' and Kathic my therapist and I just laughed. It was another new noise.

My sister-in-law, Elaine, who had been with me throughout, to make sure I understood everything and give me support, took me into Birmingham town centre so I could experience all the different sounds. We went there daily while I was in Birmingham after my switch-on. It was the start of my new life! I could hear the water running in the fountain – it was lovely. We went to the museum where there are things that you can touch that make a noise. I was like a child learning again, listening to the sounds of them and of the children playing with the games and different toys. I had come alive again. I was not on the outside looking in – I was in.

Each day brought another sound. It was wonderful. When I got back home, I heard the kitchen clock. I bent down and I could hear the freezer motor. I kept a record of all the new sounds that I heard and how I felt at the time. When I read it now, it seems so long ago and I feel so different now. I live out in the countryside and to walk along the lane and listen to the birds and animals, particularly the noisy geese who like to chase, is good. The implant has cost me money though: when I used my washing machine I could hear the bearings were very noisy, which I couldn't hear before. So I had to buy a new washing machine!

The implant has changed my life completely. I have regained my confidence. I can listen to the radio and television again. I bought talking books and listened to them on my Walkman. I found them very relaxing and good listening practice. It is so good. I go to the theatre and cinema, which I love. It just gets better; you learn something new every day. I travel quite a bit on trains. When I was deaf, I always carried pen and paper, for answers to my questions if I could not lip-read the person, which was often if it was male – I usually had difficulty then. Since the implant I don't need them. I am confident enough now to hear what is said. The implant also helps my tinnitus because I hear other sounds. Like other implantees I have had instances when the magnet has shot off onto the umbrella or the fridge door, which is quite funny.

I have now been fitted with the behind-the-ear Esprit model. I did not expect it to be as good, but it is – and no wires to bother you. I can wear clothes more comfortably now. I can hear music much better now. For me, the implant has been an outstanding success. I have tried and will go on trying to get the most out of what I have been given. It makes me feel good; it's part of me so much I went swimming and I was almost in the water before I realized I had still got it on – talk about lucky! I have had a couple of instances with the shower – you tend to forget it's there.

What I do like is you don't lose touch with your surgeon and implant team. You are not left to get on with it. You meet and can discuss things. It's all a learning curve for both of you. I can't thank everyone on the implant team enough for giving me the chance to hear again and for continuing to support me in every way and who work continually to help people like myself have a better life. To those who are considering an implant, go ahead – you are missing out on such a lot, and you have nothing to lose. It is one of the miracles of life. Pray that it happens to you. Good luck!

## TIMOTHY STANLEY

When I was born in Birmingham in 1947 it was not noticed that I had hearing impairment. When I was seven, I was given a routine hearing test at primary school and the school clinic discovered that I had nerve deafness. I was first given one of the old flat box type National Health hearing aids and, while this did not seem, to my thinking, to make very much improvement to the level of my hearing, at least it did draw people's attention to my disability. I was fortunate that during my last two years at primary school I had two very attentive teachers who ensured that my education was fully developed, enabling me to pass the 11+ and go on to grammar school.

During my grammar school days, I tended to use the hearing aid less and less as its overall effect seemed to diminish. This of course led to difficulties not only at school but later at college in following everything the teacher/lecturer said. I became very much dependent upon book learning as opposed to verbal lessons. At least one advantage of my lack of hearing was the ability to touch down at rugger quite consistently because I never heard the whistle!

My hearing did not hold me back from my social life, which seemed to be devoted mainly to outdoor activities with the Scouts, gaining my Queens Scout and gold Duke of Edinburgh award in due course.

After completing my school education, I was accepted for articles with a medium-sized firm of chartered accountants in the Midlands and at the age of 21 qualified as a chartered accountant. In the earlier days, while working, my hearing did not seem too much of a problem since I was able to use an amplifier on the telephone and to a certain extent get by. In addition it was the norm for most businesses to rely on the written word for record purposes rather than, for a deaf person, the curse of the telephone. Having remained in public practice until I was 24, I took the opportunity for a change in career and went into the shipping industry. Since this involved a certain amount of foreign travel, and in those days airports did not necessarily have visual displays, a certain amount of stress arose in ensuring that (a) I did not miss my flights and (b) I arrived at the correct destination. Over the years, my hearing gradually declined further and I found I was less and less able to cope with the telephone. I needed to concentrate more and more on my self-taught lipreading when dealing with people in general. In 1984, I decided on a further career change and acquired my own private chartered accountants practice in the Midlands. I rapidly found that I became very dependent upon Alison, my wife, to deal with telephone calls; I very quickly got to the stage where I could no longer use the telephone myself. It was also necessary when seeing clients to have Alison present to ensure I missed nothing of importance. Despite the problems of my rapidly declining hearing ability, over a period of some seven years Alison and I built the practice up from a small one with a turnover of some £35/40,000 a year to £200,000 plus by 1991. At this stage, despite having tried both state and several private hearing aids, my hearing continued to deteriorate and a decision was made to try to find a quieter practice in Devon.

We were fortunate in finding a small practice in south Devon, although one would probably not still consider it a quiet practice since it has trebled in size over the last decade. Nevertheless, with the very strong support of my wife and other members of the staff, it continues to thrive.

In 1997, I had become quite despondent about my level of hearing and after reading about cochlear implants asked my doctor to refer me to the Ear, Nose and Throat Consultant at Torbay Hospital to see if I might be a suitable candidate. After the usual tests and programmes, he referred me to Mr David Proops at the Queen Elizabeth Hospital, Birmingham, as a possible candidate for a cochlear implant. My initial consultation turned out to be a little disappointing. It was decided that before any decision could be made further tests with more powerful hearing aids would be carried out by the Audiology Department. However, I would have been grateful for any improvement in my hearing. I persevered with these more powerful aids but, after a period of eighteen months or so, I think it was accepted by all parties that the best way forward would be the implant. In

November 1999, I attended the QE Hospital for the implant to be carried out. Prior to the operation I was warned that there could be some adverse side effects, mainly of a short-term nature rather than long-term, and obviously I went into the operating theatre rather apprehensively. Coming around after the operation and in the following few hours I felt some pain and certainly a fair amount of discomfort from having to sleep with dressings the size of a motorcycle helmet on my head. Fortunately, other than these minor inconveniences no other adverse effects seemed to be present and within twenty-four hours I was on my feet able to walk around the ward. At the end of five days, I was discharged from the hospital into the tender care of my wife, relatively fit and suffering only the inconvenience of a long row of metal staples down the site of the operation, which were painlessly removed after another week or two. There were no physical side effects from the operation and, probably against the doctor's advice, I was back in my office within ten days. Then began the wait of some four weeks for the scar to heal and I was deemed fit until the 'switch on' at Selly Oak Hospital.

The initial switch on and testing proved to be rather disappointing, despite the warnings I had been given by the team. I was probably expecting to be able to run before I could walk, and it was not until a few days later that the full impact of the implant began to surface. Probably the first and most startling effect came when I happened to be standing close to a water tank after someone had flushed the cistern. The noise of the water, which I had never heard before, convinced me that something had gone seriously wrong with the operation and it was only the detective work of my wife that prevented me from returning to the hospital poste haste.

I continued to be monitored by Huw Cooper and his team at the Hearing Assessment and Rehabilitation Centre at Selly Oak Hospital, and mostly this took the form of sound and speech recognition. Speech recognition was no problem at all; I either heard and understood or I did not – it was very simple. Sound recognition, however, proved a bigger problem. When we first began assessments, many of the sounds that were used for testing I had never heard before, such as a cockerel crowing (there weren't many in Birmingham in 1950!), raindrops falling or footsteps. I was concerned at the time about my inability to say what these sounds were or even to be able to describe them. Of course, as my experience of the hearing world grew, I found these tests easier.

Very quickly, the improvement to my hearing manifested itself and I was constantly asking, 'What's that sound?' The sound and volume of everyday things that so many people take for granted and are so diverse – such as the birds, the noise of the sea, cars passing by or cats mewing – I was hearing again for the first time in many years and with some sounds for the first time ever. The sounds I do recollect hearing in my younger days now sound vastly different, partly due to modern technology as in the case of a vacuum cleaner and also probably due to the fact that my hearing was poor. I have found dealing with individuals on a face-to-face basis certainly less stressful than it has been in the past, although far from perfect. I can now distinguish what people are saying without the need to lipread, which I had depended upon for a very long time.

One of the biggest changes my wife noticed was that at last, if she wanted my attention, she could call me instead of having to find me before speaking to me. Unfortunately, with the one implant I still was not able to use the telephone and this was obviously a great disappointment. Over the following months, there was a slow but steady improvement in hearing quality and I was very pleased with the end result. Initially, I was a little self-conscious about the wearing of the speech processor but this feeling wore off quite quickly. It became important that I remembered to carry a supply of batteries with me as these tended to last some four or five days and I would only have a warning of a few minutes before they cut out entirely. This could prove embarrassing when it happened during the course of an ongoing conversation.

The main problem I discovered with one implant was when the sound source was not visible, in which case, unless I had a directional microphone fitted, my hearing would suffer. This particularly applied in the case of car travelling and during meetings involving several people when the speaker was on the opposite side to the implant. It would often happen at meetings that by the time I had sourced the person speaking, the conversation would have moved on to another person and so on. It was still important that someone sat beside me making notes of the conversation so that I could follow the discussions.

Some twelve months after my first cochlear implant was switched on I was contacted by the cochlear implant team at the Queen Elizabeth Hospital and asked if I was interested in taking part in a trial to assess the effect of bilateral implants as opposed to single ones. Volunteering for a second implant took no thought at all. If a second gave me even a fraction of the benefit I had received from the first, then I would have been delighted. After various meetings and tests, I received my second implant in May 2001. The procedure was very similar to the first, again carried out by the capable hands of Mr David Proops, Consultant ENT Surgeon. The big difference this time was that I knew what to expect and this seemed to make the operation certainly less stressful and probably a little less painful. 'Switch on' again came some four weeks after the operation. The difference in the second switch on was quite remarkable. Instead of having several weeks of 'running in' for the sound quality and recognition of sounds, the benefits were instantly noticeable. As soon as the processor was switched on, I was able to distinguish the speech of a person standing behind me with the new implant alone.

While the impact of the second implant was not as great as the first, nevertheless I found a distinct improvement in the quality of my hearing. I now make very few mistakes by missing words, I can hear inflections in speech and so do not misunderstand the meaning. Far more importantly, the use of a second ear definitely gives a clearer picture of the location of sound. It gives all-round hearing for situations such as in the car or multiple-people meetings and probably not quite so important but it is comforting to have an automatic backup should I have battery failure on one side.

A word of warning to prospective users: the processor is anchored by means of quite a powerful magnet which has meant at different times I have found my processor stuck to the garage door, clamped to the side of a removal van and, probably the most unusual circumstance, when my cat became the first feline with a cochlear processor after walking past my head wearing a metal-studded collar! Luckily, the doors were closed and so neither cat nor processor disappeared over the back hedge.

Having had the second implant for some two years, I can now look back and see what a big difference not only one but, because of the fortunate circumstances, two cochlear implants have made to my life. Without these implants I have no doubt that I would not be working as I do now and the consequences of this would have been the loss of revenue to the government in the form of tax and national insurance and in addition I certainly would not have been running my own firm which would have meant a reduction in the local employment.

I myself feel that I have grown considerably in confidence. I am now slowly getting used to using the telephone again, except in the rarest of cases do I now need my wife to be with me when meeting clients and this additional confidence is gradually leading to a more fulfilling social life. I can also now attend board meetings and am able to follow, quite often without any prompting, the matters that are being discussed around the table even at the largest of meetings.

In conclusion, my first implant made a vast difference to my life. Not only was I able to more conveniently communicate with my fellow men but hearing everyday sounds helped to establish a useful level of normality in my life. The second implant, while not of such significant impact, nevertheless heightened my hearing awareness and perception, not to mention being a useful backup should there be any failures such as batteries etc. on the first implant. The second implant greatly improved the directional sense of my hearing, enabling me to more fully participate in business meetings, social gatherings and community programmes. I feel that the combined impact of the implants has given me confidence to continue my self-employment for the indefinite future and indirectly not only benefit myself but also the economy in providing continued employment and taxation inputs. My grateful thanks to David Proops for his surgical skill and care, and also to Huw Cooper and Louise Craddock for their continued support and assistance.

# CHAPTER 18

# A parent's perspective

JENNIE CLEWES

## My son Matthew

I was delighted to be asked to present my perspective as a parent of a child receiving a cochlear implant. As I sit here now, I can hear Matthew saying to Phil, 'Dad, that's cheating – you're not allowed to press restart!' as they laugh and play together on the PlayStation. What a lovely, natural string of words that is. Looking back on the early years of Matthew's life, we have come a long way.

It is now March 2004, exactly four years since Matthew received his cochlear implant. He is our second child, brother to Sam who was almost two when Matthew was born. To say that we were shocked when we got Matthew's diagnosis of a profound hearing loss is putting it very mildly. With no family history of hearing impairment, no illness while I was having him and an uncomplicated birth, we just enjoyed him. I can honestly say that there was not one instance in his first nine months when I ever even thought for one moment that he had a hearing loss. I went along to his nine-month check with the health visitor with no concerns over his development.

I thought the health visitor was crazy when she shook her head and said, 'Matthew should have turned to that.' I said, 'He wouldn't turn to a bang on the window – we have got Sam at home so Matthew is used to noise,' but still the health visitor was concerned. I can hear myself now telling my Mum on the telephone, 'They've only referred him on to a Hearing Centre!' and Mum's reply, 'Well, I know he can hear. Whenever I say all gone when he's finished his meal, he lifts his hands up and down.'

So began five months of inconclusive visits to the Hearing Centre. The trouble was Matthew did appear to turn to some sounds some of the time. I was completely convinced that he could hear and there was always a good reason for his lack of reaction. If he wasn't teething, he'd be tired, he'd have a cold or be hungry, and there was always some reason to cast doubt on the results of the tests. Meanwhile at home, we all drove Matthew and probably ourselves mad by constantly making noises behind him, shouting from behind doors ringing the doorbell to see if he reacted to the sound. Now I realize that there were so many visual clues to what we were doing that of course some of the time he turned. I was even driven to bang saucepans over his cot while he was asleep and, of course, he began to wake up. Well, now I realize that I cast a shadow, he would smell me and you just do wake up when someone is looking over you in the night, with or without saucepans, don't you?

I went to my GP and told him that Matthew had been referred to the Hearing Centre and he said, 'Mrs Clewes, if Matthew couldn't hear, you as his mother would know. Trust me – you would know.' I felt like a weight had been lifted off when he said that. I thought, 'Well, I think he can hear; so I'll trust my instincts.'

Consequently, Phil and I had thought no further ahead than grommets. We were sure his hearing came and went, and how many children have had grommets once you start asking around? Eventually, brainstem tests were undertaken at the hospital. We were met at the Hearing Centre a couple of days later by an ENT consultant who delivered the news: 'Matthew has a profound hearing loss in both ears and will need to wear hearing aids.' He was surprised by my reaction of complete disbelief and did say that we should have been better prepared for the news.

Do you know, we were nearly all the way home before it even occurred to me that he wouldn't be able to speak, that was how little we knew. On that same journey Phil said, 'I think I'd rather have hearing aids than glasses.' From that day onwards I had an ever-present knot of worry in my tummy over Matthew. Would he ever hear my voice, birds singing, would he ever be able to order a McDonalds or chat with his mates on the telephone?

Referred by the Local Education Authority, a visiting teacher of the deaf and a speech therapist started weekly visits. My sister and I embarked on sign language lessons and began to teach it to Matthew and the rest of the family.

When we eventually got Matthew's hearing aids some six months after that visit to the health visitor, there was absolutely no reaction. He was as good as gold at wearing them, which made this all the more disappointing, really. At the very least I thought he would begin to recognize my voice or Sam calling him, but there was nothing. I can see now Matthew sitting on the lawn at home and Phil was right behind him with the lawn mower, wanting him to move out of the way and Matthew didn't even realize he was there. Phil had to go over and pick him up out of the way.

We went privately to see an ENT consultant, who advised us to give the hearing aids six months and then go back and see him again.

As he was now eighteen months old, Matthew was growing up to be the most insecure child. I would just dread being invited to anyone's house because he hated being anywhere other than home. If we visited a friend, he would not leave my lap. If I went to the bathroom, he would follow me. I felt smothered by him. Even at home I had to be in his sight or he would just cry and look for me. He was completely bewildered when people came to the house and even more so when they left. Unless you got his attention and waved goodbye, he wouldn't understand why visitors had just disappeared. The only sound from him was a high-pitched squeal, which he used for everything. When shopping, if there was something he saw on a shelf that he wanted he would scream for it, thus drawing everyone's attention to us. I hated going to the supermarket because with Matthew in the trolley it made him more on eye-level with everyone and just about every visit someone would ask about his hearing aids. Whenever he woke in the night, he would immediately scream, waking up the entire household. I just used to feel sick with worry for him.

This was the worst time for us as a family. Phil was really too embarrassed to use sign language and tended simply not to speak to Matthew. Sam found him a complete pain; the double standards between the two children were dreadful. When Sam would ask for another biscuit, it would be, 'It's too close to teatime, Sam.' When Matthew squealed for one, I'd just give it to him because he wouldn't understand anything else.

I felt so angry that this had happened to Matthew and to the whole family. In fact, I'm still angry about it now. It just seemed so unfair when he hadn't even had a chance yet. I was angry with every mum who said, 'Shut up!' to their child who wouldn't stop talking. I was angry with anyone who said, 'Are you deaf?' when their child wasn't listening. I was angry with all mums who had so much time to spend with each other just chatting and drinking coffee while their children played, when I always seemed to be in a rush to see the speech therapist, the education officer or to re-visit the Hearing Centre.

When we went back after this dismal six months to see the ENT consultant, for the first time a cochlear implant was mentioned. Right out of the blue he said, 'I'm going to refer you on to the Cochlear Implant Team in Birmingham.' Now Matthew was just two.

I was on the telephone to the Implant Team before they even received his letter of referral. We went for our first meeting early in January 2000. From then on we felt like we were in safe hands. All the people who we met were positive, enthusiastic, kind and up to date.

The assessment procedure involved numerous meetings at the Implant Centre. To manage our expectations, we were given a contact list of other families with implanted children at various stages of progress, several of whom I called. Matthew had an MRI scan at the Children's Hospital for which he had to be sedated, which gave us a good idea of hospital procedures to follow. Staff at the Implant Centre advised us that this was not a miracle and nor was it a cure. We never felt pressure to go ahead. We were given all the facts, information and contacts to make an informed decision. We attended for several sessions at the Children's Hospital for distraction tests to ascertain what Matthew could hear with and without his hearing aids. We met the whole team and the surgeon. When the opportunity for an implant was offered, the decision to accept was not a hard one. We had nothing to lose. The concern over losing residual hearing was not a consideration for us, as Matthew had none.

Our referral to the Cochlear Implant Team seemed to generate 'opinions' from family, friends, even Matthew's teachers of the deaf. I was told, 'Jennie, you're going at things like a bull at a gate.' 'Give his hearing aids more time.' 'I don't know how you could consider invasive surgery.' 'Matthew was born deaf and always will be.' 'You're forcing him to hear when he wasn't made to.' 'Give his hearing aids more time.' One very good friend of mine who I used to meet up with every week said, 'If Matthew was born to me, I would learn sign language and leave him alone.' That's fine in theory, but what about grandparents, aunties and uncles; they wanted to speak to Matthew too. We simply wanted Matthew in our world and this well-meant advice was coming from people who had never been in our situation.

Matthew received his implant on 27 March 2000. Surgery was completed without any complications. After the operation, the surgeon told us that the device was in place and working and that Matthew now had every opportunity to learn to hear. He stayed in hospital for only one night. Just three hours after leaving the operating theatre, he was up and about as if nothing had happened. He didn't take any medication after the second day.

The following month we were all just counting the days to his first switch-on appointment in early May. We continued with visits to the Implant Team even when he wasn't switched on, to keep the routine and familiarity with the people going. That was a particularly long month for me. People thought that now that he'd had his operation Matthew was 'better', and I got totally fed up with explaining that all the plumbing was in place but he hadn't been switched on yet. However, it was all worth the waiting for when the first switch-on day arrived. We've got the moment on video when Matthew heard sound for the first time and he reacted immediately. The audiologist said, 'I'm switching you on now, Matthew,' and he immediately looked up and around. It was the first time, ever, we had seen him acknowledge hearing anything.

Auditory verbal therapy sessions continued at the Implant Centre until Matthew started school. These were really sessions to teach me how to teach Matthew at home. I would be given specific goals to incorporate into our play. Listening was emphasized, and Matthew was soon pointing to his ear to acknowledge that he could hear something. The speech therapist would send me away with 'homework' most weeks. Starting with the six Ling sounds, Matthew quickly caught on to the idea of connecting sounds, then words to objects.

His first word was 'open' during a 'shake, shake, shake' game only four months after switch-on. In that time he changed from hearing and saying nothing to saying 'Mum', 'Dad', 'Sam', 'no' and 'open'.

It's amazing how much speech Matthew has learnt through just chatting with him about daily experiences and routines. Explaining why we do what we do enables you to bring so much other language in. Repetition is also valuable: I go over the same words and sentences again and again. I would go charging into my session gushing with the news that Matthew could discriminate between 'coat' and 'goat', and the speech therapist would say, 'Great, but does he know what a coat is? Does he know that a goat is an animal? Jennie, bring in the wider picture.' I could have given up, more than once, but I always managed to rise to the challenge and do my homework. I had no idea, then, of how well he would be able to hear. Matthew can hear a clock ticking, a whisper and a distant plane flying overhead.

Matthew has learned to listen and talk in much the same way as Sam did, but we have moved things along at an accelerated rate, trying to close the gap, as he heard nothing until he was two and a half. Today, I think his vocabulary is pretty much age-appropriate and his speech is intelligible to all.

At the moment we all ask a lot of 'why' questions: 'Why do you wear shoes, Matthew?' 'Why do you clean your teeth?' I talk to him constantly, using different words for the same thing, eliminating even natural gesture from our conversation so that he has to listen to understand what's being said, repeating, explaining and modelling questions and answers. It just goes on. Sam chats constantly to him in a far more natural way and now they are the best of buddies.

After much deliberation, I opted to send Matthew to the same preschool as Sam. They overlapped for six months and so Matthew was happy to go as his big brother was there. Although the manager had concerns, she was keen to include Matthew and learn through him. He settled right in and made good progress.

From there, against much advice and after lots of thought, we opted to send Matthew to mainstream school. This was not an easy decision. I visited the specialist unit local to us where there are a couple of implanted children and many with hearing aids, signing children and teachers and I was totally impressed. It was obviously a happy school, but Matthew expected to go to the same school as Sam.

He was familiar with the place, the uniform, the routine and I was sure that if Matthew felt safe and secure in his school environment that was half the battle to helping him to learn. After a meeting with the statement officer and all involved in Matthew's education, we spoke to the school, who were happy to give it a go. Matthew's Additional Needs Statement recommended fifteen hours' support from a special needs teacher.

The move from pre-school to mainstream was seamless. On his first day he was happy to go; he looked proud to be a part of the class and he has been learning from day one. He is now confident, solid, self-aware and his own little person. He has opinions, preferences, likes and dislikes and he can let us and his teachers know them all. His speech is slightly immature and he finds background noise and locating sound a problem, but thanks to the help of his support teacher he is doing more than getting by: he's flying by. We have a home-to-school diary, which is so helpful for the teacher to just note things that she thinks he may have not understood and I just bring that subject up while we chat in the evenings. Do you know he even went to a friend's house for tea the other week? He just passed me by on the playground all full of his own self-importance as he marched off with his buddy. I was a nervous wreck and really wanted to give the other Mum a cochlear implant awareness session, but Phil said, 'Let him go; he can speak for himself now,' and he did.

Matthew has the confidence now to say 'pardon' and 'talk louder'. He automatically sits close to the teacher when it's story-time in the classroom; he fetches his radio-aid himself when it's time for assembly. He is only six but already seems aware of what a benefit he gets from making these small adjustments to his surroundings to enable him to hear more clearly. He has always told me, and now his teacher, if the batteries have gone in his processor.

I can have a conversation with Matthew without him even looking at me. I ask him what he's done at school today and he replies, 'Oh, this and that.' We even have lovely arguments about bedtime, vegetables and what he's going to wear. Our whole family life seems so 'normal'.

I know that Matthew's story is far from over and we have a long way to go, but I can only sing the praises of everyone who works with cochlear implant technology. Although I was told over and over again not to expect a miracle, it's exactly what we've got. That knot of worry I had in my tummy over Matthew has long gone. I don't worry about him any more. He's part of our world and we just enjoy him again. As far as ordering his own McDonalds goes, there's just too much choice, he'll change his mind three or four times in the queue. He calls it McDonalds, the Chip Monster, Old McDonalds, McDs or the café, take your pick. I now am working on trying to remove all these words from his vocabulary! Without his cochlear implant, Matthew would not be who he is today. With the implant, his life is in full swing and the sky's the limit.


Tricia Kemp

# Ending the silence

In writing this, I have deliberately not named professionals. Many have been truly fantastic throughout; some I am proud to now class as friends. My heartfelt thanks go to all those who have helped us. To the very few who were unhelpful and condescending, I would say: a child may just be another patient, but please remember that to the parents that child is the most precious thing in the world. And never underestimate the lengths to which parents will go for their children!

I would like to start this chapter by stating that our story is certainly not typical of a family seeking a cochlear implant for their child. I hope that most families have not had to go to the lengths that we have, but, on the other hand, I hope that ours is an inspiring and encouraging tale. I know that it has changed me for ever but, on the whole, for the better.

Let's go back to 1988. Meet the Kemp family. Nothing particularly unusual about us: my husband, Steve, was a chartered accountant, we owned our house in a lovely part of south-west London and had a son, Jamie, who even at the tender age of three was already a high achiever. And then there was me, Mrs Average Middle Class, expecting my second child and anticipating a mother's life of coffee mornings, playing tennis and comparing my children to my friends' children. None of us had any idea of just how much our lives were about to change, especially me. My cosy existence with very few worries was soon to be turned upside down and I would no longer be a part of that comfortable existence. We would no longer be 'the family at number Four'; we would now be 'the family with the deaf child'. We were about to enter a new world, one that we knew nothing about, but which would ultimately be the most interesting and rewarding part of my life.

Jamie's fourth birthday was on 22 October 1988 – his brother, arriving two weeks early was an unexpected birthday present! Fortunately, I am a well-organized person and everything was ready for Jamie's party. Steve was able to attend the birth, get home and cope with the party (with help from some of the mums!) and come back to visit Alex and me in the hospital that evening.

We suspected immediately that Alex had a hearing difficulty. Jamie had needed grommets as a baby, after which he was a changed person. We weren't looking for problems with Alex, but the fact that he never responded to any sound led us to assume, naively, that grommets were needed. We made an appointment to see the consultant, who confirmed that there was something wrong, but it was not the same as Jamie's problem. He made an appointment for Alex to have some tests. We didn't really think much of it, and I took Alex to the hospital a few days later. I watched the flat line being produced on the screen. Logic told me that this was not how it was meant to be, but if I needed confirmation of this I only needed to look at the audiologist's face. I pressed for information. She told me politely, but firmly, that I would need to see our consultant who was not at the hospital that day. I refused to leave until I could see someone who could give me the information. Finally, another consultant arrived and gave me the news.

'Your son is profoundly deaf. He can be fitted with hearing aids in a few days' time, and a local teacher of the deaf will visit you at home.' Poor man was having a bad day: he was running late for his clinic, had been asked to take a phone call, was signing a letter as he walked along the corridor and now had to see this insistent mother whom he had not met before. It was probably just another busy day in his clinic and I expect he soon forgot all about us, especially as we weren't even his patients, but that day brought devastation for me and I would remember it for ever.

There was so much I wanted to ask; but it didn't take long before it dawned on me what the million-dollar question was: 'Well, how will he learn to talk?'

'Oh, the teacher of the deaf will tell you where you can learn to sign.' And that was it.

I don't know how I drove home. I cried the whole way. I collected Jamie from the friend who had looked after him. She was a busy mum with two children:

'Is everything OK?'

'Alex is deaf,' I blubbed.

'That can't be right; I'm sure he'll be fine,' she responded. Little did she know!

The next few days were a blur. Things like this just didn't happen to people like us. I couldn't stop crying; it all seemed so negative. We didn't even know any deaf people. Alex couldn't hear, wouldn't be able to speak and couldn't enjoy music. It seemed to me, at that time, that deafness could only mean misery. (I hasten to add that I know better now.)

We gathered some information and went to see the consultant together. We had seen a glimmer of hope in a newspaper.

'What about these new "bionic ears" – could Alex have one of these?'

'No, they are not for born-deaf children.'

'Not now; not ever?'

'I'm afraid not. He has the best hearing aids possible and that's all we can do.'

Well, now what? Clearly, we had to move on and start getting to grips with the situation. The message seemed to be: 'Go away and get on with it.' But get on with what? Where could we begin?

Having spent a few days trying to explain to family and friends what we couldn't even understand ourselves, the initial shock and grief started to subside and we began to realize that we were lucky. We had a lovely son whose only problem was his deafness – it could have been much worse. Maybe he was just another case to the medical profession but he was the most precious thing in the world to us, and we would go anywhere and do anything that would help him and above all would give him the most love, support and encouragement that any child could have. It wasn't that we were denying his deafness; we simply wanted to do everything we could to ensure that he would lead as full a life as possible.

To find out how we could best help Alex, we clearly had to understand exactly what we were dealing with and we needed to learn more about deafness. We joined the NDCS (National Deaf Children's Society), the BDA (British Deaf Association), the RNID (Royal National Institute for Deaf People), the NAG (National Aural Group, now known as Delta) and the FYD (Friends for Young Deaf People, now merged with NDCS) and enthusiastically read all their booklets. We started the John Tracy correspondence course. Each day I sat down with Alex, doing some set activities and giving him the language to go with them. He loved the attention and was very responsive. He watched my face, giggled a lot and started to babble – but he never actually responded to any sound. At that time, children were often put in a playpen while Mum did the washing up; not Alex: he sat in a rocker chair on the draining board and watched me talking about the dirty plates, soap bubbles and clean plates. A fly on the wall would have thought I was completely mad. Everywhere I went, he went with me. I was amazed how many opportunities there were for language in everyday objects and chores. His hearing aids were worn every minute of the day, but I was certain he was not hearing a thing. I was doing all I could, but it just didn't seem to be enough.

Alex had always vocalized well, but the hospital seemed to think that speech was going to be out of the question. Realizing that he had to have a language for communication purposes, we decided to go to a signing class. We were amazed that we were the only parents in the class. Some were professionals, some were learning 'for fun' and one lady told us her department had funding and she could go on any course she wanted, so she decided to try signing as it was something 'completely different'! We felt we were the only ones who *had* to learn and we both found it very difficult. The language taught in the class was mostly aimed at adults, but our teacher, who was a very kind deaf lady, gave us a few minutes at the end of each class to show us particular signs we wanted to know which were relevant for a baby.

While we were accumulating knowledge, Alex was having all sorts of X-rays and tests to ascertain whether there were any other problems. At the age of seven months he had his first general anaesthetic to insert a grommet in his right ear.

As time went on, I became frustrated with badly fitting earmoulds, the time it took to get hearing aids repaired, the lack of spares and with being kept waiting for up to an hour for routine appointments which were only to last for five minutes. As a parent starting on this long road, these routine appointments seemed vital. Each time I somehow expected something magical to happen, something to be different, just a glimmer of hope. But it never came. In the hospital he was just another deaf child attending a clinic. But he was my child, and so special to me; I just could not rest until I had explored every avenue and was satisfied that everything possible was being done.

I also believed that the more knowledge we had and the more we put in, the more we could help Alex, but one thing was painfully obvious: he did not hear anything at all, and it seemed that there was nothing that could be done about that.

Our local teacher of the deaf started visiting us. As the hospital had told us that Alex would need to learn signing I assumed that our teacher would help us with this, but initially she was not at all in favour of signing as we lived in an 'oral area'. I began to realize just what a contentious issue this was: to sign or not to sign. To me, communication, in any form, was what mattered. However, it seemed that the system was so inflexible that communication was more likely to be determined by where a child lived rather than by what his needs were! The teacher was just as much a victim of the system as we were, and once Alex started to sign she did too.

I had the good fortune to meet an extremely experienced speech and language therapist who suggested that I visit some schools for the deaf. My first visit was to a secondary school for the deaf. I had never seen a group of deaf children together and was quite apprehensive. A girl who must have been about fifteen came and signed to me, 'He's got hearing aids; is he deaf?'

I was pleased with myself that I understood her signing and signed back, 'Yes, he's deaf like you.'

'Wonderful,' she signed back enthusiastically.

I had got used to responses such as 'What a shame' or 'Oh well, the other senses will compensate' or just embarrassed silences when I had told people that Alex was deaf. It was a revelation that someone, especially of that age, would think it was 'wonderful' to be deaf. Perhaps it wouldn't be so bad to be part of this community.

However, when I left the school, I went to the supermarket, to our GP and to collect Jamie from school. The reality hit me in the face. None of these people in our community could sign. Perhaps if we were a deaf family already in the deaf community things would be different, but we were a hearing family; we could never be part of that world. Yes, I could accept that sign would be Alex's first language, but for him to have access to the hearing world at large, let alone be part of it, he would really need to develop some speech. Surely, if he had sign and some speech, he could be part of both communities?

We started seeing a private teacher of the deaf just before Alex's first birthday. Here, at last, I had found someone who did not seem to be confined in a 'system', was enthusiastic about the future and was truly gifted in working with children. I told her we were using sign at home; she did not sign, but respected our decision to do so. At her house we met several families with deaf children, some of whom are now our best friends. There is a natural and strong bond between families who are facing the same issues with their deaf children.

Gaining more confidence in dealing with professionals and realizing that they were only human beings (not the gods that some would have you believe) and still feeling that there must be more we could be doing, I started to telephone anyone whose name I came across in the field of deafness. We had been told that Alex was not suitable for a cochlear implant, but I telephoned Nottingham where they had implanted a boy deafened by meningitis. I was told that implants for congenitally deaf children were still a long way off in the UK, although they had started overseas. I was given some addresses, and duly wrote to hospitals in New York, Iowa, Hannover, Melbourne and Israel. They all replied promptly and all confirmed that congenitally deaf children were being implanted. At that time, the youngest child to have been implanted was two years three months. Alex was just one year old so time was on our side, although it seemed logical to me that if a born deaf child was to have an implant, the younger the better so as to maximize the possible benefit.

Alex was still showing absolutely no response to sound. He had more powerful hearing aids and had grommets inserted in both ears. I decided to approach a different consultant at another London hospital who had finally agreed to see me privately. She was clearly interested in Alex (who was a very engaging toddler) and felt it would be worth doing some more tests and scans. She did not dismiss, as others had done, the possibility of an implant. A few weeks later, Alex had various tests, including a CT scan. This proved to be quite a stressful experience. On the first occasion we went to the hospital the bed had been booked, but not the scan and so we had to go home. On the second occasion they tried to sedate him to avoid him having a general anaesthetic. This had the opposite effect and he became completely hyperactive! Yet again we went home without the scan. On the third and final attempt it was decided to use a general anaesthetic, but as Alex was being given the 'pre-med' injection the needle snapped in his hand! The nurse was very upset, but it didn't seem to bother Alex who giggled and signed, 'Broken!' Fortunately, the CT scan finally went ahead and we were told that either of Alex's ears would be suitable for a cochlear implant. Well, it was a start.

We now needed to obtain a lot more information; so I contacted the UK representative of Cochlear AG (manufacturer of the Nucleus 22 device) who was extremely helpful and provided me with masses of reading material. I wrote to Nottingham again, hoping their policy might have changed, and enquired whether, if Alex had an implant overseas, Nottingham would agree to do the rehabilitation. In June 1990, we had a reply that they were not yet in a position to implant a congenitally deaf child and neither could they fragment their programme. It is one of the very few occasions that a letter has reduced me to tears. Here was a young boy with no residual hearing, who had had all the necessary tests and scans, with a supportive family who would do anything for him. Why wouldn't they help us? It was a setback, but not entirely unexpected. However, we had received many knocks before and in a way it made me more determined than ever. If it was the right thing for Alex, we would get it one way or another.

We decided to spend our summer holiday in the USA so that we could combine it with a visit to an Implant Centre in New York. This was easier said than done. They said they did not implant children from overseas and it would be a waste of time for us to see them. I replied that IF we decided on an implant and IF they agreed to do it, we would move to New York, but that we couldn't make that decision without seeing them first. I also sent a photo of Alex, copies of all his medical tests and the CT scan and finally they agreed to see us. They soon realized that we had done a

good deal of research and that Alex was a suitable candidate. The programme director referred to him as being 'very stimulable' – rather an
'Americanism', but nonetheless an accurate description! They gave Alex a
vibrotactile device consisting of an electrode on his chest that vibrated to
sound. Nobody in the UK had suggested this device, but immediately Alex
responded to 'sound'. Alex clearly enjoyed the sensation and started
experimenting with his voice. He soon began signing for it each morning.

We were given contact details for several families who had congenitally deaf children with implants. We spent a whole day with one of them
and were delighted to see how well their daughter was doing: signing and
speaking and, in particular, really enjoying her 'hearing'. Her parents
were fantastically informative about issues that could only be learned
from other parents, and we left their house knowing that we wanted Alex
to have the same opportunity as their daughter had.

We returned to the UK feeling really optimistic. I kept in touch with
New York and, in spite of what they had previously said, they did offer to
implant Alex, but said we would have to move to the USA for a couple of
years for the ongoing rehabilitation.

At least we had one firm offer. However, with an older hearing child
just settled at school who had already put up with considerable disruption on account of his younger brother, we were not keen to move to the
USA unless there was no alternative. We had tried New York first because
they were English-speaking, but we now turned our attention to
Hannover, where, at that time, there was the most experience of implanting young children. I sent all of Alex's details, and one of their surgeons,
who happened to be coming through London, kindly offered to meet us
at Heathrow to discuss matters. It transpired that they wanted Alex to
have an MRI, and so this was the next thing to organize at yet another hospital. The film was sent to Hannover and we waited anxiously for their
verdict. It seemed satisfactory, but they then wanted us to go to Hannover
so that they could confirm the presence of a main auditory nerve.

In November 1990, we made our first trip to Medizinische Hochschule
and, after the test under general anaesthetic, they offered to implant Alex
as soon as we liked after Christmas. I went home, discussed it with Steve
and we booked a date during February.

Having spent a few days in Hannover, there was no doubt in my mind
as to the competence of their team, but, even just for three days, it was
very lonely being in a general ward of a German-speaking hospital.

I decided to have a final attempt at finding a team to do the implant in
England. I visited Cambridge, Manchester and Southampton, all of whom
were interested in Alex but were hesitant about implanting a congenitally deaf child, even though they agreed he was a good candidate. In my
heart I felt that Nottingham was the only possibility. They had already got
a 'team' and seemed to be warming to the idea of implanting congenitally deaf children, but their final answer around Christmas time was 'No'. It
was clear that when (and now it was 'when' rather than 'if') they started

implanting congenitally deaf children, they would prefer to start with a child from their own clinic.

Around this time, a London hospital indicated that they would be starting a programme soon and that Alex would be high on their list. It seemed too good to be true and, sure enough, a lack of funding then prevented the programme from starting. Another hospital offered to help us, but the cost was as much as Hannover with a tiny fraction of the experience, so we ultimately decided that Hannover was the best choice. Surgically and medically, it was an excellent option. But the thought of being away from home for two weeks in a huge hospital where very few people spoke English was daunting, as was making arrangements for Jamie while we were away. Was this really the right thing to do anyway?

The issue of a congenitally deaf child being born to the deaf community was (and still is to some extent) a huge one that had weighed heavily on my mind for months. I know that Alex will always be a deaf person and I accept that. I was not trying to change him into a hearing child. However, it is a hearing world and Alex was born into a hearing family. Surely even the smallest amount of sound would make life easier for him as an adult in the world at large, even if only from a safety point of view? If we waited until Alex was old enough to make the decision himself, he would have lost all the formative years when language can be acquired more easily. We were carrying out our role as parents – trying to do what would be best for him. It was better to give him this opportunity now and know that we had done all we could, and accept the possibility of him rejecting it, rather than face the situation of him asking us when he was older, when it might be too late, why we had not given him the opportunity when he was younger. He had no residual hearing. He was a bright, responsive child with a loving and supportive family. We had found an excellent team to carry out the implant and had an experienced private teacher who would help Alex to make the most of any 'hearing' he gained. There seemed nothing to lose. If Alex did not like the sound, he would take off the device. We would not stop him signing. It didn't seem to be an 'either/or' situation to us. The most important thing was communication. Access to sound, which an implant might provide, would be a bonus. (By today's standards, this is, of course, a very low expectation!)

We had done as much research as possible and were convinced not only that Alex was a good candidate for an implant but also that there was no reason to wait. What encouraged me the most, however, was our conversations with the family in America and my many telephone calls with Marion Batt, mother of the first meningitic child to be implanted at Nottingham. Professionals simply cannot provide the emotional support or the insight into everyday life with an implanted child that other parents can. It was experience of this kindred spirit support which, eighteen months later, led Marion and I to set up the Cochlear Implanted Children's Support Group ('CICS') to provide contact, information and support for families whose children have implants and for those who are considering an implant for their child. (CICS is now a registered charity and has a membership of around 650 families.)

Alex's implant took place on 26 February 1991. Steve and I sat in the very clinical room that was to be home for Alex and me for the next two weeks and waited. It took much longer than we had been told, but there were no English-speaking staff around to ask what was happening. Finally, we were called to the recovery room to see a pathetic little creature wearing what looked like a white helmet (very different from today's procedures), desperately trying to stand, but not having the strength, and clutching Stripy, the bunny who had been with him through thick and thin. His adenoids had also been removed and he had blood pouring from his nose. He looked utterly miserable, far from our happy little boy who was always smiling and giggling.

Steve returned home the next day to look after Jamie, and I felt totally alone and exhausted, having been up most of the night with Alex. There was no one to talk to. The doctors breezed in and out, gabbled away to each other in German, said a few sentences to me in English and rushed out again. It took a whole morning to arrange to have a telephone in our room. The girl in the office spoke only German, and I spoke only English and couldn't understand the formalities she wanted me to complete. It nearly defeated me, but I got the phone and thus had contact with home, which made life much better.

The next day Alex cheered up immensely and was soon charging up and down the corridors moving all the food trolleys in his path and causing chaos. We were on a general ENT floor. There was a centre for implanted children but, as foreigners, we could not use it. The nurses were soon won over by Alex's charm, and I began to appreciate some of the difficulties that deaf people must experience – mouths gabbling away at me and I couldn't understand a word – it was an isolating and, at times, frightening experience.

The food was ghastly and arrived at the most odd times. We walked up and down endless corridors to kill time. But Alex was fine and I knew he was feeling better when he started pulling off the bandage. We went through several, but in the end it was taken off completely much earlier than planned, and Alex started wondering what had happened to his hair (in those days, of course, half the head was shaved).

Once the stitches had been removed, eight days after surgery, we could go outside. We played football in the grounds and, even though we were told not to leave the hospital, we sneaked out one day to visit the zoo, which Alex loved. There were no taxis for the return journey and, just as I was starting to wonder if we would ever find our way to the hospital, some very kind British soldiers came to our rescue and drove us back.

Two weeks after surgery we went home, and soon got used to people staring at Alex's rather odd half-bald head and scar. The time seemed to go very slowly as we anxiously waited for switch-on.

The whole family and Alex's private teacher went to Hannover for the switch-on, which took place on 15 April 1991 and was to be the most emotional experience I have ever had. We arrived at the hospital in an excited, but nervous, state. We didn't know what to expect. We had been working towards this moment for so long but had been trying not to have any expectations of the outcome. It had been a mission, and I felt as if I had won a battle, a triumph for determination over 'the system'. But that didn't really matter now. The struggle we had had to get to this point was of no consequence. What mattered was what this switch-on would mean for Alex. He sat in the clinic sucking his thumb, clutching his bunny and clearly wondering what was happening. He didn't seem to be bothered by the presence of the coil on his head, but found the cable leading from it to the computer equipment very irritating. We, of course, were eager for a response and scrutinized his every move. The emotional strain and tension was enormous. Would there be any response? It certainly wasn't immediate. The beeps seemed to go on for ever. The change was so subtle that had we not been so desperate for a response it would have been easily missed. It was just a stilling, but it was a response. Something at last! Then he looked at us and looked around the room as if he was looking for the sound. At this point I knew he could hear. The tears welled up inside me. It had all been worthwhile.

The audiologist tried to interest Alex in dropping marbles down a tube. Although he was initially unenthusiastic, he did finally join in and realized that he was supposed to drop the marble when he heard a beep. However, two hours was enough for the first session. He was exhausted, pulled off the coil and made it clear that enough was enough. We were so relieved to have got through the first session and to have seen Alex respond to sound. It hadn't been a tremendous response, but he had definitely heard something. He was desperate to get out of the clinic and refused to put the coil back on until we got outside the hospital. We made our way to the noisy railway station, and Alex, who was always unsteady on his feet, lurched along looking at the people, the shops and the trains. As one started up he pointed at his ear and signed, 'Train noisy.' Wow! This was the best! Alex's journey into the exciting world of sound was beginning.

This time we had stayed with a wonderful family who really made us feel at home – much better than having to be in the hospital. We were able to relax at the end of the day and our boys loved playing with the go-karts in their lovely garden. Alex wore the device happily and even on the first evening was already indicating an awareness of certain sounds. But the following three days at the hospital were exhausting, frustrating and not very exciting. Alex did not like the surroundings and was not particularly co-operative with the audiologists. We had been booked in for the whole week, but by the Thursday morning he had clearly had enough and, as soon as we got to the hospital, he ripped off the coil and refused to wear it. We were all absolutely exhausted. We just wanted to go home to our family and friends. We left Germany in a despondent and emotionally drained frame of mind. The next morning we put on the device and crossed our fingers. No problem! Alex took to hearing like a duck to water, and it was an absolute joy watching him delight in exploring the world of sound. I honestly believe that his hearing is the greatest gift he has ever received.

At this point, I must mention how very fortunate we are as a family in that we were able to raise the vast amount of money required to take the 'private route', not only in paying for Alex's implant but also in seeing a private teacher of the deaf and obtaining speech and language therapy of which there was never enough within 'the system'. An enormous amount of stress and disruption to the family could have been avoided if we had been able to get advice, tests and an implant in one centre, instead of having to scratch around organizing it ourselves, but it did prove that perseverance, determination and belief in ourselves to make the right decision paid off. My only regret is that Alex was not able to have his first implant in the UK. I certainly don't regret having gone to Hannover; the team were very experienced and took excellent care of Alex. Given the same circumstances, I would do it again. We had no way of knowing how long we would have had to wait for an implant in the UK and, as it happened, six months after implantation, Alex was rushed into hospital for emergency bowel surgery, so dealing with an implant during the following few months would have been too much – even for the Kemp family!

The next few months were fascinating. The difference in Alex was truly amazing. He loved any sound, and I was forever trailing round the house after him as he showed me all the things he could hear, even the taps running. He would turn on the water, giggle, point to his ear and sign 'water'. He had quite a good sign vocabulary. The acquisition of each new sign had always given me great joy, but when the spoken words started to come I have to admit that it was an even greater joy. The thrill of hearing each new word he spoke was just wonderful, especially 'Mummy'. As I put him to bed each night I marvelled at the pleasure he got from listening to his music box. It had been a present before we knew he was deaf. I had put it away as it was just a painful reminder of his deafness. In fact, I don't even know why I kept it, but I was glad I had and I got it out when we returned to England following switch-on. I had often cried over this silly music box but, whereas before they were tears of sorrow, now they were tears of joy.

The Hannover Implant Team and Cochlear were very good to us. They minimized the number of trips we had to make to Germany for mapping by seeing Alex in London whenever they could, but we did have to make some trips to Hannover. It was stressful enough travelling with a three-year-old, but the added strain of hoping that Alex would be co-operative when we got to the clinic made it even worse. Although I looked forward to the improvement in hearing which a new map might bring, I dreaded coping with making arrangements for my older son, the packing, the journey and managing in a country where I couldn't speak the language.

However, it had to be done, I was utterly committed and I would have gone on doing it for ever had it been necessary; but I couldn't help thinking how much easier life would have been if Alex's implant had taken place in England.

We carried on with a Total Communication approach and Alex started at a Hearing Impaired Unit following the same method. Listening and comprehension seemed to come quite quickly, but the spoken word was frustratingly slow at times. Of course, Alex was the first child with an implant to attend the Hearing Impaired Unit, and it was at this point that it became clear to me that the school would benefit from contact with an implant team. This would clearly not happen with Hannover and it was going to be disruptive for us travelling there for mapping. I approached Nottingham again and to my relief and delight they offered to take Alex into their programme in August 1993. Finally, I had achieved exactly what I wanted!

A year later, progress with speech was still rather slow, but just when we started to think that perhaps we should stick to sign, Alex changed to a Spectra processor and the map changed from common ground to bipolar plus 1. A week later his spoken language took off, and he went from two- and three-word utterances to sentences of about ten words. Gradually, we dropped the sign support at home and when it was time to move to secondary school we chose an oral school for the deaf. The school places strong emphasis on developing spoken language and has helped Alex to become a very effective oral communicator. I think I could write a book about the issues surrounding educational provisions for deaf children, but that, as they say, is another story!

There have been many issues to be dealt with along the way – provision of speech therapy, finding the right school, getting support in social activities etc. It's funny how with some children it seems to be one thing after another ... all the time! It appears that this is particularly true for children with a special need. However, some of the 'things' are much bigger than others and the one that I am going to write about now is one of the biggest and perhaps the one that I, as a parent of a child with a cochlear implant, dreaded the most.

Things were moving along steadily until November 1995, when he didn't seem to be as responsive to sound and he kept taking the coil off his head, putting it back on and 'singing' to himself as if he was testing the sound. We went to Nottingham where they found that four of the electrodes were only working inconsistently. This was, of course, a tremendous shock. However, the audiological scientist remapped the processor and, although initially Alex did not like the new sound very much, after a few days of complaining, he got used to it. Unfortunately, worse was to come. A month or so later he put on his processor one morning and screamed in pain: 'It hurts, it hurts.' My heart sank and I flew into a panic. At times like these it is so important to have an implant team in whom you have every confidence. We had an emergency appointment and were told that two more electrodes had failed. During the following two years, Alex's response to sound became somewhat variable. He was still doing quite well but, on occasions, appeared to be struggling to hear, and could often be heard doing his 'singing tests'. We were going to Nottingham every few months and the map seemed to need changing each time. Alex has always liked consistency in everything in his life, and I started to dread the visits to the Implant Centre because I knew the following few days would bring complaints from him about how he was hearing after the latest change.

In July 1997, he complained of pain and would not wear the processor. Although no further faults showed up on testing at the Implant Centre, it was decided to change his map into 'common ground'. During the next two years' progress was rather patchy, and I felt that he was not hearing as well as he had four years previously. At the Implant Centre he continued to produce a good audiogram, but listening for 'beeps' from a machine in an acoustically treated room is not the same as hearing in everyday life.

In February 2000, Alex started to complain of 'popping and crackling' in his head. More electrodes were switched off and he was now down to twelve. Alex hated the new map and became moody, which was unusual for him at that stage. I started to think seriously about re-implantation. The strain of continually worrying what each day would bring was immense. Would it be a good or bad hearing day? Would we be rushing off to Nottingham, yet again missing more school? On the other hand, I did not like the thought of going through the surgery again, and anyway would it even be possible to remove the existing implant and insert a new one?

We discussed the possibility of keeping the failing implant and having a new implant in the other ear. Alex absolutely refused, his reasons being that he regarded the other ear as his 'deaf ear', and he wanted to keep it until there is a totally implanted device which can be used in water so that he can hear while swimming. I could see the logic in this and, in any event, his mind was made up, and that was that.

In June 2000, events took a strange turn. Having had the processor at maximum sensitivity and still not hearing properly, we made another trip to Nottingham. Alex tried three different processors, each with the same map. With two of them he could hardly hear anything, but with the third it was just about acceptable. We couldn't understand what was going on. We struggled through the next six months taking the rough with the smooth, and looked forward eagerly to Alex trying the new Esprit 22 ('behind the ear' processor), which at least would be much easier to wear.

He was very excited to be given one in January 2001 and naively expected to hear better with it. However, the excitement was short-lived. It was wonderful to be free of wires, but the sound kept cutting out. A month later another electrode failed, leaving eleven functioning. The audiogram deteriorated and we noticed that Alex was saying 'what' more and more and was becoming very bad-tempered and frequently accused us of 'whispering'.

In May 2001, Nottingham and Cochlear advised us that no more could be done with this device and that re-implantation was now necessary. We spent the summer discussing the procedure with Alex making sure he understood exactly what would happen. We returned to Nottingham in September to discuss the surgery and met with an unexpected turn of events. It was felt that Alex's audiogram was still too good to be considering re-implantation and more evidence of the difficulties being caused by the situation was required.

Alex was asked to keep a diary of problems he experienced with his implant. He started this, but soon became disillusioned with it because it didn't change anything for him; he wanted a solution. I was exhausted and fed up with the whole situation. It was an emotional rollercoaster existence. Most of all I was annoyed and disappointed that I had put so much energy into preparing Alex for the re-implantation. He and I had assumed he would be having it that autumn and now it was not to be. Alex had believed that I could fix anything for him, and now, in his eyes, I had let him down. All I could do was to keep taking him to Nottingham to check that there was no more they could do and keep in touch with Cochlear on any new developments.

A few weeks later another type of interference began. Alex reported that he was hearing helicopter noises all the time. It was these helicopters which signified the last chapter for Alex's 22. Alex prepared a written list of questions for the Implant Team. After discussion of these, at long last, everyone was agreed that he should have a re-implant.

Alex was adamant that he wanted the same ear re-implanted, he did not want to have any hair shaved and he must have the new 3G processor straight away. He also wanted a guarantee that the noises and interference he was experiencing would stop. It was quite difficult persuading him to accept that it was probable, but not definite, that the same ear could be re-implanted. No guarantee could be given about the noises either, as Cochlear was not able to confirm exactly what was causing the interference, and it was even suggested that it could have been physiological. For a thirteen-year-old deaf boy, these were unsatisfactory responses to his requests for reassurance. However, at the end of the day it was Alex who made it very clear that he wanted a re-implant come what may, and he would not take 'no' for an answer.

At about this time, Alex's best friend was undergoing assessment for a cochlear implant. Alex had been wanting him to have an implant for some time and it was interesting that, even with the difficulties he was experiencing with his device, he was still actively encouraging his friend to go ahead because he wanted him to hear better.

It was very stressful having to wait a few months for the surgery. Knowing that it was finally going to happen, I just wanted to get on with it. The situation was complicated by a sudden improvement in his hearing a month before the surgery. This presented a great dilemma. Could we really be certain we were doing the right thing? This situation must be similar for those families whose children are on the borderline for implantation. It is not a happy place to be. Certainly, the decision to have Alex's first implant was much easier. He heard nothing; so there was nothing to lose. This time there was a lot to lose. Although he was having to put up with an inconsistent level of hearing and intermittent interference, he could still hear. I found it very difficult to sleep during the weeks leading up to the surgery date. I just couldn't switch my mind off. I worried about whether we should wait until the 22 failed altogether, by which time there might be another new and improved device. I worried about the surgery. I worried about whether I should have tried harder to persuade Alex to have a second implant in the other ear instead of a re-implant. However, on the other hand, he needed the best possible hearing he could have now while he is at school and still has so much to learn and, as he refused to consider an implant in the other ear, surely a re-implant must be the best option. But if something went wrong and he could not be re-implanted at all, he would be distraught. What should we do? Round and round, one minute wanting it, the next minute not.

Alex was also worried, but not about the surgery, or the pain, or the silence between surgery and switch-on, or the possibility that he couldn't be re-implanted at all; he was worried about the new sound. He really wanted the same sound but without the interference. During the week before surgery, he said he wasn't so sure he wanted it and would I mind if he didn't have the operation. I told him that it was entirely his decision, and whatever he decided I would support. He then asked me the most difficult question he has ever asked me: 'What would you do if it was you, Mum?'

I just didn't know. I felt helpless. He was looking to me for advice and all I could do was go through the facts with him (yet again) in the hope that it would make it easier for him to make the decision.

I don't suppose the hospital would have been too pleased, but the night before surgery, as he and I were going through it all for what seemed like the millionth time, I said, 'If you go into the operating theatre tomorrow and decide that you don't want it, we will simply walk out and go home.'

'Good,' he said, turned over and went to sleep. I lay awake all night and convinced myself that he was going to decide against it. I even prepared exactly what I would say to the surgeon.

In the morning, in a state of total exhaustion, I woke Alex to see whether he really did want to make the short drive to the hospital. Unusually, he got ready very quickly and said, 'Hurry up, Mum. I don't want to be late'! I could see that he had made up his mind. This was it. He was having a re-implant. The surgeon came in to see Alex and said we would be called down to the theatre shortly. Alex commented to me that he hoped the surgeon's hands wouldn't be shaking when he operated, and he wondered whether there would be music playing in the theatre like he had seen in *Casualty* (one of his favourite TV programmes). At this point I felt confident in reassuring him that, in my view, he had an excellent surgeon and fantastic Implant Team to help him afterwards. Knowing that Alex was now completely calm and at ease with his decision to go ahead, I felt as if some of the weight had been lifted from my shoulders.

As we went into the operating theatre I knew there would be no going back. Alex has had many operations and we have been in many operating theatres, but the moment he went limp under the anaesthetic just before surgery was as frightening as if it was the first time. Although he is almost the size of an adult, he looked so helpless, and I was quite overcome by the emotion of the moment. As I went back to wait for him in our room, memories of his first implant surgery came rushing back to me. I reflected that at that time I really didn't know if an implant could help at all, but that Steve and I had taken that decision for him. This time so much more was known about implants and there was every reason to be optimistic. But what really struck me was that this time it was Alex's decision. He had chosen to hear and was hoping to hear much better than before. I felt a certain relief and satisfaction that Alex was now confirming that our initial decision to take him out of a silent world had been the right one for him.

The surgery was much shorter than I expected, less than three hours, and all went well. He did not recover as quickly as he had as an infant, and was sick and exhausted for two days following the surgery. He only had two weeks to wait for switch-on, but that period served as a sharp reminder as to how life would have been had he not had an implant. We had just not fully realized how dependent Alex (and the rest of the family) was on technology. It is a frightening thought, and I was glad that we had learnt to sign. Alex is such a good listener that he has not developed his lip-reading skills to the fullest extent and, even though my signing is a little rusty now, it was good enough to help us through the silent time. Alex couldn't wait for switch-on. When I asked him how it felt to be in a silent world, he replied, 'I miss my CD player and it's lonely in my head.'

I had spent a lot of time emphasizing to Alex that his new implant would sound very different and that it might take a little time to get used to it. In true teenaged fashion he had got utterly fed up with me 'fussing' and although he kept saying, 'I know, I know', I was not certain that he had really accepted the idea.

The day we had so anxiously awaited arrived and he and I went to Ropewalk House on the morning of 10 December 2002. Alex took it all in his stride and did not seem as excited as I had expected. I was looking forward to it, but was anxious at the same time. It did not seem to be a particularly emotional experience for him, more like something he wanted to get through as quickly as possible. At the end of the morning's session he was wearing it, but I could tell he was not too happy. As it was just before Christmas, I thought we could do some shopping and go out for a meal in Nottingham to celebrate. Alex was not very communicative in the afternoon except to say that he couldn't understand anything I said. It was different, and he didn't really like it. I told him I was sure they could make it a little better for him the next day and reminded him, yet again, that it might take some time to get used to the new sound. We went to his favourite restaurant, Friday's, and as we waited for the food he started to fiddle with the controls. I suggested that it might be better to leave it alone, to which he snapped, 'It's my choice.'

He didn't say a word during the taxi ride back to the Marjorie Sherman House where we were staying, and the atmosphere between us was very tense. I made some tea and as we sat down he suddenly ripped off the processor and shouted, 'It's rubbish. I don't want it. I want my old one back.' I was shocked and distraught at this sudden outburst. Alex had always been a model implant user and had certainly never rejected his Nucleus 22 in this manner. He refused to put it back on and although he was clearly very angry I could also see that he was very upset.

Alex's class teacher had been invited to come to the tuning session the following day. We thought it would be interesting for her as she had not been to an implant centre and she was thrilled at the prospect. Now I started to dread her arrival. I really didn't want her to see Alex in such a state! However, it turned out to be a blessing in disguise. She was fresh to the situation and so enthusiastic. She sat in on the tuning session with him and he was obviously not going to vent his anger on her in the way he would have done on me!

The three of us went out for lunch, and, although Alex said he didn't understand us very well, he seemed to be coping and I became cautiously optimistic. As we got into the car he said he was looking forward to seeing his kitten, Beanie, and hoped he would be able to hear her purr. He knew that cat's purring was a sound that could be heard, but he had previously only been able to feel the vibrations of her body. Purring is a very quiet sound and I felt duty bound to warn him that he might not be able to hear it. After half an hour in the car he took the processor off and said he didn't like it. I spent the rest of the journey worrying about whether he would put the processor on again and what would happen if he couldn't hear Beanie purring.

As we arrived home Alex put on his processor and marched into the house. Beanie came to greet him and luckily started to purr enthusiastically. It was one of those tear-jerking moments for me when he said, 'I can hear her purring, Mum.' I didn't think there could ever be a moment as magical as Alex's first switch-on, but I was wrong. This was every bit as emotional for me. He could obviously hear a lot more than he did with the Nucleus 22, but as it sounded so different to him I thought it would take him quite a long time to get completely used to it and to understand our speech again. However, he spent much of the following weekend listening to his favourite CD over and over again. He already knew the words to the songs, so it was as if he was teaching himself to recognize how those words now sounded with his new hearing.

He complained that when we said 's' it sounded like 'ee' but, apart from this, he got used to the new sound much quicker than everyone expected, and just two weeks after switch-on he was trying out mobile phones. It was a great pleasure to buy him one for Christmas. As the parent of a deaf baby, it was beyond my wildest dreams that, as a teenager, he would be able to speak and hear on a phone!

Looking back, I wish Alex had been re-implanted earlier – but hindsight is a wonderful thing, isn't it? There had been ongoing problems with the device for so long, but it was very difficult to know where to draw the line. However, I am certainly glad that we did not wait any longer. It was a controversial decision to re-implant a boy whose implant aided responses were around 35 dB, and it is a tribute to the Implant Team that not only did they take the time to listen to the concerns of a thirteen-year-old boy but also to involve him in the whole process and to respect his views. If he had not been able to put forward such a strong case, I suspect he would have had to struggle on with his original implant for a lot longer.

Fourteen months later, his hearing and listening skills are greatly improved. He overhears conversations and is much more confident in group situations. His vocabulary has expanded and his word endings are much better – obviously due to the improved hearing.

It was a stressful few years, but the experience highlighted what was really important in our lives – love and support from family and friends – and was a constant reminder that technology cannot be taken for granted.

The decision to re-implant is clearly much easier if a child's implant just stops working. Our case was probably the worst scenario – a failing implant lingering on and on. It is not something one goes into lightly, but at least if a re-implantation is necessary it is reassuring to know that your child will have the latest device and that there are already many successful outcomes from the procedure. Perhaps some of you reading this may, at some stage, face the same issues over the re-implantation of a child as I have done with Alex. Each case is, of course, different, but I hope you have found Alex's story encouraging.

There is no doubt in my mind that the implant has transformed Alex's life, enabling him to leave the isolating world of silence and to enjoy sound, join in conversations with family and friends and experience more social opportunities. It has also increased his self-confidence and broadened his horizons, and will ultimately enable him to lead a more independent life and widen his employment options. He speaks by choice, but signs with some deaf peers who have less hearing than he does. When asked about himself, he says, 'I am deaf but I hear with my implant.' I am very proud of his attitude and am happy that he accepts his deafness. I would be concerned if he thought that his implant changed him into a hearing person. He can only hear with the help of technology and, as good as it is, our own experience has shown us that it can never be 100%.

Some children have achieved more with their implants than Alex and some a great deal less. I hate the use of the word 'success' when discussing the outcome of a child's implant. If anything at all is gained from the procedure then surely it is a success.

Implants are not the right option for all children, however, and parents must investigate all avenues before making such a decision. I suspect that there will always be a part of the deaf community who are opposed to implants for children, which is, of course, their right, but they must understand that an implant does not turn a deaf child into a hearing child. There should be no reason why an implanted child cannot be a member of the deaf community, unless of course that community is so narrow-minded that it refuses to look beyond an implant and see the deaf child. Similarly, if the concern is for the preservation of BSL, an implant does not prevent a deaf child from using BSL if they so choose.

When families are first thinking about a cochlear implant for their deaf child, I would not want them to think of a possible implant failure as a reason for not going ahead. However, it is important to bear in mind that the implant given to a young child may not last a lifetime. It is reassuring to know that re-implantation is possible and can be successful. Although there is a wide range of outcomes for the children who were implanted over a decade ago, it is encouraging to see that many of them have developed good speech, some manage in mainstream schools and some can use a phone. These results have led to higher expectations for the current generation of young implantees, and, together with today's improved implants and the wider experience of professionals in the field, there is every reason to expect even better outcomes for children being implanted now. Today's technology can do so much for them, and the future has never been brighter for deaf children.

However, it is not just about technology. Life-long support and people are vital ingredients. Our children need dedicated and well-trained professionals in the implant centres; they need committed teachers with high expectations in well-equipped and acoustically treated classrooms and a greater awareness of cochlear implants amongst the general public. Above all, implanted children need dedicated parents to co-ordinate their programme and to ensure that everything is in place to enable them to reach their potential.

However, the magic and most important ingredient, the one that makes the whole equation work, is the child himself, and we must never forget this.

# Index